Working in the Operating Theatre

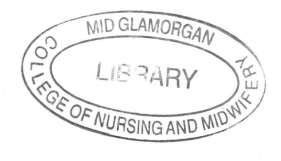

*To
Corrinne*

Working in the Operating Theatre

Bakul Kumar MB BS DA FFARCS
Consultant in Anaesthetics and Pain Relief, Dudley Road Hospital, Birmingham

Foreword by
Peter Hutton BSc PhD MBBS FFARCS
Professor of Anaesthesia, University of Birmingham, Birmingham

CHURCHILL LIVINGSTONE
EDINBURGH LONDON MADRID MELBOURNE AND NEW YORK 1990

CHURCHILL LIVINGSTONE
Medical Division of Longman Group UK Limited

Distributed in the United States of America by Churchill
Livingstone Inc., 650 Avenue of the Americas, New York,
N.Y. 10011, and by associated companies, branches and
representatives throughout the world.

First Published 1990
  Reprinted 1993

ISBN 0-443-03908-9

British Library Cataloguing in Publication Data
A catalogue record for this book is available from the British Library.

Library of Congress Cataloging in Publication Data
Kumar, Bakul.
  Working in the operating theatre/Bakul Kumar.
    p.   cm.
  ISBN 0–443–03908–9

1. Anesthesiology. 2. Therapeutics, Surgical.
3. Anesthesiology – Examinations, questions, etc.
4. Therapeutics, Surgical – Examinations, questions, etc.
I. Title.
RD81.K85 1990
617.9 – dc 20   90-1595
                                        CIP

The
publisher's
policy is to use
**paper manufactured
from sustainable forests**

Produced by Longman Singapore Publishers (Pte) Ltd
Printed in Singapore

Foreword

I was delighted to be asked to write a Foreword introducing this book. Not only does its subject area fill a very real gap in the literature, but also the selection and standard of content are ideal for its purpose.

Working in the operating theatre and its associated environments are topics which have been relatively neglected by authors. Until now, they have been covered piecemeal in a variety of texts with the consequence that a student's knowledge has often been determined more by chance than by judgement.

This problem has now been solved with the publication of Dr Kumar's book. There is much within it which will be of great value to student nurses, trainee ODAs and anaesthetic and recovery nurses. It is particularly useful because it covers a wide field to a depth which is both appropriate and sufficient for the practical and examination requirements of its intended audience. It also combines together the relevant factors of traditionally diverse subjects so as to build up an integrated picture of patient care. The MCQs at the end of each chapter allow a convenient form of self-assessment.

Recent publications on 'The Efficiency of Theatre Services' and 'Assistance for the Anaesthetist' from the Association of Anaesthetists of Great Britain and Ireland and 'The Management and Utilisation of Operating Departments' from the NHS Management Executive have emphasized the need for an up-to-date and well-informed theatre staff. This book is therefore very timely and I wish it every success.

Birmingham, 1990   P.H.

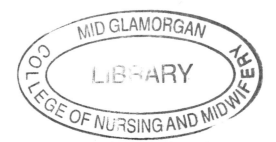

Preface

When I started teaching operating theatre personnel — anaesthetic and recovery nurses and operating department assistants — I soon realized that there was a shortage of textbooks which catered for their courses. This prompted me to take on the task of writing a text which would cover in one volume the needs of those undertaking studies in anaesthetic and operating department nursing as well as those training as hospital operating department assistants.

My aim in writing this book has been to provide a comprehensive, straightforward text, presented in an organized and systematic format, with simplified theoretical explanations. To aid the student in revision I have included multiple choice questions at the end of every chapter.

I hope this volume will be of considerable help not only to the theatre personnel mentioned above but also as a primer for medical students who are interested in basic anaesthetics and theatre work and for any other hospital staff whose role involves them in the work of the operating theatre.

I would like to thank Christopher Reay, ODA Course Coordinator, Selly Oak Hospital, for his valuable help in compiling the chapter on Surgery; Andrew Claxson for the line drawings; and Wendy Fellows, Nicola Perks and Dilys Thomas for secretarial work. I am also grateful for the constant encouragement and patience of the staff of Churchill Livingstone. Finally I would like to thank my wife Corrinne who gave me tremendous support while I was writing this book.

Birmingham, 1990   B. K.

Contents

1. Anatomy and physiology

CELL AND THE TISSUES

Anatomy is defined as the study of the form of the body.

Physiology is defined as the study of the functions of the body.

The cell (Fig. 1.1) is the unit from which tissues are made up. Cells vary in size, shape and content based on the functions they carry out.

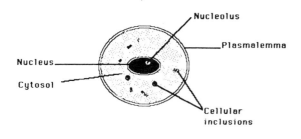

Fig. 1.1 The cell.

A cell consists of:

a. Cell membrane: a thin membrane made up of protein and lipid which encloses the cell.
b. Cytoplasm: the substance of which most of the cell is made up. It contains a fine network and granules.
c. Nucleus: a thick structure which lies within the cytoplasm. It contains chromatin and is surrounded by a membrane.
d. Nucleolus: a small circular body which lies within the nucleus. It is made up of ribonucleoprotein.

Each group of cells has a different function. For example, cells in the thyroid gland produce thyroid hormone, cells of cardiac muscle (in the heart) bring about contraction and relaxation of the heart. The cells are separated by a thin space which is occupied by a fluid which allows water and certain chemical substances to pass from fluid to cell and cell to fluid.

Cells:

(i) usually require oxygen and produce carbon dioxide;
(ii) contain enzymes (those substances which bring about a chemical reaction without themselves being altered) which have a specific action.
(iii) break down food and release chemical energy.

THE TISSUES

There are five main types of tissue (Fig. 1.2): (A) epithelial, (B) connective, (C) nervous, (D) muscular, (E) blood.

Epithelial tissue

This tissue covers the external and internal surfaces of the body and lines the ducts and glands which open onto these surfaces. The cells which make up the epithelial tissue are: squamous, or flat, cells; columnar, or tall, cells; cuboidal, or cube-shaped, cells.

Squamous, or flat, cells are again divided into three groups:

a. Simple squamous epithelium (endothelium), made up of one layer of flat cells, e.g. the cells that line the inside of blood vessels, alveoli (air sacs) of the lungs, and heart.
b. Stratified epithelium, made up of more than one layer of squamous cells, e.g. skin.

1

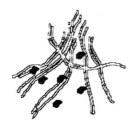

Connective tissue

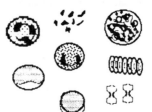

Red and white blood cells
and platelets

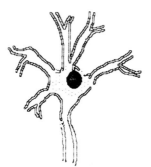

Nerve cell

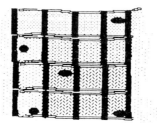

Muscle cells

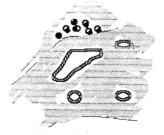

Kidney tissue

Fig. 1.2 Types of tissues: connective, blood, nervous and muscle.

c. Transitional epithelium made up of three to four layers or more of squamous epithelium, e.g. the inner lining of the uterus, bladder and part of the female urethra.

Columnar epithelium lines the inner surface of the stomach and intestines. One of the groups included in this section is ciliated columnar epithelium, which has fine cilia (cilia = movable, fibre-like structures). By constant movements, cilia keep the dust out of the lungs and move an ovum (egg) along the uterine tube.

Connective tissue

The connective tissue helps in binding together or supporting or protecting structures. It can be either dense or soft.

Dense connective tissue

This includes:

a. Tendons. These are made up of fibres packed closely together. One end of the tendon is attached to the end of a muscle and the other to the bone.

b. Bone, made up of bone cells and a matrix. Bone cells are again divided into two groups: osteocytes, which form new bone; osteoclasts, which destroy the bone. Matrix is made up of ground substance, salt and fibres.

c. Cartilage, made up of cells and fibres enclosed in a solid matrix. It is elastic in nature and has no blood vessels, lymph vessels nor nerve supply. There are three different types of cartilage:

(i) Hyaline cartilage, which is present in the larynx and rings of the trachea, the cartilage at the anterior ends of the ribs, the articular cartilage within the joints, and the cartilage in which most bones are formed.

(ii) Elastic cartilage, which is present in the epiglottis, pinna of the ear and auditory tube.

(iii) Fibrocartilage, which contains many collagen fibres and is seen in the discs of the sternoclavicular and temporomandibular joints and in the pubic symphysis.

Soft connective tissue

This is made up of:

a. Ground substance (cells, fibres)

b. Fibres. Cells could be: plasma cells, which are oval cells; fat cells; mast cells; fibroblasts; histocytes.

Soft connective tissue is divided into: (i) areolar tissue, a loose tissue with few fibres as seen under the mucous membranes, skin and surrounding blood vessels and nerves; (ii) fat, consisting of a large number of fat cells as seen below the skin and between the layers of the peritoneum in the abdomen.

Nervous tissue

This tissue type is made up of nerve cells with their attached fibres. It is found in the brain, spinal cord and all the nerves.

Muscular tissue

Muscle cells and tissues take part in contraction and relaxation.

There are three types of muscles (Fig. 1.3): Skeletal, Smooth, Cardiac.

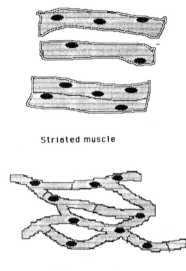

Striated muscle

Cardiac muscle

Fig. 1.3 Types of muscles: striated (skeletal), cardiac.

Skeletal muscle, is also called striated, or voluntary, muscle. It assists in voluntary movements and forms about 40% of the total body weight. It is found in the muscles attached to bone, skin or cartilage. The fibres show cross striations, and the movements are controlled by the central nervous system.

Smooth muscle is also called unstriated, or involuntary, muscle. This type is found in the walls of blood vessels and viscera. The fibres do not show cross-striations and are controlled by the autonomic nervous system (see p. 17).

Cardiac muscle is found in the heart. The fibres are striated and connected to one another by muscular branches.

Blood cells

There are three main types:
Red blood cells (RBCs)
White blood cells (WBCs)
Platelets.

BODY FLUIDS

In the human body, fluids and electrolytes are present in certain proportions in the various tissues. The quantity varies depending upon the age of the individual.

Water makes up 70% of body weight in an adult man. (For example a 70-kg man has 50 litres of water in the body.) Adult women have 10% less water than men because they have more fat. (Fat is water-free.)

In an infant, water forms 75% of the body weight.

In an old person water forms 55% of the body weight. This water is maintained in two 'compartments' of the body: extracellular fluid (ECF), and intracellular fluid (ICF).

Extracellular fluid (ECF) means water present outside the cells. It makes up 30% of the total body water and is seen in: plasma of the blood, cerebrospinal fluid, fluids in cavities and joints, lymph and interstitial fluid (fluid present in the tissue spaces between cells).

Intracellular fluid (ICF) means water present inside the cells. It makes up 70% of the total body water.

ECF helps in the transport of chemical substances from one cell to another, whereas in the ICF chemical changes of the cell take place.

A continuous exchange of chemical reactions takes place between ECF and ICF to maintain a normal electrolyte and acid base balance. The normal electrolytes in the body are:

Electrolytes	Symbol
Sodium	Na
Potassium	K
Calcium	Ca
Magnesium	Mg
Chloride	Cl
Bicarbonate	HCO_3
Phosphate	PO_4
Sulphate	SO_4

The maintenance of acid base balance is described on p. 233.

RESPIRATORY SYSTEM

ANATOMY

The respiratory system begins at the nose and ends at the alveoli of the lungs. For simplicity, the respiratory system can be divided into:

Nose
Pharynx
   Nasopharynx
   Oropharynx
Larynx
Trachea
Bronchi   (both right and left bronchus)
Lungs   (both right and left lung)
Pleura   (covering both lungs)

The nose is made up of the external nose and the nasal cavities behind the external nose.

The external nose is made up of cartilage below and the nasal bones above, covered inside by the mucous membrane and outside by the skin. It has nostrils, or external openings.

The nasal cavities begin at the nostrils in front, and extend to the posterior openings of the nose which open in the nasopharynx. They are lined by mucous membrane.

The nasal septum is a thin structure made up of bone and cartilage, lined by mucous membrane; it separates the two nasal cavities. The lateral wall of the nasal cavity is formed by the parts of the sphenoid, palatine and maxillary bones. The floor of the nasal cavity is formed by the palatine and maxillary bones. The roof of the nasal cavity is formed by the sphenoid and frontal bones.

The paranasal sinuses are those spaces in the cranial bones which open into the nasal cavity. They are lined with mucous membranes. The sinuses which open into the nasal cavity are:

Sphenoid sinus
Ethmoid sinus
Frontal sinus
Maxillary antrum

Other structures which open into the nasal cavity are the nostrils and the nasolacrimal duct.

The pharynx is divided into the nasopharynx and oropharynx.

The nasopharynx opens into the nasal cavities in front and into the oral pharynx below. The eustachian tubes (auditory tubes) open into its lateral wall on each side.

The oropharynx is common to the respiratory and alimentary systems as air enters it from the nasopharynx and lungs, and food from the mouth.

Larynx (Fig. 1.4). This is made up of cartilage, membrane, mucous membrane, muscles and vocal cords.

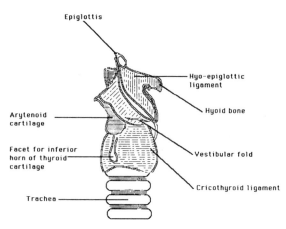

Fig. 1.4 The larynx.

A. Cartilage is made up of:
  — *Thyroid cartilage*, a 'V'-shaped cartilage with the 'V' projecting into the neck prominently as Adam's apple.
  — *Cricoid cartilage* is a signet ring-shaped piece of cartilage which is bony both anteriorly and posteriorly. It lies below the thyroid cartilage and is connected by the cricothyroid membrane. The advantage of this complete ring is made use of in cricoid pressure (Sellick manoeuvre). Here, the posterior part of the cricoid cartilage presses on the oesophagus, thus preventing food from being regurgitated upwards (see p. 194). The cricothyroid membrane is used for cricothyroid puncture, either in awake intubation or high frequency jet ventilation.
  — *Epiglottis* is a leaf-shaped piece of cartilage which extends upwards behind the base of the tongue. It is attached to the back of the hyoid bone and the thyroid cartilage. It is very small in children, and infection by *Haemophilus influenzae* (see p. 81) can cause swelling of the epiglottis (acute epiglottitis), which makes breathing very difficult and needs endotracheal intubation in an emergency.
  — *Aryepiglottic folds* stretch from the side of the epiglottis to the arytenoid cartilages.
  — *Arytenoid cartilages* are two small, pyramid-shaped pieces of cartilage which sit on the cricoid cartilage.
B. Membrane. This connects the cartilages to one another.
C. Mucous membrane. The larynx is lined by ciliated columnar epithelium.
D. Muscles. Small muscles attached to the thyroid, cricoid and arytenoid cartilage assist in the opening and closing of the vocal cords by contracting and relaxing. All the muscles are supplied by the vagus nerve (10th cranial nerve).
E. Vocal cords. These are two thin sheets of mucous membrane lying over the vocal ligaments. The vocal ligaments are attached to the inside of thyroid cartilage in front and the arytenoid cartilages behind. The vocal cords assist in making sound by vibrating during expiration. There are two folds of mucous membrane just above the true vocal cords. They are called *false vocal cords* and are not involved in making sound.

Trachea. This is a cylindrical tube about 10 cm long and 2.5 cm in diameter. It lies in front of the neck, starting at the cricoid cartilage and ending behind the manubrium sterni dividing into right and left bronchus. In the neck, the isthmus of the thyroid gland and veins run in front of the trachea. The trachea divides into two main bronchi at its carina.

Bronchi. The right and left bronchi run outwards and downwards from the trachea to their respective lungs. The right bronchus is wider, shorter and straighter than the left bronchus. For this reason, during endotracheal intubation, if the tube is pushed pass the carina it may lodge in the right main bronchus, leading to collapse of the left lung and to one-lung ventilation.

Lungs. Each lung is cone-shaped and is covered by a closed sac of pleura. The right lung consists of an upper lobe, middle lobe and a lower lobe. The left lung consists of an upper lobe and a lower lobe. At the root of the lung, one of the two bronchi which arise from the bronchus enters the lung.

A *bronchiole* is one of the smaller branches which further divides into smaller branches. An alveolar duct is the smallest of these branches; each one of these ends in a cluster of alveoli. An alveolus is a thin-walled air-containing sac through whose walls gaseous exchange occurs.

The structures which enter or leave the lung at its root are:

Bronchus and its main branches
Pulmonary artery
Pulmonary veins
Lymph drainage
Nerves.

Blood supply

Each lung receives the *pulmonary artery*, which brings deoxygenated blood (from the right ventricle of the heart). The terminal branches of this artery end in a network of capillaries on the surface of each alveolus. Here, gaseous exchange occurs and the capillaries drain into the *pulmonary veins*, which carry oxygenated blood to the left atrium.

Nerve supply

Sympathetic nerve supply is derived from the sympathetic chain (see p. 17), while the parasympathetic nerve supply is from the vagus nerve.

PHYSIOLOGY

Respiration is the transfer of gases between body cells and the environment.

Mechanics of breathing

Air moves into the lungs during *inspiration* and out during *expiration* owing to changes in pressure within the chest. During this period, the lungs expand and shrink passively.

During inspiration, the diaphragmatic muscle contracts and the dome of the diaphragm descends. At the same time, external intercostal muscles (present on the chest wall) contract, thus increasing the space in the chest and allowing air to enter the lungs.

During expiration, the diaphragm and external intercostal muscles relax, the diaphragm rises and the air moves out of the lungs.

An adult breathes between 12 and 16 times/min, while a newborn baby can breathe up to 40 times/min.

During respiration, oxygen is absorbed by the alveoli and carbon dioxide is breathed out into the atmosphere.

The composition of gases in the atmosphere are as follows:

Oxygen	20.98%
Carbon dioxide	0.04%
Nitrogen	78.06%

Gas exchange in the lungs. Oxygen diffuses out of the breathed air into the alveoli and from there enters the bloodstream, and carbon dioxide diffuses out into the alveoli from the blood. The volume of gases transferred depends on the surface area of the alveoli and the thickness of the alveolar wall.

Transport of gases in the blood. Oxygen combines with haemoglobin in the red blood cells to form *Oxyhaemoglobin*. Each gram of haemoglobin carries between 1.34 and 1.39 ml of oxygen. Plasma carries oxygen in a dissolved form (0.003 ml/100 ml of blood per mmHg P_{O_2}). The arterial blood thus contains 19.8 ml of oxygen (in a person with a haemoglobin concentration of 15.0 g/100 ml).

Oxyhaemoglobin dissociation curve. This is a curve which relates the percentage saturation of the blood with oxygen, to the oxygen-carrying potential of the haemoglobin. It has a characteristic sigmoid shape.

Carbon dioxide is transported by plasma proteins, haemoglobin and bicarbonate.

Gas exchange in the tissues. Oxygen. When oxygenated blood reaches the tissue fluid, oxygen which is at a higher partial pressure diffuses out into the tissues. From the tissue fluid, oxygen passes into the cells according to the requirement.

Carbon dioxide is produced in the cells at a higher pressure; this is released into the tissue fluid, and from there into the blood.

Control of respiration

Respiration is controlled by the nervous system and by chemical factors.

a. Nervous system. Respiration is regulated by a respiratory centre located in the medulla oblongata of the brain.
b. Chemical factors. The *carotid bodies* (which are present at the bifurcation of each common carotid artery) and the *aortic bodies* (which lie on the arch of the aorta) are tiny organs made up of nerve cells and blood vessels. They are connected to the respiratory centre in the medulla oblongata. The carotid and aortic bodies sense changes in the carbon dioxide tension and hydrogen ion concentration in the blood passing through them. An increase in carbon dioxide and a fall in pH causes the respiratory centre to send impulses to the respiratory muscles, which in turn contract with greater frequency (increased breathing), thus expelling carbon dioxide from the lungs and restoring the pH to normal.

Tests of lung function

Tidal volume is the amount of air that moves into the lungs with each inspiration. (Normal value is 7 ml/kg body weight. Thus a 70-kg man has a tidal volume of 490 ml, of which 2 ml/kg body weight is the dead space.) Dead space gas does not take part in gas exchange.

Residual volume is the air left in the lungs after a maximal expiration (normal value 1.2 litres).

Vital capacity is the greatest amount of air that can be expired after a maximal inspiration (normal value 4.8 litres).

Forced expired volume at 1 s (FEV1) is the fraction of the vital capacity expired in one second.

CARDIOVASCULAR SYSTEM

ANATOMY

The cardiovascular system is made up of: heart, arteries and arterioles, capillaries, venules and veins.

Heart (Fig. 1.5)

The heart is the size of a clenched fist and lies in the chest. Its relations are:

Above	Aorta, pulmonary trunk
Below	Diaphragm
Behind	Descending aorta, oesophagus and spinal column
On either side	Lungs

The heart has four chambers: right atrium, right ventricle, left atrium, left ventricle.

Right atrium. This lies on the right side of the heart, behind the sternum. The deoxygenated blood enters it via: superior vena cava at the upper end; inferior vena cava at the lower end; coronary sinus, a small vein through which blood comes from the heart; right auricle, a small projection from the atrium which lies in front of the aorta and pulmonary artery.

Right ventricle. This forms a major portion of the front of the heart and has a thick-walled chamber. It consists of:

a. Right atrioventricular valve (also called tricuspid valve), which guards the opening between right atrium and the ventricle (right atrioventricular opening). This valve is made up of three flaps. The base of each flap is attached to the atrioventricular opening and its free border is attached by *chordae tendinae*. Chordae tendinae are small cone-like projections of muscle arising from myocardium and projecting into the ventricle.
b. Pulmonary opening, which opens into the pulmonary artery at the upper end of the ventricle.

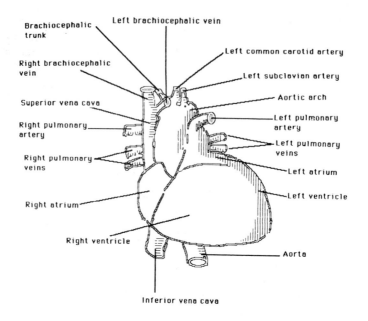

Fig. 1.5   The heart.

The left atrium is a thin-walled cavity, which lies at the back of the heart. Two pulmonary veins bringing oxygenated blood enter the left atrium on each side. The atrium opens below into the left ventricle via the left atrioventricular opening.

The left ventricle, situated at the left and back of the heart, is thick-walled compared with the right ventricle. It consists of: (i) the left atrio-ventricular valve (also called mitral valve); this surrounds the left atrioventricular opening and has two flaps, which are attached to the chordae tendinae; and (ii) an opening into the aorta at the upper end of the ventricle.

The heart is made up of three types of tissue: pericardium, myocardium, endocardium.

Pericardium is a fibrous bag in which the heart is enclosed. It is a double-layered sac with fluid between the layers.

Myocardium forms the greatest part of the wall of the heart. Myocardium is made up of cardiac muscle fibres which are striated and connected to one another by muscular branches.

Endocardium lines the inside of the chambers of the heart and covers the valves on both sides.

Blood supply to the heart

The wall of the heart is supplied by two coronary arteries (right and left), arising from the aorta immediately above the aortic valve. They supply the respective sides of the heart.

Arteries (Fig. 1.6).

The arteries are hollow tubes through which blood flows to the tissues and organs. They are made up of: an outer layer of connective tissue; a middle layer of elastic tissue; an inner layer of intima.

The major arteries in the body are listed below.

Aorta. The aorta is the major artery of the body. It is divided into the thoracic aorta, which lies in the chest, and the abdominal aorta, which lies in the abdomen.

The thoracic aorta begins at the aortic orifice of the left ventricle. It consists of three parts: the as-cending aorta, the arch of the aorta, and the descending aorta.

The abdominal aorta begins at the termination of the descending aorta; this occurs where the vessel passes through the diaphragmatic opening.

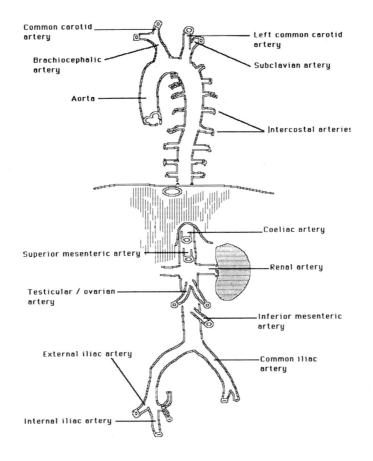

Fig. 1.6 Principal arteries in the body.

The main branches of aorta are:

In the thorax:
— right and left coronary arteries
— brachiocephalic artery
— left common carotid artery
— left subclavian artery

In the abdomen:
— coeliac artery
— right and left renal arteries
— right and left testicular arteries (in males)
— right and left ovarian arteries (in females)
— superior and inferior mesenteric arteries
— right and left lumbar arteries
— right and left common iliac arteries.

Blood supply to the organs

The head and neck are supplied by the common carotid arteries. The common carotid artery on the right side arises from the brachiocephalic artery.

The common carotid artery divides into external and internal carotid arteries.

The external carotid artery supplies various organs in the head and neck through its branches:

— lingual artery to the tongue
— facial artery to the face
— superior thyroid artery to the thyroid gland.

The eye is supplied by the ophthalmic artery, a branch of the internal carotid artery.

The brain is supplied by the right and left internal carotid arteries and right and left vertebral arteries.

The upper extremity is supplied by the subclavian artery and its branches. The right subclavian artery is a branch of the brachiocephalic artery, whereas the left subclavian artery is a branch of the aorta. The subclavian artery continues into the axilla as the axillary artery. The axillary artery runs in the arm as the brachial artery, which then divides into radial and ulnar arteries at the wrist.

In the abdomen the following arteries supply the various organs.

Organ	Artery
Stomach	Splenic artery, hepatic artery and the left gastric artery
Spleen	Splenic artery
Liver	Hepatic artery
Kidneys	Renal arteries
Testes	Testicular artery on each side
Small intestine	Superior mesenteric artery
Large intestine	Superior and inferior mesenteric arteries
Rectum	Inferior mesenteric artery and internal iliac artery
Uterus	Uterine artery
Ovary	Ovarian artery

Blood supply to the pelvic organs and lower extremity

The common iliac arteries divide into right and left branches. Each common iliac artery also divides into an external and internal branch.

The internal iliac artery supplies blood to the bladder, the lower end of the rectum, uterus and vagina, and the gluteal muscles.

The external iliac artery continues into the thigh as the femoral artery. The femoral artery gives off branches to the muscles of the thigh and femur.

The femoral artery continues as the popliteal artery below the knee, and divides into the anterior and posterior tibial arteries, which supply the ankle.

Arterioles are blood vessels with thick walls and like muscles they can contract and relax. They are present in the abdominal organs and skin. Arteriolar dilatation (also called vasodilatation) is facilitated by carbon dioxide, adenosine monophosphate (AMP), and bradykinin. Arteriolar contraction (vasoconstriction) is facilitated by adrenaline, noradrenaline and angiotensin.

Veins and venules (Fig. 1.7) Venules are small veins formed by the union of capillaries.

Veins are formed by the union of venules. They are made up of three layers: an outer layer of collagen fibres; a middle layer of muscle and elastic fibres; and an inner smooth layer of endothelial cells.

Valves are present in many veins, to prevent the back-flow of blood.

Venous drainage of organs

Brain. Veins in the brain form venous sinuses which drain into the internal jugular vein.

Head and neck. The veins of the head and neck enter the internal jugular vein. The internal jugular vein starts at the inferior surface of the skull. It joins the subclavian vein from the arm to form the brachiocephalic vein. The two brachiocephalic veins unite to form the superior vena cava, which empties into the right atrium.

Upper extremity. Veins from the hand travel upwards in the forearm as the cephalic and basilic veins. The basilic vein continues in the axilla as the axillary vein, which in the neck becomes the subclavian vein. The superior vena cava is formed by the union of the two brachiocephalic veins. It receives blood from the head, neck, arms and upper thorax.

Lower extremity. The long saphenous vein begins on the dorsum of the foot and passes upwards to join the femoral vein. The short saphenous vein starts at the back of the calf and

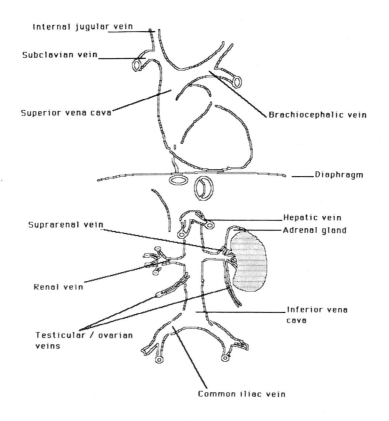

Fig. 1.7 Principal veins in the body.

ascends upwards to join the popliteal vein. The popliteal vein passes upwards to the front of the thigh to become the femoral vein. The femoral vein continues as the external iliac vein. The internal iliac vein which drains blood from the pelvic organs (bladder, rectum) joins the external iliac vein to form the inferior vena cava.

PHYSIOLOGY

The parts of the heart normally beat in an orderly manner. Atrial contraction (also called atrial systole) is followed by the contraction of ventricles (also called ventricular systole). During diastole all four chambers of the heart are relaxed.

The heart beat begins in a specialized conduction system such as sinoatrial node (SA node), atrioventricular node (AV node), the bundle of His and the Purkinje system.

Heart beat

The SA node is the normal cardiac pacemaker and its rate determines the heart beat. At the beginning of systole, a wave of contraction starts in the SA node, spreads through the walls of both atria and reaches and stimulates the atrioventricular node (AV node).

The AV node lies in the wall between the right atrium and the right ventricle. The bundle of His is a band of muscle which runs in the septum between the two ventricles and reaches the apex of the heart. Here it divides into two main branches, one for each ventricle. The wave of contraction which begins in the SA node causes atrial contraction and from there reaches the two ventricles via the AV node, to cause ventricular contraction.

The cardiac cycle is the sequence of events during one heart beat. It occurs in two phases: diastole and systole. Each cycle lasts for 0.8 s when the heart rate is about 75 beats/min.

Diastole is the period of relaxation which follows the contraction and it lasts for 0.5 s. During this period the following events take place. Initially:

a. Venous blood enters the right atrium from the superior and inferior vena cava, and oxygenated blood enters the left atrium from the pulmonary veins.
b. Blood is prevented from entering the ventricle from the atrium by the closure of the two atrioventricular valves (tricuspid and mitral, see p. 8).
c. Similarly, blood is prevented from entering the ventricles from the aorta and the pulmonary artery by the closure of the pulmonary and aortic valves. Later:
d. As the blood enters the atria, the pressure rises. When it exceeds that in the ventricles, the AV valves open and blood flows from the atria into the ventricles.

Systole is the period of muscular contraction and lasts for 0.3 s. During this period the following events take place:

a. The walls of the atria contract, following stimulation by the SA node, thus expelling blood into the ventricles.
b. As the pressure in the ventricles exceeds that in the atria, the AV valves close and the aortic and pulmonary valves open.
c. Blood from the right ventricle is expelled into the pulmonary artery and from the left ventricle into the aorta.
d. When the blood is fully expelled, the muscular contraction stops and the relaxation phase (diastole) begins.

Cardiac output. The blood expelled from the heart during each minute depends upon stroke volume and heart rate.

a. Stroke volume. This is the amount of blood expelled from a ventricle at each beat. At rest it is about 70 ml; this can increase to 125 ml with mild exercise. The stroke volume is controlled by changes in the length of cardiac muscle fibres. The greater the length of the muscle fibres, the greater the contraction.
b. Heart rate. At rest this is usually about 70 beats/min. It is controlled by (i) reduction in stimulation of vagus nerve fibres (parasympathetic) and (ii) to some extent by stimulation of the sympathetic fibres.

Cardiac output is the product of heart rate and stroke volume, as shown below.

Heart rate $\times$ Stroke volume
70 beats $\times$ 75 ml
= approx 5 litres/min

Nerve supply to the heart

Although the heart can beat on its own, it is normally influenced by two sets of nerve fibres:

a. Parasympathetic fibres, which arise from the vagus nerve (10th cranial nerve). When these fibres are stimulated, they slow down the heart rate and decrease the force of contraction.
b. Sympathetic fibres. These arise from the ganglia on the cervical part of the sympathetic trunk (see p. 17). When the fibres are stimulated, they increase the heart rate and the force of contraction.

Heart sounds. The heart, when it is contracting, produces sounds which can be heard with the help of a stethoscope. Usually, two heart sounds are heard, but on some occasions a total of four heart sounds can be heard.

First heart sound: This is produced by the closure of the mitral and tricuspid valves at the beginning of the ventricular systole. It sounds like 'lub' when spoken softly.

Second heart sound is produced by the vibrations caused by the closure of the aortic and pulmonary valves. It sounds like 'dub'.

Third heart sound is due to sudden tightening of the mitral valve cusps. It is a low soft thud, audible in most children.

Fourth heart sound is produced when either atrium (right or left) contracts with more force than the other. It is a low soft sound which precedes the first heart sound.

Electrocardiograph

An electrocardiograph (ECG) is a recording of the

electrical changes that occur in the heart during each beat. A normal ECG shows:

P wave, produced by the contraction of the atria. It lasts for 0.10 s.

QRS complex, produced by the contraction of the ventricles. It lasts for up to 0.09 s.

T wave, produced by ventricular relaxation.

PR interval, the time taken for the impulse to pass down the bundle of His.

The ECG is recorded using 12 different electrode positions.

Arterial pulse

This is a wave transmitted through the arteries as a response to the ejection of blood from the heart into the aorta. It is best felt when an artery is compressed lightly against a bone.

Sites at which pulses can be felt easily are:

Wrist	Radial artery and ulnar artery
Anticubital fossa	Brachial artery
In front of the ear	Superficial temporal artery
On the dorsum of the foot	Dorsalis pedis artery

Pulse rate

is decreased (also called bradycardia) in:
— heart block
— rest

is increased (also called tachycardia) in:
— exercise
— hyperthyroidism
— anxiety
— anaemia

is weak in:
— shock

is strong in:
— excitement
— hyperthyroidism
— raised blood pressure

is absent in:
— cardiac arrest
— complete obstruction of an artery.

Arterial blood pressure

Blood pressure (BP) is the pressure exerted by blood within a blood vessel. It depends upon: cardiac output and resistance to the flow by the diameter of the arterioles.

There are two measurements: systolic pressure—the pressure at cardiac systole; diastolic pressure—the pressure at cardiac diastole.

Blood pressure is measured in millimetres of mercury (mmHg) or kilopascals (kPa). The normal pressures are:

In aorta and large vessels	Systolic	120 mmHg
	Diastolic	80
In small arteries	Systolic	110
	Diastolic	70
In arterioles	Systolic	40
	Diastolic	insignificant

Pressures in various chambers of the heart:

	Systolic	Diastolic
Rt Atrium	5 mmHg	0 mmHg
Rt Ventricle	25	0
Lt Ventricle	121	0
Aorta	120	80
Pulmonary artery	25	12

Normally the blood pressure is raised by emotion and exercise. It tends to fall during sleep.

Hypertension is a sustained rise in blood pressure for which there may or may not be a cause.

Circulation through special organs

The following table illustrates the blood flow to various organs in the body:

Organ	Blood flow (ml/min)
Brain	750
Heart muscle	250
Liver	1500
Skin	460
Kidneys	1260
(Whole body	5400)

Cerebral circulation. The blood flow to the brain is kept fairly constant by the process of autoregulation. The factors which affect the cerebral blood flow are:

a. arterial blood pressure
b   intracranial pressure
c. viscosity of the blood
d. constriction or dilatation of cerebral blood vessels.

Coronary circulation. The two coronary arteries which supply the myocardium arise from the sinuses at the root of the aorta. Blood flow in the coronary arteries occurs during diastole of the heart. Coronary blood flow at rest in man is 250 ml/min, or 5% of the cardiac output.

Pulmonary circulation. Deoxygenated blood from the right ventricle passes via the pulmonary arteries to the capillaries which surround the alveoli in the lungs, and back to the left atrium of the heart. The pulmonary artery arises at the upper end of the right ventricle.

CENTRAL NERVOUS SYSTEM

ANATOMY

The nervous system is made up of: neurones (nerve cells and fibres), neuroglia (cells with no function).

The neurone is the basic unit of the nervous system. Each neurone consists of a nerve cell and its fibres. Each cell has a nucleus and a number of granules and fibrils in its cytoplasm.

Dendrites are short, brush-like fibres attached to the outside of a cell, through which impulses enter the cell from other cells.

The axon is a fibre through which nerve impulses leave the cell to be transmitted to other cells. Most of the axons are covered with a sheath of myelin, a lipid material; these types of axons are called myelinated. This myelin sheath is not present at the nodes of Ranvier.

Transmission of nerve impulse. This occurs in one direction: into the cell through the dendrites and out through the axon. The nerve impulse is an electrochemical change. As a wave of impulse passes along the axon, potassium (K^+) ions leave the axon and sodium (Na^+) ions enter. The nerve impulse occurs as a result of the difference in electrical potential between potassium and sodium. After the wave has passed along the axon, potassium and sodium ions return slowly to their original position.

A synapse is the point of contact between one neurone and another. At this point, transmission of the nerve impulse occurs chemically, the chemicals liberated being acetylcholine, noradrenaline and dopamine.

Neuromuscular junction (Fig. 1.8)

The neuromuscular junction consists of an axon supplying a skeletal muscle which at this point loses its myelin sheath and divides into a number of terminal buttons, or end feet. The end feet contain small clear vesicles which store acetylcholine, the chemical transmitter. These end feet fit into the thickened muscle membrane (also called motor end-plate). The whole structure is collectively called the neuromuscular junction. The nerve impulses arriving at the neurone cause liberation of acetylcholine from the vesicles in the nerve terminals. The acetylcholine increases the permeability of the underlying membrane, and entry of sodium produces a potential which in turn stimulates the adjacent muscle membrane to send the impulses.

The function of the neuromuscular junction is to transfer nerve impulses from small motor neurones to the large muscle fibre and cause it to contract.

Parts of the nervous system

The nervous system is divided into:

A. Central nervous system, which includes the brain and spinal cord.
B. Peripheral nervous system, which includes the cranial and spinal nerves.
C. Autonomic nervous system, which includes the parasympathetic and sympathetic systems.

White matter is the nervous tissue in which there is a high proportion of nerve fibres.
Grey matter is the nervous tissue in which there is a high proportion of nerve cells.

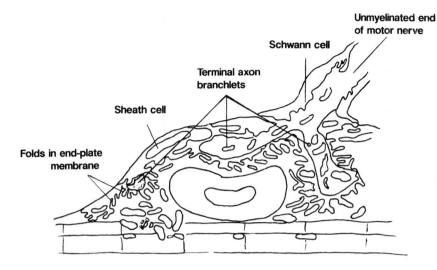

Fig. 1.8 Neuromuscular junction.

A. Central nervous system

This consists of (1) brain, (2) spinal cord.

Brain

The brain is made up of the cerebral hemispheres (right and left), midbrain, pons, cerebellum, and medulla oblongata (which continues with the spinal cord).

Cerebral hemispheres. Together these make up the largest part of the brain, consisting of:

a. cortex (outer layer)
b. thalamus and basal ganglia
c. corpus callosum.

The surface of the cerebral hemispheres is marked by gyri (ridges) and sulci (fissures). Each cerebral hemisphere is divided into four lobes: frontal lobe, parietal lobe, occipital lobe and temporal lobe.

The midbrain is a small structure which lies between the cerebral hemispheres above and the pons below. It is made up of nerve fibres which pass up and down it.

The pons is a thick mass of nervous tissue which lies between the midbrain above and the medulla oblongata below.

The cerebellum consists of a small central lobe and large right and left lobes. It is connected by nerve fibres (in bundles called peduncles) to the midbrain, pons and medulla oblongata.

The medulla oblongata is a narrow piece of nervous tissue which lies between the pons above and the spinal cord below. It contains the cardiac and respiratory centres through which the heart action and breathing are controlled.

Ventricular system of the brain (Fig 1.9)

This is a series of chambers in the brain which are connected to each other. They contain cerebrospinal fluid (CSF). They are:

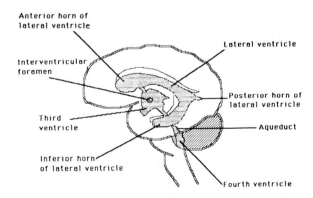

Fig. 1.9 Ventricular system of the brain.

a. Lateral ventricles, which are present in each cerebral hemisphere.
b. Third ventricle. This is present in the mid-brain and is connected to the lateral ventricles above and via a narrow tube called an aqueduct to the fourth ventricle below.
c. Fourth ventricle. This is a lozenge-shaped space which lies between the pons and medulla oblongata in front and the cerebellum behind.

Cerebrospinal fluid (CSF)

This is a clear fluid which fills the above mentioned ventricles and is formed from the blood plasma in the choroid plexuses. The choroid plexuses are whorls of capillaries which lie in the ventricles. About 500 ml of CSF is secreted daily.

Normal values for cerebrospinal fluid:

Volume	120–135 ml	
Pressure	70–150 mmHg	
Glucose	50–85 mg/100 ml	
		(2.2–3.4 mmol/l)
Protein	20–45 mg/100 ml	
		(20–45 g/l)
Sodium	147 mEq/l	(147 mmol/l)
Potassium	2.9 mEq/l	(2.9 mmol/l)
Chloride	113 mEq/l	(113 mmol/l)

Spinal cord

The spinal cord is about 45 cm long and occupies the upper two thirds of the vertebral column. It is continuous above with the medulla oblongata and ends at the level of the 1st or 2nd lumbar vertebra by tapering into a cone called the conus medullaris.

The conus medullaris is connected to the coccyx by the filum terminale, a thin strand of connective tissue.

The spinal cord is made up of nerve fibres on the outside (called white matter) and an H-shaped group of nerve cells (called grey matter) in the middle. A central canal runs through the grey matter (Fig. 1.10).

The nerve fibres are organized in three groups—anterior columns, lateral columns and posterior columns.

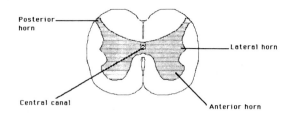

Fig. 1.10   Cross-section of the spinal cord.

Within the cord:

a. Sensory fibres run upwards in the posterior and lateral columns.
b. Motor fibres run downwards in the anterior and lateral columns.
c. Short nerve fibres interconnect at different levels of the cord.

Spinal nerves are attached by anterior and posterior roots to the whole length of the spinal cord.

The meninges are the coverings of the brain and spinal cord. They consist of the following parts:

a. Dura mater, a thick, white membrane which encloses the whole of the brain and the spinal cord.
b. Arachnoid membrane, a thin membrane which fuses in places with the pia mater and in others is separated from it by a subarachnoid space filled with cerebrospinal fluid.
c. Pia mater, a very thin membrane attached to the surface of the brain and the spinal cord.

B. Peripheral nervous system

Cranial nerves

There are 12 pairs of cranial nerves, which are nerves connected to the brain. They are numbered as follows:

1 Olfactory nerve
2 Optic nerve
3 Oculomotor nerve
4 Trochlear nerve
5 Trigeminal nerve
6 Abducent nerve

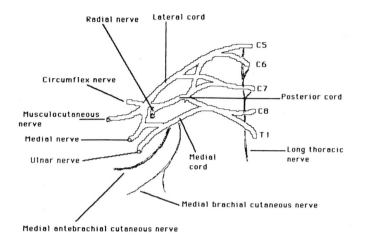

Fig. 1.11 Brachial plexus.

7 Facial nerve
8 Auditory nerve
9 Glossopharyngeal nerve
10 Vagus nerve
11 Accessory nerve
12 Hypoglossal nerve.

Brachial plexus (Fig. 1.11)

This plexus is formed by the anterior branches of cervical nerves C5 to T1. It arises in the lower part of the neck and passes behind the clavicle into the axilla. The major nerves which arise from this plexus are:

Radial nerve
Median nerve
Ulnar nerve
Musculocutaneous nerve
Circumflex nerve.

Lumbar plexus

This plexus is formed by the anterior branches of the 12th thoracic nerve and the first and second lumbar nerves (T12, L1–L2). The nerves which arise from this plexus are:

Femoral nerve
Obturator nerve.

Sacral plexus

This is formed by the anterior branches of L4, L5, S1 to S4 nerves. From this arises the sciatic nerve, which further divides into lateral and medial popliteal nerves which supply the hamstring muscles at the back of the thigh and all the muscles below the knee.

C. Autonomic nervous system (Fig. 1.12)

The autonomic nervous system is made up of two parts: the parasympathetic system and the sympathetic system.

The autonomic nervous system (ANS) supplies the nerves to blood vessels, internal organs (stomach, oesophagus) and endocrine glands. Its functions are integrated with the central nervous system. The actions of parasympathetic and sympathetic systems are opposite in nature.

Parasympathetic system

This is made up of the following parts:

a. Cranial part, which has connections with the cerebral cortex and the hypothalamus. Fibres from these connections are distributed to the oculomotor, facial, glossopharyngeal, vagus and accessory nerves.
b. Sacral part, from which the pelvic organs like the bladder and rectum get their nerve supply.

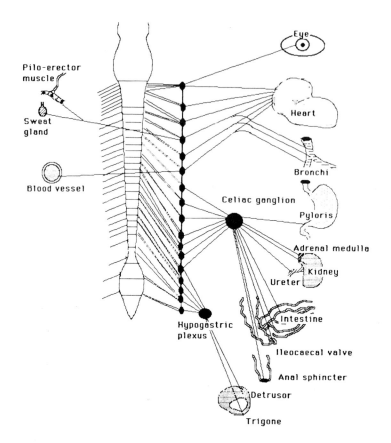

Fig. 1.12 Autonomic nervous system.

Sympathetic system

This system is made up of:

a. Controlling centres in the cortex, hypothalamus and medulla and lateral horn of the grey matter in the spinal cord.
b. A number of ganglia which run down from neck to the abdomen. Fibres which arise from these ganglia supply arteries and other organs.

There are three major ganglia:

(i) cervical ganglia which distribute nerve supply to the carotid arteries, larynx, trachea, thyroid gland and heart;
(ii) thoracic ganglia, which distribute nerve supply to the heart, lungs, aorta and its branches, and the abdominal organs;
(iii) lumbar and sacral ganglia, which distribute nerve supply to the iliac arteries and to the pelvic organs such as the rectum and urinary bladder.

The sympathetic system comes into action during an emergency. For example, during shock, fright, etc. the heart rate and cardiac output are increased, along with a rise in the level of adrenaline. The bowel and bladder movements are decreased.

PHYSIOLOGY

The main functions of the nervous system are to:

a. Receive impulses from inside and outside the body and act accordingly. For example, if a person touches a hot object, the cerebral

Table 1.1 Summary of the functions of the autonomic nervous system.

Body organ	Parasympathetic	Sympathetic
Skin	—	Stimulates sweat glands Erection of hair
Heart	Heart rate and cardiac output decreased	Heart rate and cardiac output increased
Coronary arteries	—	Dilated
Blood pressure	Lowered	Raised
Respiratory bronchioles	Constricted	Dilated
Gastrointestinal tract	Increased peristalsis Sphincters relaxed	Decreased peristalsis Sphincters closed
Liver	Converts glucose to glycogen	Converts glycogen to glucose
Urinary bladder	Sphincters relaxed Muscle tone decreased	Sphincters closed Muscle tone increased

cortex receives the sensations via temperature receptors in the skin, which ascend the spinal cord, and promptly send messages down to the hand to withdraw it.

b. Store memories and express emotions such as anger, or depression.
c. Coordinate the activity of various parts of the body.

Sensory pathways to the brain

Receptors in the skin for temperature, touch, pain, pressure relay their signals via the tracts in the spinal cord to the post-central gyrus of the cerebral cortex.

Cerebral cortex

Large areas of the cerebral hemispheres are concerned with sensory motor functions and some parts are concerned with hearing and vision. The right cerebral hemisphere recognizes various objects and expresses emotions, whereas the left cerebral hemisphere controls the activities of the right side of the body.

There are two major systems by which signals are transmitted from the brain to the spinal cord to produce movement. These are: the pyramidal system (corticospinal system) and the extrapyramidal system (extracortical system).

Cerebellum

The cerebellum is involved in the production of coordinated rapid movements.

Reticular activating system

This is made up of large interconnected neurones in the brain stem. The reticular system is involved in setting the level of consciousness and in the regulation of respiration, heart rate and blood pressure.

Limbic system

This is made up of cortical tissues in the cerebral cortex encircling parts of the hypothalamus, thalamus, the amygdaloid nucleus and hippocampus.

Hypothalamus

The hypothalamus is an extremely important brain centre. It controls body temperature, appetite and the release of a number of hormones from the pituitary gland.

SPECIAL SENSES

EAR AND HEARING

The ear is made up of: external ear, middle ear and inner ear.

External ear

The external ear is composed of: the auricle (pinna) and the external auditory meatus.

The auricle (pinna) is made up of elastic cartilage covered with skin.

The external auditory meatus is the tube leading from the auricle to the tympanic membrane. The outer one third of this meatus is cartilaginous and the inner two thirds made up of bone.

Wax is formed by ceruminous glands in the cartilaginous part.

Middle ear (Tympanic cavity)

This a small, oblong-shaped cavity in the temporal bone. It consists of tympanic membrane and the ossicles.

The tympanic membrane (ear-drum) occupies most of the lateral part of the middle ear and is tightly stretched except in the upper segment.

The ossicles are three little bones: malleus, incus, and stapes, which occupy much of the tympanic cavity.

Inner ear (Fig. 1.13)

Situated in the petrous portion of the temporal bone, the inner ear consists of two organs: the organ of hearing and the organ of balance.

The labyrinth is made up of vestibule, cochlea and three semicircular canals. It is divided into the bony labyrinth, which is a series of interconnected

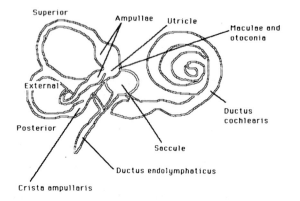

Superior
Ampullae   Utricle
Maculae and otoconia
External
Ductus cochlearis
Posterior
Saccule
Ductus endolymphaticus
Crista ampullaris

Fig. 1.13   Inner ear.

cavities, and the membranous labyrinth—a closed sac within the bony labyrinth.

The perilymph is a clear fluid occupying the space between bony and membranous labyrinths, while the endolymph is a fluid lying within the membranous labyrinth.

The vestibule is a small chamber which communicates anteriorly with the cochlea, posteriorly with the semicircular canals and laterally with the middle ear by two openings—the oval window and the round window.

The cochlea is shaped like the shell of a snail. It is hollow with a cochlear canal running in the tube. The ascending tube begins at the oval window and is called the scala vestibuli; the descending tube is called the scala tympani and ends at the round window.

The organ of Corti is a complicated structure which runs spirally up the cochlea and has about 15 000 hair cells.

The semicircular canals are set at right angles to each other and consist of a superior canal, a lateral canal and a posterior canal. They contain endolymph and open into the posterior wall of the vestibule. Nerve endings of the vestibular branch of the 8th cranial nerve (see below) are connected to hair cells projecting into the endolymph. The utricle and the saccule are parts of the membranous vestibule.

Eighth cranial (auditory) *nerve*. This is the cranial nerve of the internal ear. It is made up of a vestibular part and a cochlear part.

Hearing is the ability of the ear to detect pressure vibrations in the air and to interpret them as sound. The ear converts the energy of the pressure waves into nerve impulses, which are carried to the cerebral cortex and perceived as sounds. The human ear can pick up frequencies ranging from 20 to 16 000 hertz (Hz). One hertz is equal to one cycle per second.

Sound transmission in the ear. Sound waves are received by the auricle and transmitted to the tympanic membrane via the external auditory meatus. The tympanic membrane vibrates and its amplitude is proportional to the intensity of sound. From here, the sound is picked up by the ossicles (malleus) and transmitted through the incus to the stapes. The stapes transmit this sound to the oval window. The sound vibrations within the cochlea stimulate the hair cells in the organ of Corti, which then transmit impulses into the nerve fibres of the cochlear nerve. The cochlear nerve transmits these impulses to the brain.

Balance. The semicircular canals and the saccule and utricle are responsible for maintaining balance.

EYE AND VISION

The eye consists of: transparent cornea, lens, retina, pupil, iris, aqueous and vitreous humour.

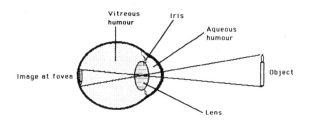

Fig. 1.14 Perception of light.

Perception of light (Fig. 1.14)

The light enters the eye through the transparent cornea and the lens inverts the image. The amount of light entering the eye is regulated by the iris, which acts as a diaphragm, the size of the pupil being controlled by the circular and radial muscles of the iris.

The pupil enlarges in darkness and constricts in bright light.

The rods and cones are light-sensitive cells in the retina. Rods are used for seeing in dark or dim light, whereas cones are used in bright light and to appreciate colours.

THE ALIMENTARY SYSTEM

ANATOMY

The alimentary system (Fig. 1.15) begins at the mouth and ends at the anus. The structures which lie between these two organs are: the pharynx; oesophagus; stomach; small intestine; large intestine.

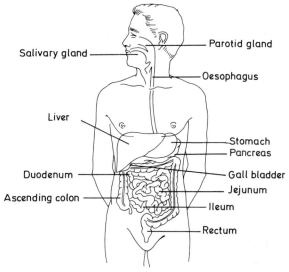

Fig. 1.15 Alimentary system.

The mouth is surrounded by the hard and soft palate above, laterally by the cheeks, by the mandible and tongue below and by the opening into the pharynx behind.

The tongue is made up of muscle enclosed by a mucous membrane. Taste buds are specialized cells which lie at the junction of the anterior two thirds and the posterior third of the tongue.

Blood supply to the tongue is from the lingual artery (a branch of the external carotid artery).

Nerve supply. The motor nerve supply to the tongue is derived from the hypoglossal nerve (12th cranial nerve). The sensory nerve supply to the anterior two thirds of the tongue is derived from the lingual nerve (a branch of the 5th cranial nerve) and the facial nerve (7th cranial nerve). The 5th cranial nerve identifies the touch sensation whilst the 7th nerve identifies taste. The posterior third of the tongue is supplied by the glossopharyngeal nerve (9th cranial nerve) which identifies touch and taste.

Salivary glands are made up of specialised secretory cells. The human salivary glands are: right and left parotid glands, right and left submandibular glands, right and left sublingual glands.

The pharynx is a fibromuscular tube attached to the base of the skull above, and continuous with the oesophagus below. It is made up of three parts: the nasopharynx, the oropharynx, and the laryngeal pharynx—the part of the pharynx which lies behind the epiglottis and the larynx. Food passes through the oropharynx and laryngeal pharynx to enter the oesophagus.

The oesophagus is a muscular tube, about 25 cm long, which begins in the neck as a continuation of the pharynx, passes down the neck and thorax, and then through the left crus of the diaphragm to enter the stomach. The oesophagus is surrounded: in front by trachea and heart; on either side by lungs and pleurae, and behind by the vertebral column. It is slightly narrower at its upper end and also where the left bronchus crosses it and when it passes through the diaphragm.

The stomach (Fig. 1.16) is a wide, dilatable part of the alimentary tract. Its position and shape vary according to the amount of food in it, the presence of peristaltic waves and respiration.

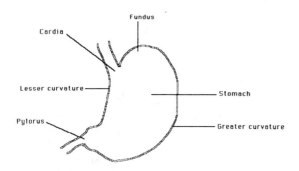

Fig. 1.16   The stomach.

It is a J-shaped organ which lies in the upper left quadrant of the abdomen. It has: an anterior and a posterior surface; a greater curvature on the left side and a lesser curvature on the right side; a cardiac orifice, where the oesophagus joins it; a fundus (dome-like), which lies above the level of the cardiac orifice; a body which forms a large part of the stomach; a pyloric canal; a narrow tube below the body; and a pyloric opening into the first part of the duodenum.

The pyloric opening is surrounded by the pyloric sphincter, which is formed by the thickening of the circular muscles of the stomach. The cardiac orifice has no special sphincter, but is closed by the mucous membrane and muscle fibres at the bottom of the oesophagus.

Structure of the stomach. From inside out, the stomach is made up of: a mucous membrane with the ducts of millions of glands; submucous coat of loose areolar tissue; muscular coats of circular, oblique and longitudinal muscle fibres; peritoneal covering.

Blood supply is from the gastric and coeliac arteries.

Venous drainage is into the portal system.

Lymph drainage is into the lymph nodes along the lesser and greater curvatures.

Nerve supply is from parasympathetic (vagus nerve) and sympathetic nerves.

Small intestine

This is the part of the alimentary system which lies between the stomach and large intestine. It is made up of: duodenum, jejunum, ileum.

The duodenum is a C-shaped tube, about 25 cm long, which lies at the back of the abdomen, curved around the head of pancreas. It is divided into four parts and the pancreatic and bile ducts open into the second part by a common opening. This opening is controlled by a sphincter called the sphincter of Oddi.

Jejunum and ileum. Their combined length varies from 300 to 900 cm. The jejunum is slightly bigger, with a thicker wall, more folds of mucous membrane and fewer Peyer's patches than the ileum.

Blood supply of the small intestine is from the branches of the superior mesenteric artery.

Venous drainage is into the superior mesenteric vein, which drains into the portal vein.

Lymph drainage is into the nodes in the mesentery.

Nerve supply is from the parasympathetic (vagus nerve) and sympathetic nerves.

Structure of the small intestine. From inside out, the layers of small intestine are:

a. Mucous membrane, which is coiled into a number of circular or spiral folds. The surface of the mucous membrane is covered by a large number of villi. (A villus is a tiny projection covered with a single layer of cells. This layer surrounds blood vessels, nerves, and lymph vessels.) Peyer's patches are patches of lymph tissue in the mucous membrane; they are more common in the ileum than in the jejunum.

b. Submucous coat.
c. Muscular coats of circular and longitudinal fibres.
d. Peritoneal coat.

Large intestine

The large intestine has an average length of 150 cm. It is differentiated from the small intestine by its large diameter and the presence of taeniae coli and appendices epiploicae (Fig. 1.18). The taeniae coli are three bands of longitudinal fibres on the outside of the colon, giving the bowel a puckered appearance. The appendix and rectum do not have taeniae coli. The appendices epiploicae are tags of fat-containing peritoneum which lie on the surface of the caecum.

The large intestine is made up of: caecum, appendix, ascending colon, transverse colon, descending colon, sigmoid colon (pelvic colon), rectum and anal canal.

The caecum is a wide sac lying in the right iliac fossa. The ileum enters into the caecum at the ileocaecal opening, and the appendix opens into it below the ileocaecal opening. The caecum is continuous above with the ascending colon (Fig. 1.17).

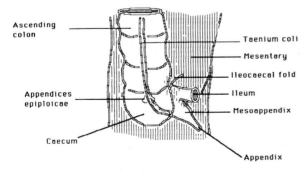

Fig. 1.17 The caecum.

The appendix is a worm-like diverticulum up to 18 cm long which opens into the caecum about 2.5 cm below the ileocaecal valve. It has a narrow lumen and its position is variable, lying either behind the caecum or hanging into the pelvis or in front of the caecum.

The ascending colon extends from the caecum, in the right iliac fossa, up the right side of the abdomen to the right colic flexure under the right lobe of the liver.

Transverse colon. At the right colic flexure the colon bends sharply to the left and passes, as the transverse colon, across the abdomen. It ascends on the left side to end in the left colic flexure under the spleen.

Descending colon. At the left colic flexure the colon bends to pass downwards, on the left side of the abdomen, to the brim of the pelvis, where it continues as the sigmoid colon.

The sigmoid (pelvic) colon has several loops within the pelvis and becomes continuous with the rectum opposite the middle of the sacrum.

The rectum is about 12 cm long. It begins at the middle of the sacrum and ends at the anal canal.

The anal canal, about 3 cm long, runs downwards and backwards and ends at the anus. On either side of this canal are the ischiorectal fossae. An internal and an external sphincter muscle control the opening and closing of the anus.

Blood supply of the large intestine. This is from the branches of the superior mesenteric artery up to the left colic flexure, and then by the branches of inferior mesenteric artery.

Venous drainage is into the superior and inferior mesenteric veins.

Lymph drainage is into lymph nodes in the peritoneum and finally into the aortic glands.

Nerve supply from the parasympathetic and sympathetic nerves.

Structure of the large intestine. From inside out, the layers of the large intestine are: mucous membrane, submucous coat, muscular coat, peritoneum.

Pancreas. This is a long organ which lies at the back of the upper part of the abdomen. It consists of a head (which lies in the curve of the duodenum), neck, body and tail (which reaches the spleen). The pancreas is made up of (a) cells which secrete pancreatic juice and (b) intraalveolar islets, also called islets of Langerhans.

Liver and biliary system

The liver is the largest gland in the body, weighing about 1300–1500 g. It is soft, vascular and wedge-shaped, with its base to the right and apex to the left. It lies in the right upper quadrant of the abdomen, protected by the ribs. Its smooth, rounded upper surface lies below the diaphragm. Its visceral (postero-inferior) surface lies above the stomach, duodenum, colon and right kidney.

Lobes of the liver. The liver is divided into: large right lobe, small left lobe, quadrate and caudate lobes, smaller lobes.

Structures which enter or leave the liver are: right and left branches of the portal vein, right and left branches of hepatic vein, right and left hepatic ducts, lymph vessels and nerves.

Blood supply. About 80% of the blood to the liver passes through the portal vein. About 20% of the blood passes through the hepatic artery, which is a branch of the coeliac artery.

Venous drainage: From the liver is by two large hepatic veins, which enter the inferior vena cava at the back of the liver.

Structure of the liver

The liver is made up as follows:

a. Lobules. There are a large number of very small lobules, each composed of hepatic cells arranged in columns.
b. Sinusoids. These are channels between the columns of cells through which blood passes from the portal vein and the hepatic artery. They are lined by endothelial cells and the cells of the reticulo-endothelial system (see p. 29).
c. A central vein in the middle of each lobule.
d. Canaliculi which run between adjacent columns of hepatic cells and unite to form the hepatic ducts.

The biliary system is made up of: common hepatic ducts, hepatic ducts (right and left), cystic duct, gall bladder, and bile duct.

The right and left hepatic ducts arise from the visceral surface of the liver and unite to form the common hepatic duct. The cystic duct runs from the end of the common hepatic duct to the gall bladder. The bile duct, which is formed by the union of the common hepatic and cystic ducts, joins the pancreatic duct and opens into the second part of the duodenum. This opening is controlled by the sphincter of Oddi.

The gall bladder is a pear-shaped sac which can hold up to 50 ml of bile. It lies in the groove between the right lobe and the quadrate lobe of the liver. It consists of a fundus (rounded end), a body and a neck. The neck of the gall bladder is continuous with the cystic duct.

PHYSIOLOGY

Food is digested to smaller molecules at different points in the intestinal tract, especially in the small intestine. Enzymes, the substances which are involved in the breakdown of food molecules, are found in the secretions of the salivary glands of the mouth, gastric juice, bile from the liver, pancreatic juice and secretions from the mucous membrane of the small intestine.

The salivary glands secrete an enzyme called ptyalin which digests carbohydrates. Saliva also moistens the food, enhances chewing and allows food to be swallowed easily.

Swallowing. After the food has been chewed and mixed with saliva it is formed into a small bolus which is then swallowed. During swallowing contraction and relaxation of voluntary and involuntary muscles takes place. As the tongue pushes the bolus of food backwards, respiration is inhibited, the larynx raised and the glottis closed to prevent food entering the trachea.

The process of swallowing relaxes the oesophageal sphincters, allowing the food bolus to pass down into the oesophagus. As the bolus enters the oesophagus, a wave of contraction passes along the oesophageal wall. This wave of contraction is immediately followed by a wave of relaxation, resulting in the food bolus being pushed through the cardiac sphincter into the stomach. This process is called peristalsis.

Function of the stomach. The stomach acts as a receptacle, collecting food which is then passed on to the duodenum at a controlled rate for digestion and absorption. The stomach helps in mixing the swallowed food with gastric secretions, forming a semi-liquid substance called chyme. The mixing process is associated with rhythmic contractions of the gastric smooth muscle. The peristaltic waves push the liquid contents through the pylorus into the duodenum.

Gastric secretions. Gastric secretions consist of mucus, pepsinogen, hydrochloric acid and intrinsic factor, all of which arise from cells in the gastric mucosa. The main enzyme in gastric juice, pepsin, is secreted as inactive pepsinogen from serous, or chief cells. Hydrochloric acid is secreted by the parietal, or oxyntic, cells. The neck cells of the gastric glands secrete both mucus and intrinsic factor. The mucus protects the gastric mucosa from digestion by gastric juice. The pepsin digests protein.

Control of gastric secretion. Gastric secretions are produced continuously, and increase markedly during a meal. The first phase of increased secretion is called the cephalic phase because it is regulated from the brain via the vagus nerve. The second phase of increased secretion, called the gastric phase, occurs when the food arrives in the stomach. The presence of food in the stomach causes the release of a local hormone, gastrin, from the antral mucosa. The presence of proteins (polypeptides) and alcohol acts as a stimulus for the secretion of gastrin.

Intestinal absorption. The small intestine is the main site of digestion and absorption. Enzymes which break down carbohydrate and protein are located in the brush border of the epithelial cells. In the duodenum, further breakdown of carbohydrates occurs. Proteins in the duodenum are broken down by the pancreatic enzymes, trypsin and chymotrypsin, into dipeptides and amino acids. The amino acids are absorbed into the bloodstream from the lumen of the gut. The fat is digested and absorbed in the small intestine.

Bile salts break down large fat droplets, which arrive from the stomach, into smaller size. These small-sized fat droplets are broken down by the enzyme lipase into free fatty acids and glycerol. Free fatty acids and glycerol, in combination with bile salts, result in the formation of even smaller droplets, called micelles. The micelles come into contact with intestinal mucosa, allowing the free fatty acids and monoglycerides to pass into the epithelial cells. Within these epithelial cells, triglycerides are formed from fatty acids and glycerol by the activity of the endoplasmic reticulum. These triglycerides form chylomicrons, which are then released into the bloodstream.

Pancreatic secretion. The exocrine secretions of the pancreas are of two types: a watery solution with high bicarbonate content secreted by the cells lining the ducts of the glands; and a secretion rich in enzymes which comes from the acinar cells at the base of the glands. The pancreatic secretions are increased by the presence of food in the stomach, and the main secretions from the glands occur when the gastric contents (chyme) enter the duodenum. If the chyme is acid, then the pancreatic secretion is rich in bicarbonate which neutralizes the acid. This response is mediated by the release of secretin from the duodenal mucosa. The presence of fatty acids and amino acids in the duodenum results in pancreatic juice rich in enzymes being released, the mediating hormone in this case being cholecystokinin-pancreozymin.

Biliary secretion. Bile is required for the digestion and absorption of fat and it is secreted by liver cells into small ducts which open into the duodenum via the common bile duct. Owing to the presence of the sphincter of Oddi, bile does not enter the duodenum regularly; it is diverted into the gall bladder. Here, sodium is absorbed and the concentrated bile is made up of: (i) bile salts, (ii) bile pigments, (iii) cholesterol, (iv) lecithin-A (a phospholipid). The bile pigment is yellow in colour, but is chemically altered in the intestine, resulting in the brown colour of normal faeces. Approximately 1000 ml of bile is secreted daily and is stored in the gall bladder until it is required for the digestion of a meal.

Motility of small intestine. The aim of the movement of the small intestine is to mix the food contents with digestive secretions, allow the digested end-products (of proteins, fat, carbohydrates) to come into contact with the mucosa so they may be absorbed; and to move the residue towards the large intestine. The mixing movement is called segmentation, in which rings of intestinal wall contract, dividing the contents into segments. These rings of wall then relax and adjacent rings contract, breaking up the first segments.

In addition to segmentation, peristaltic waves are seen in the small intestine proceeding towards the large intestine. This movement is controlled by parasympathetic nerves (increase the movement) and sympathetic nerves (decrease the movement).

Absorption of water, electrolytes and vitamins. The average intake of water is 1200 ml/day and the average content of water in the faeces is 100 ml/day. A large quantity of water is absorbed in the small intestine. Sodium ions are absorbed actively, and chloride and bicarbonate ions may be actively absorbed or follow other ions passively. Water-soluble vitamins are rapidly absorbed in the small intestine. Fat-soluble vitamins are absorbed along with fats in the jejunum.

The large intestine absorbs water and electrolytes from chyme and stores the resultant faeces until the time is convenient for excretion. Active absorption of sodium is associated with removal of water. The potassium content of the faeces is higher than the plasma level. Peristaltic waves travel for a greater distance than in the small intestine, propelling the contents into the sigmoid colon.

Defaecation. The contents of the sigmoid colon reach the rectum by peristalsis and distend the rectal walls, which act as a stimulus for defaecation. If the conditions are suitable, further peristalsis occurs in the sigmoid colon, the rectal walls contract and both the internal and external anal sphincters relax, resulting in the elimination of faeces through the anus. Defaecation is assisted by the inhalation of a deep breath, closure of glottis and an increase in the intra-abdominal pressure owing to the forced contraction of abdominal muscles.

METABOLISM AND NUTRITION

Consumed food provides energy for the maintenance of vital functions, growth and for physical activity. When the food is converted into energy and heat, oxygen is utilized and carbon dioxide produced.

Energy requirements. The basal metabolic rate (BMR) is the energy requirement under basal conditions. The basal conditions are that a person must be resting and not have had a meal for at least 12 hours. Energy is measured in megajoules (MJ) (Table 1.2). The BMR is increased in hyperthyroidism and decreased in cretinism and myxoedema.

Table 1.2 Energy expenditure in the average man and woman.

	Man	Woman
Sedentary work	10.5 MJ	8.7 MJ
Light work	12.5 MJ	9.6 MJ
Moderate work	–	10.5 MJ
Heavy work	17–20 MJ	14–16 MJ

Food is made up of: carbohydrates, proteins, fats, vitamins, minerals, water.

Carbohydrates. The average intake by an adult is 300–450 g. The carbohydrates are present in food as: monosaccharides (glucose, fructose, galactose), disaccharides (sucrose, lactose, maltose) and polysaccharides (starches).

Sources: Wheat, barley, maize, rice, potatoes.

Digestion: Disaccharides and polysaccharides are converted into monosaccharides, as only the monosaccharides are absorbed by the small intestine.

Absorption and fate: Glucose is the end-product of digestion and absorption of all carbohydrates. Glucose passes freely in and out of cells. It is converted to glycogen by insulin and stored in the cells of the liver. Glycogen is converted back to glucose by the action of glucagon (pancreatic hormone) and adrenaline.

Proteins. The average daily intake of proteins is between 40 and 60 g.

Sources: Milk, fish, meat, peas, lentils and eggs.

Proteins are necessary for the growth and replacement of damaged tissues. A protein is a complex molecule made up of simpler substances called amino acids. Some amino acids are called 'essential' because they cannot be synthesized in the body and must be made available in the diet. They are: phenylalanine, valine, histidine, isoleucine, leucine, threonine, methionine, arginine, lysine, tryptophan. The 'non-essential' amino acids are just as important, but they can be synthesized in the body.

Digestion: Proteins in the food are acted upon by pepsin in gastric juice, chymotrypsin and trypsin in pancreatic juice. By the action of these enzymes, proteins are broken down into amino acids.

Absorption and fate: Amino acids are absorbed through the wall of the small intestine into the bloodstream. Excess amino acids are converted into proteins by the liver and some are broken down into urea and excreted by the kidneys.

Fat. The average daily intake is between 90 and 120 g.

Sources: Butter, margarine, cream, cheese, fatty meat.

Fats are made up of glycerol and fatty acids. Lipid is a term used to describe fats and sterol.

Digestion: As the fats are not soluble in water, bile salts convert them into small droplets. Lipase (an enzyme in pancreatic juice) helps the bile salts in their action and breaks down some of the fatty acids into free fatty acids, monoglycerides and diglycerides.

Absorption and fate: The small fat droplets pass into the lymph vessels of the small intestine and reach the bloodstream via the thoracic duct. Some fats pass into the capillaries of the small intestine and through the portal vein into the liver. Fat is stored or converted into energy. The fat which is not required for energy is deposited in the fat depots of the body (which lie within the abdomen and under the skin). When the need arises, fat is converted into glycerol and fatty acids in the liver. The glycerol is converted into glycogen and used. The fatty acids are oxidized into heat and energy, or into water and carbon dioxide.

VITAMINS

Vitamins are substances which are necessary in small amounts for the health of the body. They are:

| Water-soluble: | Vitamin B complex and Vitamin C |
| Fat-soluble: | Vitamins A, D, K |

Vitamin B complex. The most important of the B complex vitamins are thiamin, niacin, riboflavin, B12 and folic acid.

Thiamin. Lack of this vitamin produces beriberi (peripheral neuropathy, cardiac failure). It is found in liver, kidney, eggs, pork and beans.

Niacin. Lack of this vitamin produces pellagra (diarrhoea, dermatitis, dementia). It is found in cereals, meat, liver, yeast and fish.

Riboflavin. Lack of this vitamin produces degeneration of the cornea, of the mucous membrane of the mouth, and dermatitis. It is found in milk, cheese, green vegetables, liver and eggs.

Vitamin B12 (Cyanocobalamin) is necessary for red blood cell formation and its deficiency leads to pernicious anaemia. It is found in the liver, kidney and muscle. Vitamin B12 is absorbed in the small intestine in the presence of intrinsic factor (which is a constituent of gastric juice).

Folic acid is necessary for the formation of red blood cells. It is found in liver, yeast and green vegetables.

Vitamin C. Vitamin C is necessary for the health of capillary walls and for prompt wound healing. Lack of it causes scurvy (leading to haemorrhage and anaemia). It is found in fresh fruit and vegetables, especially tomatoes, grapefruit and blackcurrants.

Vitamin A is necessary for healthy epithelium and visual purple, and for the growth and development of new bone. It is present in fish-liver oils (such as halibut liver oil and cod liver oil), butter, milk, cream, liver and eggs. Carotenes, which are present in green vegetables and carrots, are converted into vitamin A in the body.

Vitamin D. Necessary for bone formation, its deficiency leads to rickets in children and osteomalacia in adults. It is found in liver, cheese, eggs, butter, fish-liver oils.

Vitamin K. This vitamin is necessary for the formation of prothrombin by the liver and thus for the clotting of blood. It is found in green vegetables (e.g. spinach) and meat.

MINERALS

The essential minerals are:

Sodium	Iodine
Calcium	Magnesium
Potassium	Cobalt
Iron	Zinc
Phosphorus	Copper

Sodium is an important constituent of cells and tissue fluids. It is found in common salt (sodium chloride), fruits and vegetables. The amount required by the body is less than 1 g daily; requirements increase during sweating and dehydration.

Calcium is necessary for the ossification of bone and teeth, coagulation of the blood, cardiac contraction, and transmission of nerve impulses. It is found in most foods, especially milk, butter and cheese.

Potassium is important in cell membrane activity and muscle contraction. It is present in most foods, especially fresh orange juice.

Iron is the essential part of the haemoglobin molecule and thus is necessary for the formation of red blood cells. It is found in liver, beef and spinach.

BLOOD

ANATOMY

Blood is an important transport system within the body. In a man weighing 70 kg the total amount of blood is approximately 5 litres.

Blood is composed of: red blood cells (RBC), white blood cells (WBC), platelets and plasma.

Red blood cells (RBC)

Also called red corpuscles, or erythrocytes, red blood cells are biconcave discs with a diameter of 8.5 μm. They do not have a nucleus and consist of: an outer membrane, haemoglobin (an iron-containing protein), and carbonic anhydrase—an enzyme involved in the transport of carbon dioxide.

The normal ranges of RBCs are:

Male	$4.5–6.5 \times 10^{12}$/litre
Female	$3.9–5.8 \times 10^{12}$/litre

The red blood cells live for a period of up to 180 days. At the end of this period they are destroyed by the cells of the reticulo-endothelial system. Haemoglobin is broken down into: haem, which contains the iron and is used in the manufacture of new red cells; and porphyrin, which is broken down into bilirubin. This bilirubin is removed by the cells of the liver.

White blood cells (WBC)

Also called leukocytes, the types of white cells are: granulocytes (neutrophils, eosinophils, basophils), lymphocytes, and monocytes.

The average values are given in the Appendix.

Granulocytes have small granules in their protoplasm. Based on the staining properties of these granules, the cells are divided into three groups:

Neutrophils	Granules that do not stain
Eosinophils	Granules that stain red with acid dyes
Basophils	Granules that stain blue with basic dyes

The granulocytes are about 10–12 μm in diameter. As the cell matures, the nucleus divides into several lobes, hence the name polymorphonuclear leukocytes (polymorphs). These develop in bone marrow and are discharged into the circulation as and when required.

Lymphocytes have a large, round and slightly indented nucleus which occupies most of the cell.

They vary in size from 7 to 15 μm. They develop in lymph tissue.

Monocytes are large cells, up to 20 μm in diameter, with an oval or kidney-shaped nucleus. They are formed in the bone marrow.

Platelets

These are round or oval, biconvex, non-nucleated discs and number between 150 000 and 400 000/μl. They are part of some large cells in the bone marrow and have a life of about 10 days.

Plasma

Plasma is the fluid part of the blood, which forms 5% of body weight. Plasma provides the medium in which the formed elements of blood (RBC, WBC, platelets) circulate; it also transports organic and inorganic substances from one organ or tissue to another.

Plasma is made up of:

Water—91–92%
Plasma proteins: albumin, globulin, fibrinogen, prothrombin
Inorganic compounds such as sodium, potassium, calcium, magnesium, iron and iodine
Organic compounds such as urea, uric acid, creatinine, glucose, lipids, amino acids, enzymes, hormones.

The functions of plasma proteins are:

a. They maintain the osmotic pressure of plasma—necessary for the formation and absorption of tissue fluid.
b. Prothrombin and fibrinogen are necessary for the clotting of blood.
c. They act as buffers and maintain the normal pH of the body.
d. They transport immunoglobulins which help in the defence of the body against infection.

Reticuloendothelial system (RES)

This system consists of a number of cells of similar structure with common functions, situated in various organs. The RE cells are present in spleen, liver, thymus, lymph nodes, bone marrow, blood, and vessel walls.

A common function of all RE cells is the removal of particles of foreign matter and the destruction of ageing red cells.

PHYSIOLOGY

Red blood cells. Haemoglobin present in the RBCs carry oxygen. The rate of production of RBCs depends on the level of the oxygen supply to the kidney. If it is low, as seen in hypovolaemia, RBC production is increased owing to the release of erythropoietin.

Blood pigments. Haemoglobin, the pigment found in RBCs and the carrier of oxygen, has a molecular weight of 65 000. It is made up of four subunits, each consisting of a pigment part (haem) joined to a polypeptide part (globin). The haem part is an iron-containing porphyrin, which combines reversibly with oxygen. Owing to differences in amino acid composition, haemoglobin can be classified as adult haemoglobin, fetal haemoglobin, and sickle cell haemoglobin.

Formation and destruction of haemoglobin. Haemoglobin is formed by the developing RBCs within the bone marrow; the substances essential for its formation are amino acids, iron, vitamin B12 and folic acid. When the RBC is broken down, the haemoglobin is split into haem and globin. The haem molecule is split open and iron removed for recycling. The remaining pigment is called biliverdin, which in man is converted to bilirubin and then transported to the liver where it is made water-soluble and excreted via the bile. In the gut, the bile pigments are converted to stercobilinogen which colours the faeces.

White blood cells. These are the main agents in the body's defence against infection. This is carried out by either: (i) scavenging (phagocytosis), in which a foreign body is ingested and retained; or (ii) production and distribution of antibodies—molecules which combine with foreign bodies to inactivate them.

The granulocytes are produced in the bone marrow and remain there in store. They enter the circulation for a few hours and are destroyed while performing body defence functions (see p. 85).

Neutrophils are active phagocytes and remain the body's first line of defence against bacterial invasion.

Eosinophils increase in number with parasitic infection.

Monocytes act as scavengers and help in the immune response.

Haemostasis. (Fig. 1.18) If a small blood vessel is cut, repair processes are activated which seal off the vessel. A number of factors are involved in this mechanism of clotting, which converts fibrinogen to fibrin in the blood and forms a clot at the site of the injury.

The clotting factors are:

Factor	
I	Fibrinogen
II	Prothrombin
III	Thromboplastin
IV	Calcium
V	Proaccelerin
VI	—
VII	Proconvertin, Stable factor
VIII	Antihaemophilic factor
IX	Christmas factor
X	Stuart-Prower factor
XI	Plasma thromboplastin antecedent
XII	Hageman factor
XIII	Fibrin stabilizing factor

The series of events leading to clotting are:

a. Constriction of the blood vessel to narrow the lumen
b. Formation of plug of platelets
c. Conversion of this plug into a clot of fibrin.

URINARY SYSTEM

ANATOMY

The urinary system is made up of: kidneys (right and left), ureters (right and left), bladder, urethra.

Kidneys

Each kidney is about 12 cm long, 7 cm wide and 2.5 cm thick and lies at the back of the abdomen in the gutter that runs alongside the vertebral bodies. The right kidney lies slightly lower than the left owing to the presence of the liver on the right side. An adrenal gland sits on the top of each kidney.

The renal artery and vein, lymphatics, nerves and the upper end of the ureter join the kidney at the hilum.

Blood supply is from the renal artery which arises from the aorta.

Venous drainage is by the renal vein into the inferior vena cava.

Structure of the kidney. The kidney is made up of: (i) a fibrous capsule on the outside; (ii) a cortex, made of glomeruli; (iii) a medulla, made up of a number of conical renal papillae which project into the pelvis.

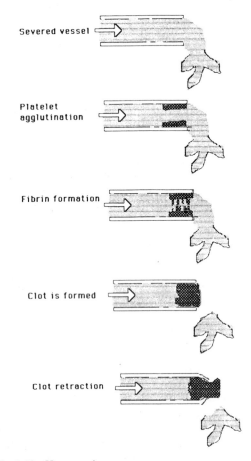

Severed vessel

Platelet agglutination

Fibrin formation

Clot is formed

Clot retraction

Fig. 1.18   Haemostasis.

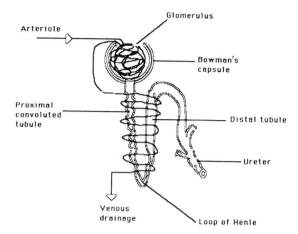

Fig. 1.19 Nephron.

Nephron (Fig. 1.19)

This is the functional unit of the kidney. Each kidney is made up of approximately one million nephrons.

Each nephron is made up of a renal tubule and a glomerulus.

The renal tubule is a long tube which is bent and lined by a single layer of cuboidal cells. It begins at Bowman's capsule, which encloses the glomerulus; then the tubule twists on itself to form the proximal convoluted tubule (PCT). The PCT runs from the cortex to the medulla and back again, forming the loop of Henle. The loop of Henle leads into the distal convoluted tubule which then ends as the collecting tubule.

Each collecting tubule joins other tubules in the medulla of the kidney and opens on the surface of a renal papilla within the pelvis of the ureter.

Blood supply. The glomerulus is a whorl of capillaries enclosed within the Bowman's capsule, and an afferent arteriole brings blood to it. An efferent vessel passes from the glomerulus to the renal tubules and divides into capillaries on its surface. The capillaries drain into a vein, which joins other vein branches to form the renal vein.

Ureter

The ureter is a tube which connects the kidney to the bladder. It is about 25 cm long and starts as a dilated part (called pelvis), which is attached to the hilum of the kidney. The ureter runs down behind the peritoneum in the posterior abdominal wall. In the pelvis it turns forwards and inwards to enter the urinary bladder.

Urinary bladder

This is a muscular sac into which the ureters empty the urine. The relationship of the bladder to other organs is as follows:

> In front of the bladder lies the pubic symphysis
> In the female, the uterus and vagina lie behind the bladder
> In the male, the vas deferens, seminal vesicle and the rectum lie behind the bladder
> At the sides lie the pelvic fascia and ligaments and the levator ani muscles
> Above the bladder lie the coils of the small intestine
> In the female, the anterior vaginal wall lies below the bladder
> In the male the prostate gland lies below the bladder.

The ureters enter the bladder posteriorly and the urethra leaves the bladder anteriorly.

Structure of the bladder. From outside inwards, the bladder consists of: (i) peritoneum or pelvic fascia on the outside; (ii) a muscular coat, which forms the bladder wall; (iii) a submucous coat; (iv) a mucous membrane, which is folded when the bladder is empty.

Female urethra

This is a small tube about 3 cm long, which extends from the bladder to an opening between the labia minora about 2 cm behind the clitoris. It runs in front of the vagina.

Male urethra

The male urethra is a tube about 20 cm long, which extends from the bladder to the end of the penis. It is made up of three parts: prostatic urethra, which passes through the prostate gland; membranous urethra, which is enclosed by a sphincter of muscle fibres; and spongy urethra, which is 15 cm long and passes through the corpus spongiosum of the penis to end near the tip.

PHYSIOLOGY

Formation of urine

The kidneys are the main excretory organs of the body. They receive about 25% of the cardiac output. The glomerulus and the tubules play an active part in the formation of urine.

Glomerular function

The initial stage in the formation of urine is the filtration of almost protein-free plasma through the glomerular capillaries into the Bowman's capsule. During urine's passage through the tubular system, its composition is altered by selective reabsorption of certain substances and selective secretion of others. In a healthy adult, about 120 ml urine/min are filtered out, or about 170 litres in 24 hours.

Tubular secretion

As the filtrate passes along the tubule and collecting duct, its composition is altered by exchanges between it and the blood in the capillaries.

The substances which are reabsorbed into the blood are:

Sodium (90%)
Chloride (90%)
Glucose (100%)
Water (90%)
Amino acids, calcium and bicarbonate.

The substances which pass out of the blood into the filtrate to maintain a constant pH are: ammonium salts, hydrogen ions, phosphates and potassium.

The antidiuretic hormone (ADH), which is secreted by the hypothalamus and stored in the posterior lobe of the pituitary gland, controls the reabsorption of water in the collecting duct. Of the 23 litres of fluid which pass into the ducts, about 21.5 to 22 litres are reabsorbed. 1–1.5 litres are excreted as urine in 24 hours.

Excretion of end-products and drugs

End-products of protein metabolism such as urea, uric acid and creatinine are excreted in the urine. A number of drugs are excreted mainly through the kidneys.

Constituents of urine
Amount: 900–1500 ml/24 h
Specific gravity: 1002–1030
Reaction: Acid, pH 6.0
Uric acid: 0.6 g
Urea: 20–30 g
Water
Creatinine: 1–2 g
Ammonia, potassium, sodium, chloride, phosphates and sulphates.

Physiology of micturition

Micturition is a reflex action controlled by higher centres in the nervous system. When the urine enters the bladder it stretches the muscle fibres of the bladder wall. The afferent nerves in the bladder wall send impulses to the lumbar part of the spinal cord. From the spinal cord the impulses are transmitted to the cerebral cortex which produce a desire to micturate.

The efferent nerves pass along the sacral parasympathetic nerves to the bladder and cause the muscle of the bladder wall to contract and the sphincter of the bladder to relax. The urine is expelled, assisted by the contraction of the muscles of the abdominal wall and the diaphragm, which collapse the bladder by raising the intra-abdominal pressure.

LYMPHATIC SYSTEM

ANATOMY

The lymphatic system is made up of: lymph capillaries, lymph vessels, lymph nodes.

Lymph capillaries. These are thin-walled, blind-ended tubes which lie in the tissue spaces of various organs and tissues.

Lymph vessels. These are larger tubes, formed by the joining of lymph capillaries. They contain a number of valves which give them a beaded appearance. Superficial lymph vessels drain the skin, while the deeper lymph vessels drain the deeper organs in the body. Lymph vessels drain into lymph nodes.

Lymph nodes. These are round or oval masses of lymph cells, enclosed in a capsule. Lymph vessels enter or leave the glands, connecting one node to another.

Certain structures in the body such as the tonsils, nasopharyngeal adenoids, thymus gland and Peyer's patches in the small intestine are made up of lymph tissue.

Lymph is the fluid in the lymph vessels. It has a similar composition to blood plasma and contains lymphocytes.

Cisterna chyli and thoracic duct. The cisterna chyli is a large sac which lies in the upper part of the abdomen, behind the aorta and in front of the bodies of the upper two lumbar vertebrae. Lymph from the abdominal organs and the legs passes to the cisterna chyli via the aortic glands. The thoracic duct, which is continuous with the cisterna chyli, passes into the thorax via the diaphragm and ends in the junction of the left subclavian vein and the left internal jugular vein. It receives lymph vessels from the left arm, the left side of the head and neck, and the chest.

Lymph drainage in the body

Organ	Drainage site
Head and neck	Nodes in the neck
Breast	Nodes in the axilla, neck and in the chest
Lungs	Nodes in the hilum of lung, at the bifurcation of the trachea
Stomach	Nodes around greater and lesser curvature of stomach and the lower end of oesophagus.
Small intestine	Nodes in front of the aorta, mesenteric nodes
Large intestine	Mesenteric nodes
Pelvic organs	Nodes in front of the lower end of the aorta
Genitalia	Nodes in the groin
Legs	Nodes in the popliteal fossa, in the groin and in front of the lower end of the aorta

PHYSIOLOGY

The functions of the lymphatic system are:

a. Drainage of tissue spaces: fluids which pass out of the capillaries are removed by the lymphatics
b. Production of antibodies: the lymph nodes are sites of antibody production
c. Production of lymphocytes: lymphocytes which are produced in the lymph nodes reach blood via the lymphatic system
d. Absorption of fat: approximately 60–70% of the fat absorbed from the small intestine enters the blood via the cisterna chyli and thoracic duct.

ENDOCRINE SYSTEM

The anatomy and physiology of the endocrine glands will be described simultaneously.

The endocrine system is made up of glands which secrete substances called hormones directly into the bloodstream.

Some of the important endocrine glands are: pituitary gland; thyroid and parathyroid gland, adrenal glands, pancreas, pineal gland.

Pituitary gland (Fig. 1.20)

The pituitary gland lies in a deep depression (called the pituitary fossa) in the upper surface of the body of the sphenoid bone in the skull. The stalk of the pituitary gland connects the hypothalamus with the gland. The gland is made up of two lobes, anterior and posterior.

Anterior lobe

This consists of three types of cells: basophils, which stain blue; acidophils, which stain red; chromophobes, which stain poorly.

The anterior lobe's activities are controlled by chemical factors in the hypothalamus. The important hormones produced by the anterior pituitary are:

a. Growth hormone (GH), which is essential for growth and storage of nitrogen.
b. Adrenocorticotrophic hormone (ACTH), which stimulates the cortex of the adrenal glands to produce glucocorticoids.
c. Thyroid stimulating hormone (TSH), which stimulates the thyroid gland to produce triiodothyronine and thyroxine.
d. Gonadotrophic hormones such as interstitial cell-stimulating hormone (ICSH), which in men stimulates cells in the testes to produce androgens, follicle stimulating hormone (FSH), which ripens the ovarian follicles in women, and luteinizing hormone (LH), which completes the ripening of the follicles and stimulates the development of the corpus luteum.

Posterior lobe

The hormones secreted by the posterior lobe of the pituitary gland are produced in the hypothalamus and pass down the nerve fibres to the posterior lobe. The important hormones are:

a. Oxytocin, which is involved in controlling uterine action during the birth of a baby and in contraction of the muscle of the ducts of the breast, causing the milk to be squeezed from the deeper to the superficial ducts.
b. Antidiuretic hormone which stimulates the distal tubules of the kidney to reabsorb water from the fluid in them.

Thyroid and parathyroid glands

Thyroid gland

The thyroid gland is situated in the neck and consists of right and left lobes connected by a narrow isthmus.

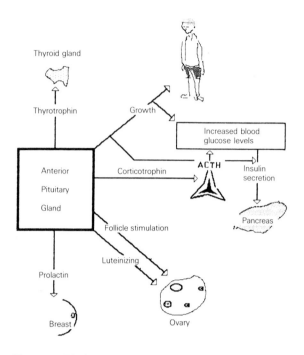

Fig. 1.20 Pituitary gland and its relation to other glands.

The thyroid gland secretes triiodothyronine and thyroxine. Both these hormones contain iodine and are essential for oxidative processes in metabolism. Whenever the blood levels of thyroxine fall, its production is stimulated by the thyroid-stimulating hormone (TSH) of the anterior pituitary gland (Fig. 1.20).

Parathyroid glands

Four in number, the parathyroid glands lie behind the thyroid. They are made up of clumps of cells, separated by connective tissue with sinusoids for blood running around the cells.

The parathyroid glands secrete parathyroid hormone, which raises the amount of calcium in the blood plasma by: (i) increasing the reabsorption of calcium by the tubules of the kidney; (ii) transferring calcium from bone to plasma; (iii) promoting the absorption of calcium by the intestines.

Adrenal glands

These glands lie at the back of the abdomen immediately above the kidneys. Each gland consists of a yellow cortex and an inner reddish-grey medulla.

Adrenal cortex

This has three zones of cells: an outer zone made up of cells in clusters; a middle one of cells in columns; and an inner layer of irregular columns.

The adrenal cortex produces three types of hormone:

a. Glucocorticoids. Their secretion is regulated by ACTH from the pituitary gland. Cortisol (hydrocortisone), the most important hormone, breaks down tissue proteins which are converted in the liver into glycogen; it causes deposition of glycogen in the liver and raises blood sugar; it also controls the exchange of electrolytes and water between extracellular spaces and cells.
b. Mineralocorticoids. Aldosterone, an important hormone, controls the sodium balance in the body by acting on the tubules of the kidneys. It causes the retention of sodium and excretion of potassium. Its secretion is regulated by the production of renin by the kidney and the level of plasma potassium.
c. Androgens. These are produced in the male and are responsible for the development of secondary male sexual characteristics (growth of hair on the face and deepening of the voice).

Adrenal medulla

The adrenal medulla is formed from the same tissues as the nervous tissue, and is made up of irregular cells surrounded by blood sinuses and innervated by sympathetic nerves.

The adrenal medulla produces adrenaline and noradrenaline. These hormones are secreted in response to stress, allowing the body to take protective action in a dangerous situation. The actions of noradrenaline and adrenaline are summarized in Table 1.3.

Pancreas

The hormone-secreting groups of cells lying

Table 1.3 Action of noradrenaline and adrenaline.

Organ	Noradrenaline	Adrenaline
Metabolism	Very little action	Increase oxygen consumption, raises blood sugar, converts glycogen to glucose
Heart	Initially, rate increased then decreased. Very little action on cardiac output	Cardiac rate and output increased
Coronary arteries	Constricted	Dilated
Blood vessels in skin voluntary muscle	Constricted Constricted	Constricted Dilated
Blood pressure	Increased	Increased initially, then decreased owing to dilatation of blood vessels in muscle
Involuntary muscles	Sphincters contracted. In the gut, tone and peristalsis decreased	Sphincters contracted. In the gut, tone and peristalsis decreased. Bronchi dilated

within the pancreas are called islets of Langerhans. They contain two cell types: alpha cells and beta cells. The alpha cells produce glucagon and the beta cells produce insulin.

Glucagon

The chief function of this hormone is to convert glycogen in the liver into glucose. The production of glucagon is stimulated by a fall in the blood sugar, which could be due to either severe exercise or fasting.

Insulin

Insulin's function is to stimulate the transfer of glucose across cells walls and to facilitate the utilization of glucose by the cells. The production of insulin is stimulated by a rise in the blood sugar, which occurs after a meal containing carbohydrates.

Normal blood sugar levels are between 4.5 and 8.5 mmol/l.

Factors which increase the blood sugar are: adrenaline, cortisol, growth hormone, glucagon.

Insulin is the only hormone which *lowers* the blood sugar.

Pineal gland

This a small oval structure lying near the midbrain. It is made up of epithelial cells. The pineal gland produces melatonin, which delays the onset of puberty.

Kidney

In addition to controlling acid-base and water balance, the kidneys produce erythropoietin and renin.

Erythropoietin

This is produced in response to hypoxia. It stimulates the formation of RBCs in the bone marrow.

Renin

Renin is produced by juxtaglomerular cells in the walls of the arterioles through which blood passes into the glomeruli. It is secreted in response to a fall in blood pressure, thus raising the pressure.

REPRODUCTIVE SYSTEM

ANATOMY

Female genital system (Fig. 1.21)

This consists of: ovaries, right and left; Fallopian tubes, right and left; uterus, vagina, external genitalia.

Ovary. There are two ovaries. Each is attached to the lateral wall of the pelvis by the broad ligament, a double fold of peritoneum. The fallopian tube arches over the ovary and ends on it.

Fallopian tubes. They are two in number, right and left. Each tube is approximately 20 cm long, extending from the lateral angle of the uterus to

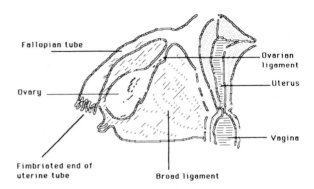

Fig. 1.21 Female genital system: uterus, Fallopian tubes and ovary.

the ovary. At the ovarian end, the tube opens by a small hole into the peritoneal cavity.

Uterus. This is a muscular, pear-shaped, thick-walled organ. It lies in the pelvis between the rectum, behind, and the bladder, in front. It consists of: the fundus, which has a rounded upper end; and the body, which forms about two thirds of the organ and is continuous with the cervix at an angle, so that the whole uterus bends forwards (termed anteversion). The uterus is hollow.

Cervix. The cervix has a cylindrical shape in the lower one third and it ends in the vagina. It has a cervical canal between the internal os (where the body of the uterus opens into the cervix) and the external os (where the cervix opens into the vagina).

Peritoneal attachments. The round ligament is a narrow, fibrous band which runs from the side of the uterus, through the board ligament, down the inguinal canal to end in the labium majora.

The broad ligament runs on each side of the uterus to the lateral wall of the pelvis. The uterine blood vessels, nerves and lymph vessels run between the two layers.

The recto-uterine pouch of Douglas is formed by the peritoneum between the rectum and the uterus.

Blood supply of the uterus. The uterus is supplied by a uterine artery on each side, which is a branch of the internal iliac artery.

Venous drainage is into the internal iliac vein.

Lymphatic drainage. From the fundus of the uterus the lymph vessels drain into inguinal lymph nodes, from the cervix they drain into the external iliac and internal iliac nodes.

Structure of the uterus. The uterus is made up of three layers: endometrium, which is the inner layer and is made up of columnar epithelial cells and glands (these undergo changes at various stages of the menstrual cycle); myometrium, which is the middle layer and is made up of plain muscle fibres; and peritoneum, which covers the uterus externally.

Vagina. This is a tube like structure which extends from the cervix of the uterus to the vulva. The cervix of the uterus extends into the upper part of the vagina. The hymen is a thin, mucosal fold at the opening of the vagina.

Structure of vagina. From inside out the layers are:

a. mucosal membrane made of squamous epithelium
b. muscular coat made up of plain muscle
c. fibrous tissue.

The vagina is continuously kept moist by secretions from the cervix and transudate from the vaginal wall.

Vulva. This is the female external genitalia. It is made up of:

Labia majora — two layers of hair-bearing folds which begin at mons pubis (pad of fat in front of the pubic symphysis) extending to the perineum in the midline behind.

Labia minora — two thin lips of skin which lie within the labia majora, enclosing the clitoris in front.

Clitoris — a small organ, equivalent to the penis in the male.

Vestibule — the area enclosed by labia minora, it contains the opening of the urethra and the opening of the vagina.

Bartholin's glands — a pair of oval mucus-secreting glands which lie deep to the posterior parts of the labia majora; they open by a duct at the side of the labia minora.

Male genital system

This consists of: testes, epididymis and other ducts, prostate gland, penis.

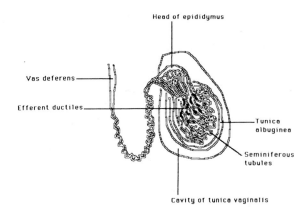

Fig. 1.22 Male genital system: testis.

Testes (testis = singular) (Fig. 1.22). The testes are oval bodies; each of which is suspended by the spermatic cord in its half of the scrotum. The tunica albuginea is the fibrous capsule of the testis, and the tunica vaginalis is a double-layered covering which encloses the testis.

Structure. Each testis is divided by septa (partitions) into 150–300 lobules. Each lobule is made up of 1–3 seminiferous tubules. Spermatozoa are produced by the cells of the seminiferous tubules. The seminiferous tubules open as efferent ducts at the back of the testis. Male hormone (testosterone) is produced by the interstitial cells.

Blood supply to the testes. Each testicular artery which supplies the testes arises from the abdominal aorta just below the renal arteries.

Venous drainage. Blood from the testes is collected by the pampiniform plexus of veins in the spermatic cord. This plexus drains into the testicular vein. The right testicular vein drains into inferior vena cava and the left testicular vein into the left renal vein.

Lymph drainage. Lymphatic vessels from the testes drain into aortic lymph nodes.

Nerve supply. Sympathetic nerves innervate the testes.

Epididymis and other ducts. The epididymis consists of a series of tubes through which the spermatozoa pass. The vas deferens is a thick walled tube, which begins at the lower end of the epididymis, passes through the inguinal canal and opens at the back of the urinary bladder. The seminal vesicle is a vessel formed of coiled sacculated tubes; one lies on each side at the back of the bladder. The ejaculatory duct is a common duct for the vas deferens and the seminal vesicle. It runs through the prostate gland to open into the prostatic part of the urethra.

Prostate gland. This is about the size and shape of a horse chestnut. It lies behind the symphysis pubis, below the bladder and in front of the rectum. The prostate gland surrounds the first part of the urethra and the ejaculatory ducts pass through it.

This gland is made up of a number of tubular glands and fibromuscular tissue, and is enclosed in a capsule.

Penis. This is made up of three cylindrical bodies: the right and left corpora cavernosa and a central corpus spongiosum. It is attached posteriorly to the perineum and the sides of the pubic bone. The glans is the tissue into which the corpus spongiosum is enlarged at the end of the penis; it is enclosed in the prepuce.

The urethra enters the corpus spongiosum posteriorly, and opens anteriorly at the external urethral opening on the tip of the glans penis.

Structure. The corpora cavernosa and corpus spongiosum are made up of sponge-like tissue, formed by connective tissue and smooth muscle. This tissue encloses vascular spaces which engorge when stimulated by parasympathetic nerves.

PHYSIOLOGY

Menstruation

This begins at puberty around the age of 11–13 years and occurs at regular intervals of 28 days until the menopause sets in at the age of 45 to 50 years.

The menstrual cycle is regular owing to ovulation at set times, and is controlled by follicle stimulating hormone (FSH) and lutenizing hormone (LH) (see p. 34).

The menstrual cycle is divided into three phases:

a. Pre-ovular (proliferative) phase. This lasts for 14 days. Oestrogen is secreted by the ovarian follicle under the influence of FSH. The endometrium grows thicker.

b. Postovular (secretory) phase. This phase lasts for 13 days. Progesterone and, to a certain extent, oestrogen, are produced by the corpus luteum in the ovary. (If the ovum is not fertilized, the corpus luteum shrinks, and from the 22nd day the progesterone secretion starts to fall.) The endometrium becomes vascular and the glands are distended.

c. Menstrual phase. This lasts for 4 to 5 days. The progesterone levels fall; the endometrium degenerates, the secretions from the gland are discharged. The unsupported capillaries break down and bleed.

Penile erection and ejaculation

Spermatozoa are formed in the seminiferous tubules which pass along the vas deferens. Under sexual excitement, impulses pass along the parasympathetic nerves to the arterioles of the penis. The arterioles dilate and the vascular spaces of the penis become swollen with blood, thus leading to the stiffening and erection of penis. During ejaculation, the semen produced by the seminal vesicles and prostate gland is discharged through the urethra.

Pregnancy

In the female, if the ovum (egg) combines with a sperm (during secretory phase), fertilization takes place. After a short delay, the fertilized egg starts dividing till it forms a fluid-filled cavity called the blastocoele. A single layer of cells called the trophoblast forms around the blastocoele. After implantation in the uterus, the trophoblast cells form the placenta and membranes. At one end of the blastocoele, there is an accumulation of cells (called the inner cell mass), which later forms the actual fetus.

The duration of pregnancy in humans averages 270 days from fertilization, or 284 days from the first day of the menstrual period before conception.

The enlarged corpus luteum of pregnancy secretes oestrogen and progesterone, and after eight weeks the placenta produces these hormones. At term, once labour begins, stimuli from the genital tract cause reflex secretion of the hormone oxytocin. This stimulates uterine contraction, which in turn dilates the cervix. The fetus descends and is expelled owing to a combination of factors such as oxytocin action and autonomic reflexes.

Lactation

Milk is formed by the cells of a glandular epithelium. Lactation occurs in two phases: milk secretion, and milk removal. The secretion of milk is controlled by prolactin and ACTH hormones. Milk removal is the transfer of milk from the alveoli to the nipple. Sensory receptors in the nipple, stimulated by the suckling infant, send impulses up the spinal cord to the hypothalamus, where they cause the release of oxytocin hormone (see p. 34). This hormone, in addition to causing uterine contraction, contracts the epithelial cells around the alveoli of the breast. This forces the milk from the alveoli to reach the nipple.

SKIN

The skin is one of the largest components of the body and forms 15% of the total body weight. It is made up of epidermis and dermis.

Epidermis, the outer layer, is made up of stratified squamous epithelium. The upper layers contain keratin. Pigmentation of the skin is due to a black pigment, melanin, which is present in the deeper layers of the skin.

The dermis is a layer made up of collagen and fibrous and elastic tissue. The superficial layer projects into the epidermis in a number of small papillae. The deeper layers contain blood vessels, lymphatics and nerves.

Nerve supply. The skin is supplied with sensory and sympathetic nerves. Sensory nerve fibres in the skin which carry impulses to the brain include:

a. free nerve endings
b. Meissner corpuscles around nerve endings in the papillae
c. Pacinian corpuscles found deep in the dermis.

Sympathetic nerve fibres supply the sweat glands and erector pili muscles.

Sebaceous glands are present everywhere in the skin except on palms and soles. A sebaceous gland is situated between a hair follicle and the erector pili muscle. It opens by a duct into the upper part of the follicle. Sebum is the collection of degenerated cells; it protects and lubricates the hair and skin.

Sweat glands. A sweat gland is a coiled tube found in the subcutaneous tissue with a long duct which opens on the surface of the skin. There are three types of sweat glands: (i) ordinary sweat glands which are innervated by sympathetic nerves; (ii) apocrine glands which are present in the axillae, nipples and vulva; they have no nerve supply and a yellowish secretion is produced following stimulation by adrenaline; (iii) ceruminous glands which are present in the external auditory meatus and produce wax.

Hair. A hair is an outgrowth from a papilla at the bottom of a hair follicle (a narrow tube which runs from the surface of the skin to the dermis).

Erector pili muscle is a bundle of smooth muscle fibres attached at one end to the dermis and at the other end to a hair follicle. This muscle is supplied by sympathetic nerves.

Nails are specialized pieces of epidermis. A nail consists of nail bed and matrix.

PHYSIOLOGY

Functions of the skin

a. Sensation. Sensations such as pain, touch, pressure and temperature changes are picked up by the receptors in the skin and transmitted through the sensory nerves to the spinal cord and brain.
b. Storage. The skin acts as a store for fat and water.
c. Protection. The skin protects the internal organs of the body against invasion by bacteria and trauma.

d. Absorption. The skin absorbs ultraviolet light and certain drugs.

Regulation of body temperature (Fig. 1.23)

While discussing the body temperature, skin, subcutaneous tissue and muscles are described as the 'peripheral shell', and the content of skull, chest and abdomen as 'the inner core'. The temperature of the inner core is maintained fairly constant by heat loss and heat gain, whereas the peripheral temperature may vary.

Heat loss occurs from the skin, expired air and faeces and urine. Heat loss occurs from the skin by conduction, convection and radiation, insensible perspiration and sweating.

Water and heat loss by evaporation. This occurs by sweating. Sweat is secreted by sweat glands, which are present all over the skin. It contains sodium chloride, urea and lactic acid, and is secreted under the control of the hypothalamus and cerebral cortex. Sweat is increased by: emotional state, exercise, a rise in body temperature, a fall in blood sugar.

In hot weather, 1.5 to 2 litres of sweat can be lost in one hour.

Heat gain occurs by its production in the body and by uptake from the surrounding environment.

Heat production is due to metabolic activity in the body. The amount of heat produced by skeletal muscle varies from minimal at rest to maximal at exercise. The internal organs such as the heart and liver produce heat at a constant rate.

Heat from the surrounding environment. The body absorbs heat from: (i) hot food, drinks and baths; (ii) hot air in hot weather; (iii) direct radiation from the sun.

Normal body temperature. The body temperature is maintained between 36° and 37°C (97–99.5°F). In every individual the temperature is low during morning and high during evening. In women, every month the temperature during the first half of the menstrual cycle is lower than the second half. The temperature rises by about 0.5°F during ovulation.

Temperature control. Body temperature is regulated by a combination of behavioural and physiological responses. In man, the behavioural responses are important. Thus if a person is hot, he moves to a cooler place and removes clothing. More blood circulates through the skin and he sweats. If a person is cold, he moves to a warmer place, puts on more clothes, blood circulation to the skin decreases and he shivers. The hypothalamus in the brain senses the temperature of the blood perfusing in the capillaries. It contains two centres for heat regulation. One responds to a fall in temperature by causing vasoconstriction and further production of heat. Another centre responds to a rise in temperature by causing vasodilatation and promotes heat loss.

The physiological responses in man are controlled by the endocrine glands.

Thyroid gland. Cold increases the production of thyroxine, which in turn increases the heat production.

Adrenal medulla. Cold increases the production of adrenaline, which increases heat production.

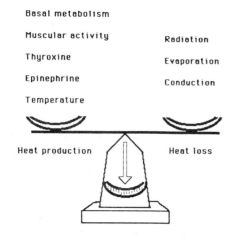

Fig. 1.23   Regulation of body temperature.

SKULL AND LOCOMOTOR SYSTEM

Skull

The skull is formed by the union of several bones, united by sutures. It protects the brain, eyes and ears. It provides attachment for muscles acting on the head and teeth.

The bones in the skull are:

Frontal
Occipital
Parietal (left and right)
Temporal (left and right)
Sphenoid
Ethmoid
Maxilla
Zygoma (left and right)
Mandible
Palatine (left and right)
Lacrimal (left and right)
Nasal (left and right)
Vomer
Conchae (left and right).

Sutures. Some of the important sutures are: sagittal, which separates the two parietal bones; coronal, which separates the frontal bone from the parietal bone; lambdoid, which separates the two parietal bones form the occipital bone.

When the skull is viewed from within, it shows: anterior cranial fossa, middle cranial fossa, posterior cranial fossa.

The anterior cranial fossa is made up of the sphenoid and temporal bones.

The middle cranial fossa is made up of the frontal, ethmoid and sphenoid bones.

The posterior cranial fossa is made up of the temporal and occipital bones.

Vertebral column and thoracic cage

The vertebral column is an important structure in the body since it carries the skull, thoracic cage, and upper limbs. It protects the spinal cord and transmits the weight of the body to the lower limbs.

The vertebral column is made up of the following bones:

Cervical vertebrae (7)
Thoracic vertebrae (12)
Lumbar vertebrae (5)
Sacrum
Coccyx.

A typical vertebra shows: a body, a vertebral arch, a vertebral foramen, an intervertebral foramen, a superior and inferior articular surface, a transverse process, a spine, and an intervertebral disc.

A number of ligaments connect the vertebrae, anteriorly and posteriorly.

The vertebral column in an adult shows: a curve forwards in the cervical region; a curve backwards in the thoracic region; a curve forwards in the lumbar region; a curve backwards above and forwards below in the sacral and coccygeal regions.

Movements of the vertebral column. The vertebral column can be flexed, extended, moved laterally and rotated by the movements between the adjacent vertebrae and alterations in the intervertebral discs.

Thoracic cage. The thoracic cage is made up of: the sternum, ribs and costal cartilage, and the thoracic part of the vertebral column.

Sternum. This is a flat bone which lies subcutaneously in the midline of the front of the chest. It is made up of: the manubrium, the body and the xiphoid process.

Ribs and costal cartilage. There are twelve pairs of ribs which encircle the wall of the chest. They articulate behind with the vertebral column and in front with the sternum.

Each rib has a head, neck, a tubercle and a shaft. The space between two ribs is occupied by the external and internal intercostal muscles.

Thoracic cage movements. The thoracic cavity increases in size during inspiration and decreases during expiration. During inspiration, the muscles of the diaphragm contract along with the external intercostal muscles, thus increasing the length and width of thoracic cavity. During expiration, the thoracic cavity returns to the normal size owing to elastic recoil.

Bones in the upper limb (Fig. 1.24)

The upper limb is made up of the following bones: scapula (shoulder blade), clavicle (collar bone), humerus, radius, ulna, carpal bones, metacarpals, and phalanges.

The scapula is a triangular bone which forms part of the shoulder girdle. It is attached to the head, trunk and arm by a number of muscles. The

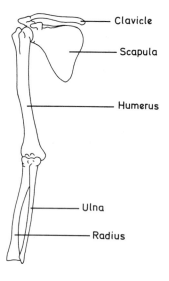

Fig. 1.24   Bone of the upper limb (excluding phalanges).

scapula has an acromion, coracoid process and a glenoid fossa. The glenoid fossa lies at the upper and outer border of the scapula and articulates with the head of the humerus to form the shoulder joint.

The clavicle is an S-shaped bone attached medially to the manubrium of the sternum and laterally to the acromion process of the scapula.

The humerus, a long bone, is made up of a head, a shaft and a lower end. The shaft has a number of muscles attached to it, including the deltoid muscle. The lower end has a lateral and medial epicondyle, along with the trochlea and capitulum.

Radius and ulna. The radius bone lies on the outer side of the forearm and has a head at the upper end which articulates with the capitulum of the humerus; a neck; a tuberosity to which the tendon of biceps muscle is attached; a shaft, to which various flexor and extensor muscles are attached; and a lower end with a styloid process and articular surface for the wrist bones.

The ulna is a long bone which lies on the inner side of the forearm and consists of an olecranon and coronoid process with an articular surface for the lower end of the humerus. At the lower end it

has a styloid process and an articular surface for the lower end of the radius.

Carpal wrist bones. The wrist consists of eight bones arranged in two rows: proximal row — scaphoid, lunate, triquetrium, pisiform; distal row — trapezium, trapezoid, capitate and hamate.

Metacarpals. There are five metacarpal bones in the hand and they have a base which articulates with the carpal bones, a shaft and a head. The head articulates with the phlanages.

Phalanges. The thumb has two phalanges and the finger three.

Bones in the lower limb (Fig. 1.25)

The lower limb is made up of the following bones:

    Hip bone (innominate), which forms part
    of the pelvis
    Femur
    Patella
    Tibia
    Fibula
    Foot
    Tarsal bones
    Metatarsal bones
    Phalanges.

Pelvis. The pelvis is formed by the hip bone in front and at the sides, and by the sacrum and coccyx behind. It is divided into the false pelvis and the true pelvis by the line joining the two iliac bones.

Hip bone. This is an irregular-shaped strong bone which articulates with a similar bone on the opposite side and the sacrum and coccyx behind. It consists of three bones: ilium, ischium and pubis.

Femur. This consists of an upper end, a shaft and a lower end. The upper end has a head, which is connected to the acetabulum of the hip bone (forming the hip joint), a neck and greater trochanter and lesser trochanter to which the muscles are attached.

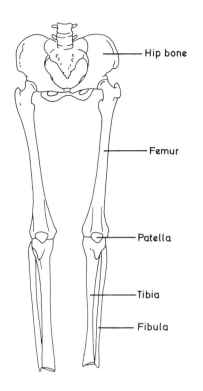

Fig. 1.25 Bones of the lower limb (excluding metatarsals).

Hip bone

Femur

Patella

Tibia

Fibula

The shaft is a long, smooth bone to which muscles attach. The lower end has large medial and lateral condyles to which the tibial bone and the patella are attached.

Patella. The patella, or knee cap, is a triangular sesamoid bone (sesamoid bones = bones formed in the tendons of muscles) situated in the tendon of the quadriceps muscles of the thigh. It glides over the articular surface on the front of the lower end of the femur.

The tibia and fibula are the two bones of the leg below the knee. The tibia lies on the medial side and transmits the weight of the body. It has an upper end, a shaft and a lower end. The upper end is wide and consists of medial and lateral condyles. The upper end of the fibula is attached to the articular surface on the lateral condyle. The shaft is thick and its anterior border forms the prominent palpable shin. The lower end has a medial malleolus and an articular surface for the lower end of the fibula and the talus.

The fibula is a long, slim bone, which lies on the lateral aspect of the leg. It has an upper end, a shaft and a lower end. The upper end articulates with the lateral condyles of the tibia, and the lower end articulates with the lower end of the tibia and talus.

Foot. The bones of the foot are: talus, calcaneum, navicular, cuboid and three cuneiform bones.

Metatarsals. There are five metatarsals, one for each toe. Each one has a base, a shaft and a head. The 1st, 2nd and 3rd metatarsals articulate with the cuneiform bones, while the 4th and 5th articulate with the cuboid bone.

Phalanges. The big toe has two phalanges while the rest have three phalanges. Each phalanx has a shaft and two ends.

JOINTS

There are three types of joints, based on their structure: fibrous, synovial, and cartilaginous.

Fibrous joints. In the lower tibiofibular joints, the bones are held together by a fibrous ligament.

Synovial joint (Fig. 1.26). Most joints are synovial, i.e. they are made up of cartilage, capsule, synovial fluid, synovial membrane and ligaments.

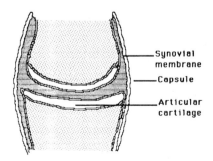

Synovial membrane

Capsule

Articular cartilage

Fig. 1.26 A synovial joint.

Cartilaginous joints. The bones are separated by cartilage; e.g. between the bodies of the vertebrae and in the manubriosternal joints.

Joints can also be classified according to their movements:

Plane joint, e.g. acromioclavicular joint
Hinge joint, e.g. elbow
Saddle joint, e.g. 1st metacarpophalangeal joint at the wrist
Condyloid joint, e.g. temporomandibular joint
Pivot joint, e.g. radio-ulnar joint
Ball and socket joint, e.g. hip joint

Movements of joints can be:

Flexion, e.g. bending the elbow
Abduction, e.g. lifting the arm away from the body
Adduction: bringing the arm to the side
Rotation: moving the part round its own longitudinal axis
Circumduction: a combination of abduction, adduction, extension and flexion.

Important joints in the body

Temporomandibular joint, formed by the articular surface of the temporal bone and the head of the mandible.

Joints of the upper extremity: Acromioclavicular joint, formed by the acromion of the scapula and the lateral end of the clavicle;
Shoulder joint, formed by the glenoid cavity of the scapula and the head of the humerus;
Elbow joint, formed by the trochlea and capitulum at the lower end of the humerus, and the upper end of the ulna and the radius;
Wrist joint, formed by the lower end of the radius and ulna with the proximal row of carpal bones;
Carpal and phalangeal joints, formed by the distal row of the carpal bones and the metacarpals. Phalangeal joints are formed by the metacarpals and the proximal phalanxes.

Joints of the lower extremity:
Pubic symphysis, formed by the symphyseal surfaces of the two pubic bones;

Sacro-iliac joint, formed by the articulation of the sacrum on each side with iliac bone;
Hip joint, formed by the head of the femur and the acetabular fossa of innominate bone;
Knee joint, formed by the condyles of the femur, the upper end of the tibia and the patella;
Ankle joint, formed by the lower ends of the tibia and fibula with the trochlea of the talus;
Joints of the foot, various tarsal bones are connected by joints.

MUSCLES OF THE BODY

Some of the important muscles of the body are mentioned below.

Muscles of the scalp and face. The frontal and occipital muscles are attached to the front and back of the skull. The orbicularis oculi and orbicularis oris muscles are seen around the eye and the mouth.

Muscles of chewing. The masseter and temporalis muscles allow the opening and closing of the mouth.

Muscles of the neck and shoulder. Sternocleidomastoid and trapezius are the main muscles.

Muscles of the upper extremity. In the arm, the biceps, brachialis and triceps, and in the forearm, the superficial and deep flexors of the fingers and the flexor of the thumb are the major muscles in the anterior aspect. On the posterior surface of the forearm, the extensor muscles of the wrist and fingers end as tendons into bones at the wrist or phalanges.

Muscles of the lower extremity. In the buttock, gluteus maximus, medius and minimus; in the anterior aspect of the thigh, quadriceps femoris, rectus femoris, vastii muscles. In the medial aspect of the thigh, the adductor group of muscles and posteriorly, the biceps femoris, semimembranosus and semitendinosus.
Below the knee joint: anteriorly, tibialis anterior, extensor hallucis longus and extensor digitorum longus; posteriorly, gastrocnemius,

soleus, tibialis posterior and flexor digitorum longus.

Muscles of the abdomen. Anteriorly and laterally, rectus abdominis; external and internal oblique muscles, transversus. Posteriorly, psoas and quadratous lumborium and iliacus.

Diaphragm. This muscular structure separates the thorax from the abdomen. Its fibres arise from xiphoid cartilage, the inner surface of the lower ribs at the sides and the bodies of the lumbar vertebrae behind. It is supplied by two phrenic nerves.

The structures which pass through the diaphragm are: the aorta, inferior vena cava, oesophagus, and the thoracic duct.

MULTIPLE CHOICE QUESTIONS

The answers to these questions can be found on page 253.

1. **The nasal cavity is lined with which type of epithelium?**
   A cuboid
   B simple
   C ciliated
   D squamous.

2. **The tidal volume is the amount of air breathed per:**
   A breath
   B minute
   C hour
   D second.

3. **One of the following structures belongs to both the respiratory and digestive systems:**
   A oesophagus
   B larynx
   C pharynx
   D bronchi.

4. **The pH of gastric juice is normally:**
   A 1.6   C 7.4
   B 5.6   D 11.0.

5. **The membrane covering the abdominal organs is:**
   A pleura
   B parietal peritoneum
   C visceral peritoneum
   D mesentery.

6. **In the heart, the valve between the right atrium and right ventricle is known as:**
   A bicuspid valve
   B tricuspid valve
   C mitral valve
   D semilunar valve.

7. **Which of the following factors is important in clotting?**
   A erythrocytes
   B monocytes
   C platelets
   D white blood cells.

8. **The coeliac artery is divided into:**
   A phrenic, gastric and hepatic arteries
   B splenic, gastric and hepatic arteries
   C splenic, renal hepatic arteries
   D splenic, pancreatic and gastric arteries.

9. **The normal white cell count is:**
   A 5000 to 10 000 cells/mm^3
   B 1000 to 5000 cells/mm^3
   C 10 000 to 30 000 cells/mm^3
   D 500 to 1000 cells/mm^3

10. **The outer layer of an artery is called:**
    A tunica media
    B tunica intima
    C tunica adventitia
    D endothelium.

11. **Which one of the following organs has transitional epithelium?**
    A uterus
    B bladder
    C skin
    D larynx.

12. The appendix is attached to the:
A colon
B caecum
C jejunum
D ileum.

13. Cerebrospinal fluid is found between the:
A pia mater and brain
B arachnoid mater and pia mater
C skull and dura mater
D dura mater and arachnoid mater.

14. Which part of the brain controls posture:
A thalamus
B cortex
C cerebellum
D hypothalamus.

15. Stimulation of the parasympathetic system causes:
A dilatation of pupil
B increased heart rate
C decreased salivation
D constriction of bronchi.

16. The second cranial nerve is the:
A occulomotor
B optic
C facial
D auditory.

17. The medulla oblongata is part of the:
A cerebellum
B cerebrum
C brain stem
D spinal cord.

18. Body temperature is controlled by the:
A pineal gland
B hypothalamus
C pituitary
D cerebrum.

19. The islets of Langerhans are found in the:
A spinal cord
B spleen
C pancreas
D kidney.

20. The loop of Henle is found in:
A pancreas
B kidney
C ovaries
D uterus.

2. Pharmacology

Drugs are chemical substances which have an effect on the tissues of the human body. Pharmacology consists of two major divisions:

(i) Pharmacodynamics, which is defined as how drugs either by themselves or in combination have an effect on the body.
(ii) Pharmacokinetics, which is defined as how the body affects drugs, in the form of absorption, distribution, metabolism and excretion.

In brief, pharmacodynamics is what drugs do to the body and pharmacokinetics is what the body does to drugs.

Pharmacodynamics

Drugs act on tissues in a number of ways, the most important being:

a. Action on specific receptors—many drugs operate by acting on specific receptors present in the body. A receptor is a small part of a cell which combines chemically with a drug.
b. Action on the metabolic process e.g. antibiotics, sulphonamides, insulin. Some antibiotics act by (i) stopping bacterial growth such as cell wall formation (e.g. penicillins), (ii) inhibition of protein synthesis (e.g. tetracyclines).
c. Action by inhibiting enzymes i.e. anticholinesterases (e.g. neostigmine which acts by preventing the destruction of acetylcholine—the effects in the central nervous system are due to its accumulation).
d. Acting on physicochemical properties (e.g. volatile anaesthetics, see below).

An important type of action is called competitive antagonism which can be against (i) a specific receptor e.g. β adrenergic blockers, or (ii) an enzyme e.g. sulphonamides.

In the following sections, drugs will be described according to the system on which they act.

DRUGS ACTING ON THE CENTRAL NERVOUS SYSTEM

The following terms are commonly used:
Hypnotic is a drug which induces sleep.
Sedative is a drug which calms or soothes without inducing sleep.
Tranquillizer is a drug which quietens a person without him losing consciousness.
Narcotic is a drug which produces sleep or drowsiness.
Anticonvulsant is a drug which prevents or controls convulsions.
Anaesthetic is a drug which induces reversible loss of consciousness.
Analgesic is a drug which relieves pain.

Hypnotics

These drugs are used in small doses to reduce anxiety and/or as a premedication drug, and in high doses to produce sleep during the night.

Chloral hydrate is given orally as a solution and is rapidly absorbed from the intestine. It produces sleep within half an hour, lasting for 6 to 8 hours.
Dosage is 50–75 mg per kg orally.

Triclofos (Tricloryl) acts in a similar manner to chloral hydrate.

Chlormethiazole (Heminevrin) is a powerful sedative, antiemetic and hypnotic with an anticonvulsant action. It is used during treatment of the initial withdrawal phase of acute alcoholism, in the control of status epilepticus and as a sedative in intensive care or in pre-eclampsia.

Dosage: it is available as a 0.8% solution in 5% dextrose and is given intravenously at the rate of 8–20 ml/minute.

Barbiturates

Barbitone, a derivative of barbituric acid (malonyl urea), was first introduced in 1903 as a hypnotic, following which a number of barbiturates were synthesized. Barbiturates are classified into long, medium, short and ultra-short acting based on the duration of action of a single dose. The examples are:

— Long acting: barbitone, phenobarbitone (8–12 hours action)
— Medium and short acting: amylobarbitone, pentobarbitone (2–8 hours)
— Ultra-short acting: thiopentone, methohexitone (act rapidly following IV injection).

They have an action on all levels of the central nervous system (especially on the cerebral cortex).

In low dosage they can antagonize analgesia, hence patients in pain when given barbiturates become restless. They prevent convulsions in epileptics or following an overdose of local anaesthetic. They produce a fall in blood pressure in large doses.

Barbiturates produce respiratory depression based on the amount of drug given.

The short-acting barbiturates are metabolized and excreted via the liver and the long-acting are removed by renal excretion.

Mode of administration: oral, intramuscular or intravenous.

Contraindications: patients suffering from acute porphyria (a congenital hereditary disorder). They should be used with great caution in patients with liver and kidney disease.

Barbiturate overdose and treatment. Signs of overdose include central depression (coma), respiratory and cardiac depression. Treatment consists of cardiac and respiratory support and forced alkaline diuresis using 10% mannitol, measuring the urine volume and pH, and replacement with intravenous fluids.

Tranquillizers

The benzodiazepines are a widely used group of tranquillizing drugs.

Diazepam is available in doses of 10 mg (in 2 ml) with solvents like propylene glycol. This preparation is highly irritant to veins, hence a newer preparation **Diazemuls** has been made available. It acts on the reticular formation and limbic system in the brain. In small doses it makes the patient less anxious but in high doses causes drowsiness, amnesia and, if given intravenously, unconsciousness. It has the ability to decrease anaesthetic requirements by decreasing the minimum alveolar concentration (MAC) (see p. 53). It has no effect on blood pressure or cardiac output other than producing a rise in heart rate for a short period.

Metabolism: it is metabolized in the liver and its breakdown product (desmethyldiazepam) is found to be active for up to 96 hours.

Indications: as a premedication drug, for induction of anaesthesia; in small doses in dental anaesthesia, for cardioversion and as a drug of choice to control convulsions.

Dosage: as a premedicant 0.2 mg/kg orally 90 minutes before surgery.

Midazolam (Hypnovel) is a rapidly-acting water-soluble benzodiazepine. It is supplied as a colourless solution of 10 mg midazolam in 2 ml aqueous solution. This drug can be used as either an IV sedating or induction agent. For sedation, a total dosage of 2.5 to 10 mg IV is required. For induction, a dosage of 0.1–0.5 mg/kg is required. The recovery from midazolam is faster because of a short half-life.

Indications: as an IV sedation drug during endoscopy and dentistry.

Lorazepam (Ativan) is presented in doses of

4 mg in 2 ml dissolved in polyethylene glycol and propylene glycol. It has actions similar to those of diazepam. It produces anterograde amnesia (loss of memory for recent events).

Indications: as a premedication drug, and also to prevent an emergence reaction (i.e. hallucinations) following ketamine anaesthesia.

Dosage: on a weight-to-weight basis Lorazepam is five times more potent than diazepam. For premedication, 1–4 mg is given orally to be effective.

Temazepam is presented as 10 mg or 20 mg capsules. It is used as a night sedative or as a premedication drug.

Dosage: 20–40 mg, 60 minutes before surgery.

Nitrazepam (Mogadon) is used as a hypnotic for night sedations.

Dosage: 5–10 mg.

Flumazenil (Anexate) is a benzodiazepine antagonist. It blocks the central effects, such as sedation and hypnosis, of benzodiazepine. Flumazenil is indicated in the reversal of general anaesthesia, induced or maintained by midazolam (Hypnovel), for the reversal of sedation due to midazolam (Hypnovel) in short diagnostic procedures such as endoscopy. It is also used in the intensive care unit.

Dosage: in adults, it is injected as 200 micrograms of flumazenil IV over 15 seconds with increments until the desired effect is achieved.

Neuroleptic drugs

These are the drugs which cause quietening of emotional behaviour and psychomotor slowing. They are also called major tranquillizers or antipsychotics. The major sub-groups of neuroleptics are:

— Phenothiazines, e.g. chlorpromazine, promazine, prochlorperazine, perphenazine
— Butyrophenones, e.g. droperidol, haloperidol.

Phenothiazines

Chlorpromazine (Largactil) produces lethargy, apathy and sleep by acting on the hypothalamus.

It has a marked antiemetic action (prevents vomiting by acting on the vomiting centre and the chemoreceptor trigger zone).

It causes tachycardia and a fall in blood pressure due to peripheral vasodilatation. It decreases bronchial, salivary and gastric secretion. It can also cause cholestatic jaundice in about $\frac{1}{2}$–1% of patients. It has a mild antihistamine action. The drug is metabolized in the liver.

Indications: as a premedicant, to treat intractable hiccup and vomiting.

Dosage: it can be given orally, intramuscularly or intravenously. A very dilute solution 1 mg per ml (10 mg in 10 ml normal saline) can be used for treating peripheral vasoconstriction in patients who have been adequately resuscitated.

For premedication 25–50 mg may be given intramuscularly one hour preoperatively with an analgesic like pethidine (50–100 mg).

Side-effects: postural hypotension, agranulocytosis.

Promethazine hydrochloride (Phenergan). Many of its actions on the central nervous system are similar to chlorpromazine, although its sedative effects are marked.

There are no other marked effects on heart, skeleton, muscle, kidneys or liver. It causes bronchodilatation and has a marked antihistamine action. It is metabolized in the liver.

Indications: it is used in premedication and to treat allergies such as hay fever, urticaria and motion sickness.

Dosage: for premedication 25 mg IM one hour before surgery along with pethidine 75–100 mg.

Side-effects: an overdose can cause circulatory collapse and central depression.

Prochlorperazine (Stemetil) is an effective antiemetic agent which does not have many side-effects.

Indications: it is used as an antiemetic during surgery, in psychiatry and in the treatment of migraine.

Dosage: as a deep intramuscular injection (12.5 mg) repeated at 4–6 hourly intervals for the antiemetic effect.

Perphenazine (Fentazin) has a number of actions similar to chlorpromazine. The hypotension it causes is insignificant. It is an effective antiemetic.

Indications: as an antiemetic, as a premedication drug and also in psychiatry.

Dosage: 4 mg orally or 5 mg intramuscularly.

Side-effects: it can cause extrapyramidal signs (see below) if used frequently.

Trimeprazine (Vallergan) is used to relieve itching, as an antihistamine and as a premedication in children.

Dosage: 2–4 mg per kg body weight one hour before surgery.

Side-effects: it can cause restlessness postoperatively associated with a flushed appearance.

Butyrophenones

These drugs, due to their specific action, induce a state in a patient whereby he looks tranquil, but can be readily awakened. High doses can cause hallucinations, restlessness and extrapyramidal side-effects. The extrapyramidal side-effects include involuntary movements. These drugs have a powerful antiemetic effect.

Droperidol (Droleptan) resembles the phenothiazines in structure. It has a quick onset and shorter duration of action. Droperidol produces a picture of mental calm in a patient and is used along with fentanyl or phenoperidine as a neuroleptic agent in procedures where the patient's cooperation is needed (cardiac catheterization, angiograms) and in certain poor risk patients. It is a powerful antiemetic, its action being mediated via the chemoreceptor trigger zone in the hypothalamus.

In high doses droperidol produces extrapyramidal side-effects.

Indications: intraoperatively as a neuroleptic agent or as an antiemetic.

Dosage: from 2.5 mg (between 15 and 20 kg body weight) to 5 mg (20–25 kg body weight) orally as a premedication for children; in adults 2.5–5.0 mg intravenously as an antiemetic and up to 10 mg IV for neuroleptic analgesia.

Anticonvulsants (antiepileptics)

Epilepsy is a sudden, excessive and rapid discharge of nervous activity in the grey matter of the brain.

There are a number of causes which can produce epilepsy, such as pathological (eclampsia during pregnancy, brain tumours), metabolic (hypoglycaemia, febrile convulsions in children), drugs, etc. Sometimes convulsions are seen in the operating theatre, either from an overdose of local anaesthetic drugs or following the administration of a large dose of ether.

The types of epilepsy usually seen are grand mal, petit mal, focal and temporal lobe epilepsy.

The treatment of epilepsy consists of: treating the cause e.g brain tumour; avoiding factors which precipitate epilepsy such as stress or alcohol; and the use of anticonvulsants.

Anticonvulsants are drugs which inhibit the discharge of nervous activity or its spread from the grey matter in the brain with an overall depressing or hypnotic effect.

The drugs of choice in epilepsy are as follows.

Grand mal, focal seizures, temporal lobe epilepsy
First choice—phenytoin
Second choice—carbamazepine, phenobarbitone, sodium valproate
Petit mal
First choice—sodium valproate, ethosuximide
Second choice—clonazepam.

Phenytoin (Dilantin, Epanutin) is an effective antiepileptic in all types of epilepsy except petit mal. It is absorbed slowly from the intestine and is metabolized in the liver.

Indications: all types of epilepsy except petit mal and in the control of digitalis-induced arrhythmias.

Dosage: in adults, an initial dose of 100 mg twice a day orally, increasing to 600 mg over 24 hours. To control digitalis-induced arrhythmia, it is given 50–100 mg IV every 15 minutes until a sinus rhythm on the ECG is seen.

Side-effects: it can cause drug interactions. It enhances the metabolism of other drugs such as steroids, warfarin, tricyclic antidepressants, thus increasing their daily requirement. It causes insomnia and gastric disturbances. In young children, prolonged treatment causes hypertrophy of the gums.

Sodium valproate (Epilim) controls fits with minimal side-effects.

Indications: petit mal epilepsy.

Dosage: 200 mg three times a day for adults, initially increased to 800–1000 mg per day.

Carbamazepine (Tegretol). In the past it was used in the treatment of temporal lobe epilepsy, but now it is used exclusively in the treatment of trigeminal neuralgia.

Indications: trigeminal neuralgia, temporal lobe epilepsy, intractable hiccups.

Dosage: 100–200 mg twice a day initially, increased to 600–800 mg daily.

Side-effects: jaundice, thrombocytopaenia.

Ethosuximide (Zarontin) is used in the treatment of petit mal epilepsy.

Dosage: 250 mg three times a day orally increased to up to 2 g a day.

Side-effects: nausea and vomiting, drowsiness.

Clonazepam (Rivotril) is a benzodiazepine.

Indications: as a second choice drug in grand mal, petit mal epilepsy and as a first choice in myoclonus and status epilepticus.

Dosage: 0.5 mg orally twice a day; in status epilepticus 1 mg IV slowly.

Status epilepticus is a condition in which epileptic fits are continuous and not controlled by oral medication; they can be dangerous to life due to hypoxia and the inhalation of stomach contents. The treatment consists of diazepam 10 mg IV over a 2 minute period or repeated, or as an infusion at the rate of 20 mg per hour (40 mg in 500 ml of 5% dextrose). An alternative to diazepam is clonazepam 1 mg IV slowly over a 30 second period.

Agents used for general anaesthesia

Anaesthesia is defined as the absence of sensation; and general anaesthetics are those agents which produce loss of consciousness and sensation in a reversible manner.

Stages of anaesthesia

The depth of anaesthesia can be interpreted with the aid of stages i.e. I to IV (see below). These stages were first described in relation to ether anaesthesia, and since then modifications have been made to these stages when anaesthesia is induced with intravenous induction agents.

The following four stages were described by Guedel in relation to ether anaesthesia.

Stage I: analgesia. This stage lasts from the beginning of induction until loss of consciousness. During this stage respiration is quiet but irregular and all the reflexes are present.

Stage II: delirium or excitement. This stage begins at the loss of consciousness and ends at the onset of surgical anaesthesia. During this stage, the patient is unconscious and respirations are irregular with episodes of breath holding. The reflexes are still active and if the stomach is not empty vomiting can occur.

Stage III: surgical anaesthesia. This stage lasts from the onset of regular respiration to the occurrence of respiratory failure due to toxic doses of the anaesthetic. It is divided into four planes.

Plane A. Respiration becomes regular and automatic. The eyelid reflex is lost; muscle tone and the laryngeal reflexes are still present but the pharyngeal reflex disappears late in this plane.

Plane B. Muscle tone decreases but the respiratory muscles are still active. The eyes are fixed centrally and the laryngeal reflexes are lost.

Plane C. Muscle relaxation is nearly complete and the intercostal muscles become paralysed.

Plane D. Muscle relaxation is full, respirations are depressed and a tracheal tug is seen.

Stage IV: medullary paralysis. The respiration becomes gasping in nature and eventually stops. Blood pressure is low and the pulse weak. The skin becomes cold and the pupils widely dilated.

The above stages were seen only when chloroform or ether were used but in the current situation all these stages seem to pass quickly. For example, if thiopentone is used as an induction agent the patient rapidly passes into stage III, plane B or C, depending on the dose of thiopentone given without showing signs of stage I or II.

Anaesthesia for surgical procedures

To allow the surgeon to perform a surgical procedure in a relaxed sleeping patient, the anaesthetist uses a technique called 'balanced anaesthesia'. Balanced anaesthesia comprises anaesthesia, analgesia and muscle relaxation.

Anaesthesia is induced with an induction agent (p. 58); in children a volatile anaesthetic agent is used (see below). Surgical anesthesia is then maintained using nitrous oxide (66% with 33% oxygen) and a volatile agent. Analgesia is provided with one of the agents suitable for the surgical procedure (see p. 56), and muscle relaxation is provided by a muscle relaxant (also called a neuromuscular blocker) (p. 72).

After the induction of anaesthesia, the patient either breathes spontaneously or is administered via an ET tube and ventilated with a mixture of oxygen, nitrous oxide and a volatile agent. All the volatile anaesthetic agents diffuse readily into the central nervous system depending on the circulation of blood in the patient. During the induction of anaesthesia, volatile agents from the anaesthetic machine enter the body tissues (against a concentration gradient i.e. from a high level outside to a zero level in the tissues). When the patient is adequately anaesthetized he is maintained with the same or a slightly lower concentration of the agent and there is no further uptake of the gases as the tissues become fully saturated. When the anaesthesia is completed, during the recovery period the anaesthestic gases are eliminated (against a concentration gradient i.e. from a high level inside the body to outside where the concentration is zero).

The amount of time taken for the induction of an anaesthetic depends on the rate at which the tension of anaesthetic agents in the lung (called the alveolar anaesthetic tension) equals the tension in the anaesthetic machine delivering it (called the inspired anaesthetic tension).

Some of the factors which play an important role in determining the alveolar anaesthetic tension are:

(i) Inspired anaesthetic tension

(ii) Solubility of the agent in blood
(iii) Lung ventilation (also called alveolar ventilation)
(iv) Cardiac output of the patient.

The above mentioned factors will be expanded further to make the understanding of uptake and elimination of anaesthetic gases a little easier.

Inspired anaesthetic tension. A high inspired anaesthetic tension shortens the time required for the induction of anaesthesia (e.g. the anaesthetist normally sets up 4% enflurane or 3% halothane on the vaporizer during the induction to hasten the patient to sleep).

Solubility of the agent in blood is also known as the partition coefficient of the agent between blood and gas at body temperature. If the blood/gas partition coefficient of an agent is high, it is removed from the alveoli in the lungs by its blood supply (pulmonary capillary blood), thus decreasing its tension in the lungs and increasing it slowly in the blood and brain. This leads to slower induction. As opposed to this, nitrous oxide which has a low blood/gas partition coefficient is taken up slowly by the pulmonary capillary blood. Thus the tension in the lung alveoli reaches the inspired tension comparatively fast, causing rapid induction.

Lung ventilation (alveolar ventilation). If the alveolar ventilation is increased (e.g. hyperventilating patient when breathing spontaneously or manual hyperventilation in an intubated patient), the uptake of the anaesthetic agent is increased considerably.

Cardiac output of the patient. If a patient has a high cardiac output (e.g. anxiety, thyrotoxicosis), a large amount of the anaesthetic agent is removed from the blood thus increasing the time taken for the induction of anesthesia. In patients with a low cardiac output (shocked, hypotensive patients) anaesthetic agents are slowly removed from the alveoli in the lungs. Thus the inspired concentration equals the alveolar concentration and the induction becomes rapid.

Another factor which contributes towards the uptake of anaesthetic gases is the rubber/gas partition coefficient (see below). Some of the anaesthetic agents (e.g. halothane, trichlorethylene) have a tendency to become soluble in rubber. This is of practical importance as all anaesthetics are delivered to the patient via rubber circuits. During the induction of anaesthesia, a large amount of anaesthetic agent will be absorbed by the rubber until it is saturated. (During this period the patient will get an inadequate amount.) This circuit, which is saturated with the anaesthetic, will give up the agent during a subsequent anaesthetic.

Anaesthetic agent	Rubber/gas partition coefficient
Trichloroethylene	830
Halothane	120
Nitrous oxide	1.2

Other factors which influence the uptake of anaesthetic gases include 'concentration' and 'second gas effects'. A description of these in simple terms is beyond the scope of this book.

Minimum alveolar concentration (MAC) is defined as the alveolar concentration of an agent which prevents response to a stimulus in 50% of subjects.

Metabolism and excretion of volatile anaesthetic agents. A large portion of the volatile anaesthetic agent is excreted via the lungs, a small amount being excreted unchanged in urine and sweat. Some of it is biotransformed in the liver with the aid of liver enzymes such as cytochrome P450. By biotransformation, these agents, which are highly lipid (fat) soluble, are converted into water soluble substances.

Biotransformation of agents such as trichloroethylene to trichloroethanol leads to a prolonged effect. Halothane, methoxyflurane and isoflurane liberate inorganic fluoride during their metabolism. The inorganic fluoride liberated by methoxyflurane can cause nephrotoxicity (kidney failure), and the metabolite of halothane has been said to cause hepatitis.

Insoluble agents (such as nitrous oxide) will be released from the blood into the alveoli from where they can be removed by ventilation. Soluble agents such as halothane will be removed slowly from the blood.

Volatile anaesthetic agents

These can be classified as either (i) halogenated hydrocarbons or (ii) ethers.

Halogenated hydrocarbons

Fluorine, chlorine and bromine are called halogens and the name for the chemical combination of hydrogen and carbon is hydrocarbon. When halogens are added to hydrocarbons steadily they develop a narcotic property. Many of the currently used anaesthetic agents are hydrocarbons with fluorine substitution. Some examples of these are given below.

Trichloroethylene (Trilene) is a colourless liquid with a strange odour. It is coloured blue (with waxoline blue) for identification purposes and is presented with thymol as a stabilizing agent (prevents its breakdown). In addition to being an anaesthetic agent, it is a powerful analgesic. It has minimal effect on the cardiovascular system. It causes an increase in respiratory rate with decreased tidal volume (shallow rapid respiration). It has no major effect on other systems. Nausea and vomiting are common after prolonged exposure. It is metabolized to chloral hydrate and trichloroethanol in the liver, thus prolonging its action.

Indications: it is used for producing light anaesthesia and as an analgesic during labour.

Dosage and administration: in obstetric analgesia, Emotril or Tecota mark VI vaporizers, when used, deliver between 0.35 and 0.5% trichloroethylene in air. For anaesthetic purposes 0.2–1.5% vapour concentration is needed.

Side-effects and precautions: prolonged trichloroethylene administration leads to a delayed recovery from anaesthesia. Extrasystoles and cardiac arrhythmias occur if the patient has carbon dioxide retention due to inadequate breathing during trichloroethylene anaesthesia. The treatment consists of either reducing the inspired concentration of trichloroethylene or controlling the ventilation (IPPV).

Trichloroethylene is converted into a toxic compound dichloroacetylene in the presence of soda lime at a temperature of 60°C. Dichloroacetylene can cause cranial nerve paralysis; hence it should not be used in a closed circuit with a soda lime absorber.

Halothane (Fluothane) is a colourless liquid with a sweet odour. It is made stable by the addition of thymol and by storing it in amber glass bottles. Like all general anaesthetics it depresses the central nervous system (CNS), and in addition causes an increase in cerebral blood flow and intracranial pressure. This agent is not used or should be used with caution in patients with head injury (with suspected raised intracranial pressure).

It causes a fall in arterial blood pressure depending on the depth of halothane anaesthesia and bradycardia. Arrhythmias such as ventricular extrasystoles or nodal rhythm are seen in patients breathing high concentrations of halothane spontaneously. The cause is retention of carbon dioxide (due to underventilation) which releases catecholamines. Halothane sensitizes the heart to the effect of the catecholamines, thus causing dysrhythmias. The treatment consists of improving ventilation, decreasing the halothane concentration and if necessary using beta blockers such as propranolol (1 mg IV).

Halothane potentiates the effect of muscle relaxants (d tubocurare). It has no effect on the renal system; it causes a fall in the tidal volume and increases respiratory rate (shallow rapid breathing). It inhibits the contractility of the uterus. The effect of halothane on the liver has gained considerable prominence in the last few years and it has been shown that halothane can cause postoperative jaundice. The usual recommendation is not to use halothane within six months of the last exposure in adults. Although a few cases of halothane hepatitis have been reported in children, repeated halothane administration in children seems to be an ongoing practice in the UK.

Metabolism: halothane is metabolized in the liver by microsomal enzymes.

Indications: as it is a potent inhalational anaesthetic agent, halothane is used for many surgical procedures. As it causes hypotension, halothane is used along with d tubocurare to induce hypotension (see p. 183).

Dosage: a vapour concentration of 2–4% is re-quired for the induction of anaesthesia and 0.5–1.5% for the maintenance of anaesthesia.

Side-effects and precautions: halothane has been known to cause hepatitis, hence precautions in the intervals between its usage need to be considered.

Other halogenated hydrocarbons

Chloroform is not available on the market. It was highly potent and able to cause death due to vagal arrest (acute episode of bradycardia) during induction, or ventricular fibrillation during maintenance of the anaesthesia. It was notorious in causing liver damage (delayed chloroform poisoning).

Ethyl chloride is stored in liquid form in a glass container under slight pressure but is converted to gas at room temperature. It is highly volatile and causes rapid induction and recovery. In the past it was used for the induction of anaesthesia by 'spraying on an open mask'. Ethyl chloride was notorious in causing breath holding when used in this way. When a child inhaled after breath holding, the high concentration of ethyl chloride caused ventricular fibrillation and cardiac arrest.

Its present use is as a topical anaesthetic for the drainage of localized abcesses.

Anaesthetic ethers

After the discovery that diethyl ether had anaesthetic properties a number of ethers were developed. All the new ethers are fluorinated ethers. Some examples of these are given below.

Diethyl ether is a colourless highly volatile liquid decomposed by air, light and heat. It produces loss of consciousness like all other volatile anaesthetic agents. During light planes of anaesthesia there are no significant changes in heart rate and blood pressure, but with deeper levels there is a considerable fall in blood pressure. At lighter planes of anaesthesia it causes an increase in respiratory rate and tidal volume, but at deeper levels it causes respiratory failure. It causes relaxation of the bronchial smooth muscle (hence it might be beneficial in status asthmaticus). Ether has a tendency to increase bronchial, salivary and gastric secretions. Patients receiving prolonged ether anaesthesia show a high incidence of post-operative nausea and vomiting. Ether causes relaxation of the uterus during deep anaesthesia. It can cause hyperglycaemia (due to mobilization of glycogen from the liver).

Metabolism: about 15% of the inhaled ether is metabolized to carbon dioxide and water.

Indications: although its use in modern operating theatres has declined it is still used frequently and successfully in the developing countries by a single operator with minimal equipment.

Dosage: diethyl ether can be given through a vaporizer (Boyle's bottle) or an open mask. Up to 15–20% vapour concentrations are required for the induction of anaesthesia. To maintain deep anaesthesia concentrations of 10% are required as compared to 5% for light anaesthesia. An EMO (Epstein, Mackintosh, Oxford) vaporizer delivers between 0 and 25% concentrations, and if a patient is paralysed with a muscle relaxant, a 2–4% concentration of ether in air maintains unconsciousness. Recovery following 2–4% ether concentration is fairly quick and the incidence of nausea and vomiting is insignificant.

Side-effects and precautions: ether should not be used in children with fever in hot operating conditions as they will be prone to develop ether convulsions; the chances become higher if atropine is used as a premedication. If ether convulsions occur, the treatment consists of stopping ether, cooling the patient with a fan or sponging with cold water. Diazepam 1–2 mg or thiopentone 100 mg IV will stop the convulsions.

The use of ether is contraindicated in patients with diabetes mellitus and severe liver disease. As diethyl ether is flammable, it should not be used along with diathermy apparatus.

Enflurane (Ethrane). This volatile anaesthetic agent is non-explosive and non-inflammable in the presence of air or oxygen. It produces loss of consciousness like any other anaesthetic agent. In addition enflurane is known to cause increased activity in the brain which is similar to an epileptic attack. Hence enflurane is not recommended in patients with a history of epilepsy. At light planes of enflurane anaesthesia, the cardiovascular system is stable, but in deep planes there is a fall in blood pressure. It has minimal effect on other systems.

Indications: because of the smooth induction and maintenance, enflurane is being used in a number of surgical procedures.

Dosage: initially 4–5% vapour concentration is required for the induction of anaesthesia followed by 2–5% for maintenance.

Precautions: it should be avoided in patients with a history of epilepsy.

Isoflurane (Forane) resembles enflurane in a number of ways with a slight difference in its chemical composition. It produces a more rapid induction of anaesthesia than halothane. It also produces a dose-dependent fall in blood pressure with less effect on cardiac output. Respiratory depression occurs in a dose-dependent manner similar to that of enflurane. A very small amount of isoflurane undergoes biotransformation, hence the chances of toxicity are highly unlikely.

Anaesthetic gases

Nitrous oxide (N_2O) is a colourless gas with a sweet smell. It is supplied in blue cylinders as liquid compressed to a pressure of 650 lb/in^2. It produces loss of consciousness like other general anaesthetics, but its effects are marked in the presence of hypoxia. It causes some increase in respiratory rate and has no effect on muscle, the liver or kidneys. It has a tendency to cause nausea and vomiting if given in a hypoxic mixture (i.e. with less oxygen in the mixture of N_2O and oxygen). Nitrous oxide causes depression of bone marrow if given over 24 hours and in the presence of hypoxia can cause atelectasis (collapse of the alveoli in the lungs) and pulmonary oedema.

Indications: as a supplement with oxygen (66% and 33%)in most surgical procedures; in a 50:50 mixture with oxygen (also called Entonox) for pain relief during labour and also during dental extraction in a dentist's chair.

Dosage: N_2O is a poor anaesthetic on its own, hence a mixture of N_2O and O_2 (1:1) is available which can be delivered from machines such as the Lucy-Baldwin apparatus which is a preset intermittent flow machine. Whatever form is used a degree of hypoxia occurs in patients so it is recom-mended that N_2O should be given with at least 20% oxygen added.

Side-effects and precautions: during recovery from N_2O and O_2 anaesthesia, hypoxia (also called diffusion hypoxia) occurs. This is due to the rever-sal phase in which large volumes of insoluble N_2O are eliminated from the blood into alveoli, thus decreasing the alveolar concentration of oxygen. This diffusion hypoxia can be prevented by giving oxygen in the period following extubation and in the recovery room. For the effects of N_2O on closed gas-filled cavities in the body, such as the middle ear, peritoneum and pneumothorax, readers are asked to seek an explanation from their anaesthetists.

Carbon dioxide (CO_2) is a colourless, odourless gas with a slightly acid taste. It is supplied in liquid form in grey cylinders at a pressure of 50 bar at 15°C. CO_2 is non-inflammable and does not support combustion.

The uses of CO_2 during anaesthesia are:

a. To induce hyperventilation to facilitate blind nasal intubation
b. To increase cerebral blood flow during carotid artery surgery
c. To bring the CO_2 levels to normal levels at the end of a period of hyperventilation.

It is important to turn off the CO_2 cylinder when it is not needed.

Air is the main source of medical oxygen. Com-pressed air is used extensively in medicine, to drive ventilators, as a source of power for pneumatic instruments or in oxygen-air total IV anaesthetic techniques, when nitrous oxide is not used.

Air is supplied in the UK in cylinders of capacities 1280, 4800 and 6400 litres (sizes F–J) compressed to 137 bars (2000 psi). Medical air cylinders are painted grey with black and white shoulder quadrants and are fitted with bull-nose valves.

Cyclopropane is a colourless gas with a pungent taste and a strange smell. It depresses the CNS like all other anaesthetic agents. During light anaes-thesia, blood pressure and cardiac output are increased with a small fall in heart rate. At deeper planes of cyclopropane anaesthesia, blood pressure falls and the heart rate rises. Cyclopropane is a marked respiratory depressant and has no sig-nificant effect on the liver, kidneys and muscular system. It does not have any significant effect on the contractility of the uterus.

Metabolism: cyclopropane is excreted unchanged by the lungs.

Indications: although its use in the UK is vir-tually non-existent, people still keep an occasional cylinder of cyclopropane for that 'special use'. Anaesthetists who have used this gas in the past reserve it for 'bad risk' patients and for inducing babies and small children. It is not suitable for major surgery without the use of muscle relaxants. As cyclopropane is a rapidly acting agent, the patient will be fully anaesthetized within five minutes without adequate muscle relaxation. Recovery from anaesthesia is fairly rapid (within a few minutes).

Dosage: a concentration of 5–10% produces light anaesthesia, 15–30% moderate to deep anaesthesia and around 30–40% total respiratory paralysis. It should be used in a closed circuit with a CO_2 absorber, because of its high cost.

Side-effects and precautions: patients breathing spontaneously can develop ventricular arrhythmias (hypoventilation leading to a build-up of CO_2). The treatment consists of decreasing the cyclopropane concentration and increasing the ventilation. To prevent hypotension or atelectasis of the alveoli at the end of cyclopropane anaes-thesia, oxygen is given in the immediate postoperative period.

ANALGESICS

Analgesics are usually prescribed to relieve pain which could be mild to severe (such as postoper-ative pain, pain due to trauma and cancer). They are either powerful narcotics or weak analgesics. Narcotic analgesics are either found naturally or prepared synthetically. One of the major problems with narcotic analgesics is their addiction potential (i.e. people get hooked on them!). A few definitions should be introduced:

Agonists are those narcotics which exert actions

such as analgesia, euphoria, stimulation of the chemoreceptor trigger zone (CTZ) (causing vomiting) and respiratory depression and addiction (e.g. morphine, diamorphine).

Antagonists are those agents which oppose agonist actions (e.g. naloxone).

Partial agonists are drugs which exhibit a few agonist and a few antagonist actions (e.g. pentazocine, nalorphine, buprenorphine). Some of the common narcotic analgesics used during and following surgery and those available in theatre will be described.

For postoperative analgesia

Morphine is obtained from opium which is the dried juice from the unripe poppy heads of *Papaver somniferum*.

It causes depression of the cerebral cortex and respiratory centre and miosis (pin-point pupils). The use of large doses of morphine produces a slowing of the pulse rate and a fall in blood pressure. Morphine can produce a fall in the respiratory rate and tidal volume, and it also causes constipation. Morphine crosses the placental barrier and causes respiratory depression in neonates.

Its peak analgesic effect is 20 minutes after IV and 90 minutes after IM injection, the action lasting for 4 hours.

Morphine is metabolized in the liver and excreted via the kidneys. People receiving morphine on a regular basis are in danger of becoming addicted to it.

Indications: it is used in the treatment of acute pain following surgery and myocardial infarction.

Dosage: 15–30 micrograms per kg body weight (approximately 8–20 mg) for acute pain and 8–10 micrograms per kg body weight (10–15 mg) as a premedication $1\frac{1}{2}$ hours before surgery.

Side-effects and precautions: the side-effects include confusion, nausea, vomiting and respiratory depression. It should be used with caution in elderly patients and is contraindicated in patients with liver failure and hypothyroidism.

Papaveretum (Omnopon) is less powerful than morphine in its sedative and analgesic properties. The papaveretum preparation consists of 50% an-

hydrous morphine with the other 50% being made up of papaverine, codeine, thebaine and narcotine.

Indications: in the treatment of acute pain following surgery and as a premedication.

Dosage: 0.2 mg per kg body weight IM repeated 4–6 hourly or as an infusion.

Side-effects and precautions: the side-effects are the same as for morphine. Papaveretum should be avoided in patients over the age of 70 years.

Pethidine is less potent than morphine in its analgesic action. It causes cerebral depression and induces nausea and vomiting. It dries secretions (atropine-like effect) and may produce a fall in blood pressure. The respiratory depression caused by pethidine is not marked. Pethidine crosses the placental barrier causing respiratory depression in a neonate. It is broken down in the liver and excreted via the kidneys.

Indications: Pethidine is used as a premedication and pain reliever in the intraoperative and postoperative period. It is also used in the early stages of labour.

Dosage: for premedication 0.5–1 mg per kg body weight IM repeated 3–4 hourly.

Side-effects and precautions: Nausea, vomiting and depression are the common side-effects. Pethidine is contraindicated in patients with liver disease. It is also a drug which causes addiction.

Pentazocine (Fortral) is a powerful analgesic. In small doses it causes sedation and in larger doses restlessness and euphoria. Respiratory and cardiovascular depression are not as marked as with morphine.

Indications: it is used in the relief of acute and chronic pain.

Side-effects are the same as for morphine except pentazocine causes dysphoria.

Dosage: 15–60 mg can be given IV or IM for the relief of acute pain.

Buprenorphine (Temgesic) is a 'partial agonist' with actions similar to morphine.

Indications: relief of moderate to severe pain.

Dosage: 0.3–0.6 mg IM or IV, action lasting from 4 to 6 hours.

Side-effects and precautions: nausea, vomiting, dizziness.

Narcotic analgesics used in theatre

Alfentanil (Rapifen) is a derivative of fentanyl. It has a faster onset of action and a much shorter duration of action (10–15 minutes). It is suitable as an IV infusion during anaesthesia.

Dosage: for spontaneous respiration in adults, 500 micrograms. In IPPV, 30–50 micrograms/kg. For IV infusion, 50–100 micrograms/kg over 10 minutes then 1 microgram/kg/minute.

Side-effects: respiratory depression and muscular rigidity.

Fentanyl (Sublimaze) is a highly potent analgesic with an onset of action in 1–2 minutes and an effect lasting for 20 minutes. In doses up to 200 micrograms it will not cause respiratory depression.

Indications: it is used as an analgesic in the intraoperative period.

Dosage: 3–5 micrograms per kg body weight.

Side-effects and precautions: nausea and vomiting, respiratory depression.

Phenoperidine (Operidine) is a powerful analgesic related to pethidine. When given IV it acts within 2–3 minutes, the effect lasting for up to one hour. It has little action on the cardiovascular system but causes respiratory depression.

Indications: as an analgesic during the intraoperative period.

Dosage: 20–50 micrograms per kg body weight when patients are being ventilated.

Side-effects and precautions: nausea, vomiting and respiratory depression.

Narcotic antagonists

Naloxone (Narcan) is the specific antagonist of all the narcotics (e.g. fentanyl, morphine, pethidine). The agonist actions (respiratory depression, analgesia) are completely reversed within one minute of IV injection, the action lasting 30 minutes.

Indications: it is used to antagonize respiratory depression caused by the narcotics. It has a definitive role: in reversing respiratory depression caused by intrathecal morphine (where analgesia is not reversed), treating neonatal respiratory depression, and in the treatment of neurogenic shock.

Dosage: in adults 0.2–0.4 mg IV for an immediate effect and a further 0.4 mg IM for prolonging the effect.

Side-effects and precautions: because naloxone has a short action it needs to be repeated, preferably given IM at the same time.

Intravenous induction agents

An ideal intravenous induction agent should satisfy the following criteria. The drug should:

a. be stable in solution, be water soluble and have a long shelf-life.
b. be non-irritant to the veins or tissues if accidentally injected outside the vein.
c. produce sleep in one arm-brain circulation time (i.e. the amount of time the drug takes to reach from an arm to the brain: in a normal fit person it is 15 seconds, but this is prolonged in the elderly).
d. produce rapid recovery with little hangover effect.
e. not produce excitatory effects such as tremor, involuntary muscle movements, hiccup and laryngospasm.
f. not cause undue respiratory and cardiovascular depression.
g. have a very low incidence of hypersensitivity reactions.

None of the currently available IV induction agents has all these characteristics. The important classes of IV induction agents are:

1. Barbiturates—thiopentone, methohexitone
2. Imidazoles—etomidate
3. Phenols—propofol
4. Phencyclidines—ketamine.

Thiopentone (Intraval, Pentothal) is a thiobarbiturate which is presented as a yellowish white powder. It is supplied mixed with sodium carbonate as thiopentone is soluble only in strong alkaline solutions (pH 10.5).

When given intravenously it produces loss of consciousness within 15 to 20 seconds (one arm/brain circulation time) in a fit adult patient. This is because thiopentone is taken up by brain tissue. When its plasma and brain concentration falls, the patient regains consciousness. Thiopentone is not metabolized completely but 'redistributed' to fat and other vascular tissues in the early stages.

On IV injection there is a fall in blood pressure due to peripheral vasodilatation, which becomes marked in patients with hypovolaemia. Thiopentone can induce laryngospasm during induction and respiratory depression (including apnoea) for a short duration. It is metabolized in the liver and excreted via the kidneys.

Indications: thiopentone is used for the induction of anaesthesia and in the treatment of status epilepticus.

Dosage: 3–5 mg per kg body weight; it is available as a single dose vial 500 mg in 20 ml.

Side-effects and precautions: laryngospasm, bronchospasm and if injected outside the vein it causes severe pain. If thiopentone is accidentally injected intra-arterially it can cause acute pain and if not treated urgently thrombosis and gangrene of the fingers occur. The use of thiopentone is contraindicated in patients with a history of porphyria, airway obstruction and pericardial effusion.

Methohexitone (Brietal) is a methylated barbiturate which causes loss of consciousness in one arm/brain circulation time. The patient recovers his consciousness in 2–3 minutes, the drug being redistributed to fat and other tissues. The arterial blood pressure does not fall as markedly as thiopentone.

Indications: as patients recover more quickly and are more alert than when thiopentone is used, methohexitone is used in outpatient anaesthesia and electroconvulsive therapy.

Dosage: 1.5 mg per kg body weight. A 1% solution is made up by adding 10 ml of water to a vial containing 100 mg of methohexitone.

Side-effects and precautions: hiccups and involuntary movements are quite often seen.

Etomidate (Hypnomidate) is an imidazoline derivative and causes loss of consciousness in one arm-brain circulation time. The patient recovers within two minutes. It does not cause a fall in blood pressure (cardiovascularly stable).

Indications: for the induction of anaesthesia in frail, hypovolaemic patients and also in outpatient anaesthesia.

Dosage: 0.3 mg per kg body weight.

Side-effects and precautions: nausea, vomiting, involuntary movements.

Propofol (Diprivan): This drug is presented in a concentration of 10 mg/ml in a lipid emulsion and is a di-isopropyl phenol. Induction occurs within one arm/brain circulation time and the recovery is rapid. Pain on injection can be prevented by mixing it with 1% plain lignocaine or injecting an analgesic before propofol.

Dosage: 1–2 mg per kg for induction of anaesthesia. For total IV anaesthesia, 6–10 mg per kg per hour is used.

Ketamine (Ketalar) is an acidic solution which can be used to induce sleep when given either IM or IV. If given IV it produces loss of consciousness in one arm-brain circulation time. It is also called a 'dissociative anaesthetic agent'. Ketamine produces intense analgesia followed by loss of consciousness. If given to adults, ketamine induces hallucinations and bizarre dreams. When disturbed patients react violently. For this reason the patient is given either lorazepam (Ativan) 1 mg or diazepam (5–10 mg) to prevent hallucinations and dreams and is not disturbed until he recovers fully.

Ketamine causes a rise in blood pressure, heart rate and intraocular pressure.

Indications: in patients with difficult airways (burns or trauma of face and upper airway) and in poor risk patients. Ketamine is used for the induction of anaesthesia in children below 10 years age for neuroradiological procedures, radiotherapy and cardiac catheterization. It is also used to treat bronchospasm in status asthmaticus.

Dosage: when given IV (2 mg/kg) it produces anaesthesia within 30 seconds, lasting for 5–10 minutes. If given IM (10 mg/kg) it produces loss of consciousness in 4 minutes lasting for 15–30 minutes. It can also be given as a continuous infusion and the anaesthetic effects can be reversed using physostigmine 0.5–1 mg without affecting the analgesia.

Side-effects: hallucinations, dreams, hypertension, vomiting. Ketamine is contraindicated in patients with hypertension, angina, and raised intracranial pressure.

DRUGS ACTING ON THE RESPIRATORY SYSTEM

In the prophylaxis and treatment of bronchial asthma

Sodium cromoglycate (Intal) does not prevent bronchoconstriction, nor does it cause bronchodilatation. It acts by preventing the release of histamine which is produced as a result of an antigen—antibody reaction. (Antigen is the allergic source from outside such as dust, feathers etc; antibody is the immunoglobulin which is produced in response to the antigen.)

Indications: as a prophylaxis against an attack of bronchial asthma.

Dosage: it is inhaled four to eight times a day from a single dose, 20 mg cartridge (Spincap) inhaler.

Salbutamol (Ventolin) has a highly selective action on bronchial musculature when given by an aerosol (inhaler or via a nebulizer). The action is immediate and long lasting; the maximum effect is seen in 5 minutes. The action lasts for 4–6 hours.

Indications: bronchospasm due to any cause including bronchial asthma.

Dosage: it is given as a metered aerosol inhaler (giving 100 micrograms during each inhalation). In the wards and recovery room a mixture of salbutamol 1 ml (2.5 mg) plus 1 ml of normal saline is given to the patient nebulized with oxygen.

In the operating theatre, during an emergency an IV injection of salbutamol (2–4 micrograms per kg) can be given. Salbutamol is also prescribed orally 2–4 mg four times a day.

Terbutaline is similar to salbutamol in action, reaching its peak effect 30 minutes after subcutaneous injection.

Aminophylline is similar to caffeine. It stimulates the respiratory centre and causes a small rise in blood pressure. It induces dilatation of the smooth muscles of the bronchioles.

Indications: aminophylline is used in the treatment of bronchial asthma and bronchospasm due to any cause.

Dosage: it can be given orally 100–300 mg three to four times a day or as a rectal suppository (360 mg).

In an emergency, a 10 ml ampoule (containing 250 mg) of aminophylline can be injected IV slowly to relieve bronchospasm.

Respiratory stimulants

Doxapram (Dopram) stimulates respiration by acting directly on the medullary centres. In low does it increases the tidal volume and with high doses it also increases the respiratory rate.

The injection of doxapram causes a small rise in blood pressure and heart rate.

Indications: it is used to reverse the respiratory depression caused by narcotics (fentanyl, papaveretum, morphine). An advantage of doxapram is that it does not reverse the analgesia caused by these drugs (as opposed to naloxone).

Dosage: 1–5 mg per kg body weight IV in the postoperative period to reverse respiratory depression, repeated at 2-hourly intervals. It can also be used in the ward in the treatment of respiratory failure as an infusion, the recommended rate being 1–3 mg per minute of a 0.2% solution.

DRUGS ACTING ON THE CARDIOVASCULAR SYSTEM

Drugs acting on the cardiovascular system will be divided into groups which are of relevance in the operating theatre and recovery area.

The efferent fibres from the cerebral cortex, hypothalamus and medulla are relayed at synapses in the autonomic ganglia, the exception being the efferent fibres reaching the adrenal medulla.

To simplify further, efferent fibres which start at the higher centres and relay at the ganglion are called preganglionic; the fibres which leave the ganglion are called postganglionic fibres. The preganglionic fibres are cholinergic in nature, i.e. they release acetylcholine which in turn excites the cells in the postganglionic fibres and relays nerve impulses. The adrenal medulla also carries cholinergic fibres.

The postganglionic fibres are either adrenergic or cholinergic in nature. The adrenergic fibres are sympathetic (releasing adrenaline or noradrenaline), and by exciting the nerve cells can increase the heart rate, force of contraction of the heart muscle and dilate or constrict the blood vessels.

In the following paragraphs drugs acting on the heart, drugs which raise blood pressure (vasopressors), and those which lower blood pressure (antihypertensives and vasodilators) will be described.

Drugs acting on the heart

Inotropic and chronotropic drugs

These terms need to be defined here before the discussion of various drugs which are included in this category.

Inotropic drugs are those which alter the force or the contraction of the heart beat. In practice, only drugs which increase the contractions are beneficial, the examples being digoxin, dopamine, dobutamine and isoprenaline.

Chronotropic drugs are those which influence the heart rate by increasing or decreasing it. A good example is adrenaline.

Digoxin (Lanoxin) is prepared from the leaf of *Digitalis lanata*. It is chemically related to steroids and sex hormones. Digitalis has no effect on the normal heart, but in patients with congestive cardiac failure, it increases the force of contraction, decreases the size of the dilated heart and increases the cardiac output. It also slows the conduction of impulses from the atrium to the ventricle, thus slowing the rate of atrial fibrillation. It increases the urinary output (diuretic effect) indirectly by increasing the cardiac output.

Metabolism: digitalis can be given orally or IV; although it is prescribed IM, the absorption of the drug is not uniform. Digoxin acts in 1–4 hours and the effect lasts for 1–2 days. It is broken down and excreted by the kidneys.

Indications: in the treatment of congestive cardiac failure and atrial fibrillation.

Dosage: orally 0.5 mg initially followed by 0.25 mg 6 hourly. In an emergency (theatre) 0.5–1 mg (diluted) IV, initially followed by 0.5–0.25 mg every 6 hours.

Precautions and side-effects: digoxin is not given after a myocardial infarction and should be given with caution in patients with renal impairment. Nausea, vomiting and bradycardia are early signs of overdose.

Isoprenaline (Saventrine) is an inotrope related to other catecholamines (adrenaline). Isoprenaline has a powerful stimulating action on the heart and increases the heart rate. It produces a fall in blood pressure by peripheral vasodilatation.

Isoprenaline causes dilatation of the bronchial smooth muscle and also inhibits the release of histamine. Hence it is more effective in treating bronchopasm caused during anaphylaxis (acute allergic reaction).

Indications: isoprenaline is mainly used in the treatment of bronchospasm. It is also used to treat bradycardia and low blood pressure following heart block and in the management of cardiogenic shock.

Dosage: in the treatment of asthma, either a sublingual tablet (10 mg) or via a nebulizer (1% spray). In the treatment of cardiogenic shock 1 mg of isoprenaline is added to 500 ml of 5% dextrose and given at the rate of 2–4 micrograms per minute.

Side-effects: tachycardia, chest pain, palpitations, headache, nausea and vomiting. It should be used with great caution in patients with thyrotoxicosis.

Dopamine (Intropin) is a naturally occurring transmitter in the brain and kidneys. Dopamine is the precursor of noradrenaline and adrenaline. It exerts an inotropic effect by increasing the cardiac output with a slight rise in systolic pressure and an increase in renal blood flow.

Indications: in the treatment of hypotension, following open heart surgery and in the early stages of renal failure.

Dosage: dopamine is available as 200 mg in a 5 ml ampoule which is added to 500 ml of 5% dextrose giving a dilution of 400 micrograms per ml. To improve the renal function, dopamine is started at the rate of 2 micrograms per kg per minute.

Side-effects and precautions: it causes tachycardia and peripheral vasoconstriction as the dosage is increased. It is not advisable to use in patients with phaeochromocytoma and cardiac arrhythmias. It should always be administered via a central vein.

Dobutamine (Dobutrex) is similar to dopamine in a number of ways, but dobutamine has a specific action in increasing the contractility of the heart.

Indications: cardiogenic shock following myocardial infarction; following cardiac surgery.

Dosage: it is available as 250 mg in a 10 ml ampoule which is diluted in 500 ml of 5% dextrose. It is given at the rate of 2 micrograms per kg per minute to 10 micrograms per kg per minute.

Sometimes a combination of dopamine and dobutamine is used; the former is used to improve renal perfusion and the latter to improve cardiac function in patients with cardiogenic shock.

Chronotropic drugs are those which increase the heart rate, the examples being adrenaline and noradrenaline. As these agents also increase the blood pressure they will be discussed under vasopressors.

Antidysrhythmics

Antidysrhythmics are those agents which are used to treat cardiac arrhythmias. They are classified according to their site of action on the action potential of a cardiac nerve fibre. It is not necessary for readers to have a detailed explanation of their mode of action.

A few antidysrhythmics which are used in the operating theatre are described below.

Quinidine (Delanide) is used in the treatment of ventricular extrasystoles and ventricular paroxysmal tachycardia.

Dosage: 300 mg three times a day.

Lignocaine (Xylocaine) is used to treat ventricular dysrhythmias following myocardial

infarction. It is one of the drugs seen in the cardiac arrest drug box.

Dosage: a loading dose of 1–2 mg per kg body weight followed by an infusion of 1–4 mg per minute for 48 hours.

Mexiletine (Mexitil) is used in the treatment of ventricular arrhythmias following myocardial infarction.

Dosage: 100–250 mg IV as a bolus followed by an infusion, the oral dose being 400–600 mg initially followed by 200 mg four times a day.

Propranolol (Inderal) is used to treat a range of supraventricular and ventricular arrhythmias.

Dosage: 1 mg IV per minute up to maximum of 10 mg followed by 1–2 mg atropine to counteract the severe bradycardia. Alternatively, practolol (Eraldin) 5 mg is given IV slowly during an emergency in the operating theatre.

See also beta blockers on page 66.

Amiodarone (Cordarone) is used to treat resistant supraventricular tachycardia.

Verapamil (Cordilox) is used in the treatment of A-V nodal tachycardias. It is given IV (during an emergency), the dose being 5–10 mg over 30 seconds.

Cardiac arrhythmias in the operating theatre

Cardiac arrhythmias are usually seen in patients who are spontaneously breathing a mixture of gases including halothane. If the patient underventilates due to pain, carbon dioxide retention occurs which stimulates the release of catecholamines (adrenaline, noradrenaline) in the body. These in turn make the cardiac muscle irritable and in the presence of halothane anaesthetic, dysrhythmias such as ventricular extrasystole and heart block are seen. The treatment consists of reducing the concentration of halothane and improving the patient's ventilation (manually or by IPPV). By getting rid of the excess of CO_2 most of the dysrhythmias disappear. If some irregularity still persists, drugs such as verapamil (Cordilox), lignocaine (Xylocaine) or practolol (Eraldin) are used.

Vasopressors

Vasopressors are those drugs which increase the blood pressure. In anaesthetic practice, sympathomimetic agents are used which stimulate the heart by causing vasoconstriction. In patients with hypotension caused by circulatory failure (spinal and epidural analgesia) or following the removal of a phaeochromocytoma tumour, vasopressors such as ephedrine and noradrenaline are used. In all these cases it is essential to treat hypovolaemia (blood loss), before giving vasopressors.

Some of the vasopressors used in the operating theatre are given below.

Adrenaline is a naturally occurring hormone which can be synthesized commercially. In small doses adrenaline has no effect but in large doses it causes excitement, headache and tremors. It induces a rise in systolic blood pressure with a fall in diastolic pressure, but with large doses it causes a rise in both systolic and diastolic pressure. Adrenaline induces relaxation of the bronchial smooth muscles.

Indications: adrenaline is used to prolong the effect of local anaesthetics by causing vasoconstriction (see Local anaesthetics); it is also used in the treatment of bronchial asthma, anaphylactic shock and cardiac arrest.

Dosage: when adrenaline is used to increase the duration of local anaesthetics, a solution (lignocaine with adrenaline) with a concentration of 1:200 000 is used. To make up the dilutions see the Appendix.

Use of adrenaline during halothane anaesthesia. Adrenaline is used by surgeons to decrease bleeding from the skin incision during surgery on the thyroid gland, mastoid region and during plastic surgery. Adrenaline solutions should have a maximum concentration of 1:100 000 or 1:200 000 and the total dose should not exceed 10 ml of 1:100 000 in 10 minutes of surgery. Patients should be breathing adequately without any signs of hypoxia or hypercarbia.

Ephedrine is a sympathomimetic amine which is produced synthetically and has both alpha and beta effects (see Beta blockers on page 66 for an explanation). It causes an increase in blood pressure and cardiac output. Ephedrine stimulates respiration and dilates the bronchial smooth muscles.

Indications: ephedrine was used in the prophylactic treatment of asthma. Nowadays, ephedrine is used to treat hypotension caused by sympathetic blockade during spinal and epidural anaesthesia.

Dosage: for the relief of asthma 30–60 mg tablets orally as required. To correct hypotension during spinal and epidural anaesthesia, 30 mg is diluted in 10 ml normal saline and bolus doses of 1–5 mg are given to improve the blood pressure.

Side-effects and precautions. Ephedrine causes anxiety, restlessness, tachycardia and hypertension. It is contraindicated in patients with coronary artery disease.

Mephentermine sulphate is a sympathomimetic amine with both alpha and beta effects. Mephentermine increases the arterial blood pressure, heart rate and cardiac output.

Indications: it has been used to treat and maintain blood pressure following the withdrawal of a noradrenaline drip in patients who have undergone removal of a phaeochromocytoma tumour.

Dosage: dose of 15 mg IM or IV of mephentermine is given to treat hypotension. When given IM it acts within 5–10 minutes lasting for up to 2 hours; when given IV it acts within 2 minutes and the action lasts for less than one hour.

Methoxamine hydrochloride (Vasoxine) is a sympathomimetic agent with an alpha effect. Methoxamine increases the blood pressure by causing marked peripheral vasoconstriction (α effect). The cardiac output and heart rate are decreased.

Indications: it is used to prevent and treat hypotension during spinal and epidural anaesthesia.

Dosage: 5–10 mg given slowly IV improves the blood pressure within 2 minutes, the action lasting for an hour.

Metaraminol tartrate (Aramine) is a sympathomimetic agent with both alpha and beta effects. Metaraminol increases the cardiac output and arterial blood pressure.

Indications: it is used in the treatment of hypotension following spinal and epidural anaesthesia.

Dosage: 1–5 mg given IV slowly restores the blood pressure within 3 minutes, the action lasting for 25 minutes. A dose of 2–10 mg given Im acts within 10 minutes and the action lasts for an hour.

Noradrenaline (Levophed) is a naturally occurring hormone which can also be synthesized. Noradrenaline has powerful alpha and weak beta effects. It produces an increase in systolic and diastolic blood pressure due to a marked peripheral vasoconstriction. The cardiac output remains unchanged with a slower heart rate.

Indications: noradrenaline is used to treat hypotension following the removal of a phaeochromocytoma tumour.

Dosage: it is given as an IV infusion. 2 mg when added to 500 ml of 5% dextrose gives a dilution of 4 micrograms per ml. The drip is started at 2 ml per minute and the rate adjusted according to the blood pressure.

Precautions: it is safer to infuse noradrenaline through a central vein because it can cause gangrene of the skin if it leaks subcutaneously.

Phenylephrine hydrochloride (Neophryn) is a sympathomimetic with strong alpha and weak beta effects. The blood pressure is increased due to peripheral vasoconstriction without any changes in heart rate.

Indications: it is used in the treatment of hypotension (following hypotensive anaesthesia) and for the relief of nasal congestion (nasal surgery).

Dosage: to correct hypotension, 0.5 mg is given IV or IM or as an infusion. To relieve nasal congestion, 1–4 drops of 0.5–1% phenylephrine are instilled into the nose.

Vasodilators and antihypertensive agents

A variety of drugs lower blood pressure. In this section a few drugs which are prescribed to lower blood pressure in daily practice (antihypertensives) and deliberately lower blood pressure in the operating theatre (hypotensive agents and vasodilators, see p. 67) will be described.

'Deliberate hypotension' is used by the anaesthetist (see p. 183) to:

a. make the operative surgical field bloodless
b. allow a better skin graft to be taken during plastic surgery
c. decrease the blood pressure in the immediate postoperative period, following coronary artery surgery.

1. Drugs acting on the central nervous system (hypothalamus)

Most general anaesthetics and barbiturates depress the hypothalamus and cause a fall in blood pressure.

Methyldopa (Aldomet) probably acts on the brainstem vasomotor centre where it causes a stimulation of alpha receptors which are inhibitory. These cause a decrease in outflow from the vasomotor centre leading to vasodilatation and a fall in blood pressure.

Indications: methyldopa is used in the treatment of hypertension with or without a diuretic.

Dosage: methyldopa is started at 250 mg three times a day orally and gradually increased to 2 g after 48 hours.

Side-effects and precautions: methyldopa produces sedation, mental depression, postural hypotension and occasionally haemolytic anaemia. It is contraindicated in patients with liver disease and phaeochromocytoma.

Clonidine (Catapres) acts by stimulating alpha receptors in the hypothalamus and causes a fall in blood pressure, heart rate and cardiac output.

Indication: hypertension.

Dosage: 200–300 micrograms per day.

Precautions: if clonidine is withdrawn abruptly marked hypertension develops. Hence a patient receiving clonidine treatment should continue it until the day of surgery.

Hydralazine hydrochloride (Apresoline) produces a fall in blood pressure by acting on the alpha receptors in the hypothalamus and directly acting on the arterioles peripherally.

Indications: in present practice, it is used in hypertensive crises and pre-eclamptic toxaemia.

Dosage: 10–40 mg IV followed by an infusion.

2. Drugs acting on the preganglionic sympathetic fibres

Local anaesthetic drugs such as lignocaine, bupivacaine and cinchocaine when used for spinal and epidural analgesia, paralyse the preganglionic sympathetic fibres, thus causing a fall in blood pressure and peripheral vasodilatation.

3. Drugs acting on the autonomic ganglion (ganglion blockers)

Autonomic ganglia carry both parasympathetic and sympathetic fibres and the drugs which interfere at this site are called ganglion blockers. These blockers have been used to produce deliberate hypotension.

Although a number of ganglion-blocking agents have been described, the only drug which is still used in the operating theatre is trimetaphan (Arfonad).

Trimetaphan (Arfonad) is a rapidly-acting ganglion blocker with an onset of action in 1–3 minutes and lasting for 10–15 minutes after one dose. The hypotensive action of trimetaphan is potentiated by a slight head-up position of the patient.

Indications: to produce induced or controlled hypotension.

Dosage: it can be given in a bolus dose of 50 mg and repeated at 10–15 minute intervals (10–20 mg). For a continuous infusion, a 0.1% solution (500 mg trimetaphan in 500 ml of 5% dextrose) is used with an initial rate of 2–4 ml per minute. The infusion is adjusted according to the blood pressure.

Side-effects: tachycardia and tachyphylaxis are seen. Tachyphylaxis is a mechanism in which repeated doses have less and less effect; this develops within minutes.

4. Drugs acting on the postganglionic sympathetic neurones

These drugs act by decreasing the sympathetic activity, thus causing a fall in heart rate, blood pressure and cardiac output. Examples in this group are guanethidine, reserpine and debrisoquine.

Guanethidine (Ismelin) is used as an antihypertensive agent. In pain relief clinics, guanethidine is used to improve local blood flow in the extremities.

Dosage: for the treatment of blood pressure, 10 mg orally increasing each week; to improve blood flow in the limbs, 10–20 mg of guanethidine, 100 IU of heparin, 1% lignocaine made up to 10 ml with normal saline is injected in the dorsum of the hand or foot, with the tourniquet left on for 20 minutes.

5. Drugs acting on the adrenergic receptors

The activity of the sympathetic nervous system is mediated by two different receptors called alpha (α) and beta (β). Adrenergic receptor-blocking drugs act by competing with adrenaline and noradrenaline for the alpha and beta receptors on the effector organs such as heart, blood vessels and bronchi. The alpha receptors are present in the peripheral blood vessels and the beta receptors on the heart and bronchus.

When the alpha receptors are stimulated, the peripheral vessels are constricted, thus maintaining the blood pressure or increasing it. Beta receptors are divided into two groups: β_1 receptors are present on the heart muscle and β_2 receptors are present on bronchi, arteries, uterus and skeletal muscle.

Alpha adrenergic receptor blockers

These drugs block the alpha responses of adrenaline, producing hypotension (due to vasodilatation), compensatory tachycardia, congestion of mucous membranes and pupillary constriction.

Tolazoline (Priscol) has powerful but brief action on the peripheral vessels. It is used as a trial drug in vascular diseases.

Phentolamine (Rogitine) is a short-acting agent,

with its onset of action in 2 minutes lasting up to 15 minutes following an intravenous injection. After an IV injection it causes a fall in blood pressure and an increase in cardiac output and heart rate.

Indications: it is used in the control of blood pressure fluctuations following open heart surgery and to control hypertension during surgery for the removal of phaeochromocytoma.

Dosage: to control blood pressure 5 mg diluted should be given slowly IV.

Phenoxybenzamine (Dibenamine) is a powerful alpha adrenergic blocking agent. It has a slow onset of action (one hour), the drug lasting for a very long time. Its action cannot be easily reversed due to competitive receptor binding. It causes a fall in blood pressure by decreasing the peripheral resistance.

Indications: it is used in the treatment of peripheral vascular disease and in the control of hypertension in phaeochromocytoma.

Dosage: it is given orally 20 mg three times a day increasing up to 120 mg a day.

Side-effects and precautions: nausea, vomiting, sedation and postural hypotension.

Prazosin is a powerful alpha adrenergic blocker which lowers the blood pressure without unnecessary tachycardia.

Beta adrenergic receptor blockers

These drugs block only the beta effects of adrenaline—the cardiac effects, resulting in a decreased heart rate and cardiac output (due to reduced myocardial contractility). Some of the beta blockers (β_1) are cardioselective and some are non-selective.

The main uses of beta blockers with their mode of action and adverse side-effects are given below. This is followed by a description of important beta blockers.

Disease	Mode of action of beta blockers
Angina pectoris	Reduce cardiac work
Cardiac arrhythmias	Decrease the drive to the cardiac pacemaker
Hyperthyroidism	Reduce cardiac output and heart rate
Phaeochromocytoma	Block beta effects of circulating adrenaline and noradrenaline
Glaucoma	Decrease the production and outflow of aqueous humour.

Side-effects: the β_2 blockers produce heart block, decreased peripheral blood flow, bronchoconstriction and hypoglycaemia.

Cardioselective beta blockers (β_1)

Practolol (Eraldin) is $2\frac{1}{2}$ times less active than propranolol.

Indications: it is used to control cardiac arrhythmias occurring during anaesthesia.

Dosage: practolol is given as 4–10 mg IV repeated at 5 minute intervals.

Atenolol is used in the treatment of hypertension.

Dosage: 100 mg once a day, increased to 200 mg after 2 weeks.

Non-cardioselective blockers ($\beta_1 + \beta_2$)

Oxprenolol (Trasicor) slows the heart rate associated with a fall in cardiac output.

Indications: it is used in the control of angina pectoris and cardiac arrhythmias.

Dosage: it is given as 20 mg, two or three times a day orally for arrhythmias and 40 mg three times a day for angina.

Side-effects: it can precipitate bronchoconstriction in patients with bronchial asthma.

Propranolol (Inderal) decreases the heart rate, cardiac output and in the hypertensive patient causes a fall in blood pressure after prolonged treatment. Propranolol abolishes arrhythmias caused during anaesthesia.

Indications: propranolol is used to control

arrhythmais during anaesthesia and manage tachycardia in patients with phaeochromocytoma. Propranolol is effective in the treatment of angina. In the operating theatre, 0.5–5 mg is given IV slowly to correct arrhythmias. In the treatment of angina pectoris it is given as 80 mg, four times a day.

Side-effects and precautions: sleepiness during the day, impotence and bad dreams are the common side-effects. Propranolol precipitates bronchospasm in patients with bronchial asthma.
The other non-selective beta blockers available are sotalol, timolol eye drops and pindolol.

Labetalol (Trandate) has both alpha and beta adrenoreceptor blocking actions. It is used when rapid control of blood pressure is essential.
Indications: in hypertensive crises and phaeochromocytoma.
Dosage: it is given initially 50 mg IV repeated after 5 minutes if necessary.
Side-effects and precautions: postural hypotension and bradycardia. It can precipitate bronchospasm in patients with bronchial asthma.

6. Drugs acting on the vascular smooth muscle

Some drugs act directly on the smooth muscle of arterioles and veins (without influencing the nerve supply), thus causing vasodilatation. Examples are given below.

Glyceryl trinitrate (Nitroglycerin, Trinitrin) is available as a tablet or solution. It produces relaxation of the smooth muscles of large veins and post-arteriolar blood vessels.

Its main use has been in the relief of the acute pain of angina pectoris. The action begins within 2 minutes and lasts for up to 30 minutes if the tablet is dissolved under the tongue.

It is also used to decrease blood pressure by causing venous pooling.
Dosage: 0.3–1 mg orally as required, the IV dose being 100–200 micrograms per minute.
Side-effect and precautions: light headedness and in overdose it causes methaemoglobinaemia.

Sodium nitroprusside (Nipride) has a direct vasodilator action on the smooth muscle of the

vessel wall. It causes a fall in blood pressure and tachycardia without altering the cardiac output.
Indications: sodium nitroprusside is used to induce hypotension during surgery. It has also been used in the control of hypertension during the removal of phaeochromocytoma.
Dosage: sodium nitroprusside is given as an IV infusion. 50 mg is dissolved in either 500 ml or 100 ml of 5% dextrose and the infusion titrated depending on the blood pressure. The maximum recommended dose is 3.5 mg per kg body weight.
Side-effects and precautions: it causes tachycardia and when the lethal dose is exceeded (7 mg per kg body weight) toxicity occurs. The signs of toxicity are acidosis and the blood pressure not returning to normal in spite of the infusion being stopped. The toxicity is treated by using vitamin B12, sodium nitrite and thiosulphate.

The sodium nitroprusside solution should be wrapped in aluminium foil during administration to avoid deterioration.

7. Drugs acting on the blood volume

Diuretics are those drugs which cause an increase in urine output. They are used in the treatment of oedema and ascites in congestive heart failure and renal failure. Diuretics act by working on renal and extrarenal mechanisms.
Extrarenal. Diuretics act by increasing the cardiac output e.g. digoxin, aminophylline.

Renal:
(i) Some diuretics such as osmotic diuretics (mannitol) act on the proximal convoluted tubule and increase the osmolality of the tubular fluid and prevent water resorption.
(ii) Drugs such as frusemide (Lasix) and bumetanide (Burinex) act on the ascending limb of the loop of Henle and actively prevent sodium resorption. This leads to the formation of a large volume of urine.
(iii) Drugs such as triamterene, amiloride and spironolactone act by preventing the resorption of sodium and chloride in the distal tubule.

Some of the common diuretics used in the operating theatre are given below.

Acetazolamide (Diamox) acts as an inhibitor of an enzyme called carbonic anhydrase which is present in the distal tubules.

Indication: in the treatment of glaucoma and oedema of heart failure.

Dosage: 250–500 mg once a day orally, the action lasting for 12 hours.

Frusemide (Lasix) see above for its mechanism of action.

Indication: it is used IV in the treatment of acute pulmonary oedema and congestive heart failure.

Dosage: in an emergency, 20–40 mg IV brings about a rapid response in 30 seconds. In the treatment of heart failure 40–80 mg is given orally on alternate days.

Side-effects and precautions: electrolyte imbalance (low potassium) and occasional deafness.

Bumetanide (Burinex) acts as a loop diuretic (see above).

Indications: same as frusemide.

Dosage: 1 mg of Burinex equals 40 mg of frusemide in potency. In an emergency 1–2 mg may be given IV.

Mannitol is used to reduce the brain volume in cerebral oedema and in the prevention of renal failure (during hepato-biliary and aortic surgery).

Dosage: mannitol is available as a 10 or 20% solution and the recommended dose is 0.5–1 g per kg body weight.

DRUGS ACTING ON THE UTERUS

Uterine stimulants

Uterine stimulants are those drugs which play an important role during labour and delivery of the fetus. The natural uterine stimulants available are the local hormones such as noradrenaline, serotonin, acetylcholine and ergot alkaloids.

Oxytocin (Syntocinon) acts mainly on the pregnant uterus causing it to contract rhythmically.

Indications: oxytocin is used to induce labour at term and contract the uterus after the birth of the fetus to prevent postpartum bleeding.

Dosage: 10–50 units are added to 5% dextrose and the rate adjusted to between 0.1 and 0.8 units per hour. 5 units can be given IV during caesarean section instead of ergometrine (see below).

Ergometrine maleate is a rapidly acting uterine stimulant which contracts the uterus in 30 seconds following an IV injection and 2–4 minutes after an IM injection. Its action lasts for 3–6 hours.

Indications: it is used to contract the uterus following the delivery of placenta or during caesarean section.

Dosage: 0.25–0.5 mg IV or 0.2–1 mg IM.

Side-effects and precautions: headache, vomiting, hypertension. It should be used with caution in patients with pre-eclampsia and hypertension.

Prostaglandins are a group of polyunsaturated fatty acids. Prostaglandins E_2 (PGE_2) and prostaglandins $F_{2\alpha}$ ($PGF_{2\alpha}$) are used to stimulate the uterus.

Dosage: labour can be induced with an infusion at the rate of 0.5 to 2 micrograms per minute. Prostaglandins can be given orally as 0.5 mg of (PGE_2) or 5 mg of ($PGE_{2\alpha}$) to induce labour.

Side-effects: nausea and vomiting.

Uterine inhibitors

Beta-adrenergic stimulant drugs such as salbutamol (see p. 68) relax the uterus. Hence this drug is used to prevent premature labour in the first trimester.

Papaverine and amyl nitrate inhibit the muscles of the cervix and halothane relaxes the uterus.

DRUGS ACTING ON THE ENDOCRINE SYSTEM

Hormones and drugs which are commonly seen in the operating theatre are briefly described here. Readers are asked to refer to a standard pharmacology textbook for details.

Pancreas

Insulin is a polypeptide which is synthesized

and stored in the β islet cells of the pancreas. It causes a fall in blood sugar by increasing the glucose uptake in peripheral tissues.

Indications: the main indication for a synthetic insulin is diabetes mellitus.

Dosage and preparation: there are three types of insulin preparations.

a. Short acting (with rapid onset): neutral insulin injections such as Actrapid, soluble or regular insulin.
b. Intermediate duration of action (with slower onset): insulin zinc suspension (e.g. Semilente and Semitard).
c. Long duration of action: insulin zinc suspension (crystalline, ultralente or ultratard).

The choice of insulin(s) and dose are adjusted to the individual patient and there is no fixed dose regimen.

Insulin and surgery: if a patient receiving a long-acting insulin is scheduled for minor surgery in the morning, his morning dose of insulin is omitted. If a patient who is on a long-acting insulin is scheduled for major surgery, he is admitted to the ward, and his insulin preparation changed to a rapid acting insulin such as Actrapid. When the blood sugar is adequately controlled, surgery is carried out.

Some diabetics are treated with oral hypoglycaemics such as chlorpropamide (Diabinese), tolbutamide (Rastinon) or glibenclamide (Daonil). If these patients are scheduled for minor surgery, the tablets are omitted on the day of surgery. If they are to undergo major surgery, some centres change the treatment from oral hypoglycaemics to Actrapid during the surgical period.

Adrenal gland

The synthetic corticosteroids which are available have an anti-inflammatory effect. The steriods which are available and used in theatre will be described.

Hydrocortisone (Efcortesol) has an immediate effect which is short lived after an IV or IM injection.

Indications: anaphylaxis, shock and as an anti-inflammatory agent. It is sometimes used to prevent laryngeal oedema after repeated attempts at intubation.

Dosage: 100 mg IV.

Dexamethasone (Decadron) is used as an anti-inflammatory agent in the operating theatre e.g. following maxillofacial surgery.

Dosage: 8 mg IV followed by 4–8 mg IM 8 hourly for 24 hours.

Methylprednisolone (Solu-medrone) is used by transplant surgeons as an immunosuppressant. Patients who are on steroid therapy when they are scheduled for surgery are managed as follows:

— Patients who are receiving oral prednisolone should receive a slightly higher dose until after surgery and the dose tapered back to preoperative levels.
— If the patient was receiving steroids until about 3 months before surgery, hydrocortisone is given as 100 mg IM before surgery and at 8 hourly intervals for 24 hours.
— If the patient was receiving a high dose of steroids for several years, until up to 6 months before surgery, a similar regime as described above is followed.

DRUGS ACTING ON BLOOD

Histamine and H$_1$ and H$_2$ receptor antagonists

Histamine is a naturally occurring amine which is released in response to injury or an antigen–antibody reaction. Some drugs such as tubocurarine and morphine also release histamine. The actions of histamine are:

a. increasing the acid and pepsin content of gastric juice
b. stimulation of any smooth muscle (e.g. bronchial muscle causing bronchospasm
c. dilating the arterioles and causing hypotension
d. dilatation of capillaries leading to the permeability of plasma.

The action of histamine can be antagonized either

by adrenaline preventing the release of histamine (e.g. adrenal steroids and cromoglycate in asthma) or by preventing histamine from reaching its site of action (receptors) e.g. H_1 and H_2 receptor antagonists. H_1 receptors cause the effects (b) to (d) mentioned above. H_2 receptors have an effect on gastric acid secretion.

H_1 receptor antagonists

H_1 receptor antagonists are also called antihistamines. These are effective against histamine-induced bronchoconstriction (except in asthma), histamine-induced capillary permeability and itch. Some antihistamines are effective in motion sickness. These are effective orally, IM or IV.

Side-effects: sedation, fatigue, tremors, dry mouth.

Some of the important antihistamines available in theatre are given below.

Chlorpheniramine maleate (Piriton) is used in an emergency (allergy to blood transfusion or penicillin) 10–20 mg IV or IM.

Dimenhydrinate (Dramamine) has a powerful antiemetic effect. It is effective against vomiting due to irradiation and the toxaemia of pregnancy.

Dosage: 50 mg diluted given IV slowly in an emergency or 50–100 mg tablets 4 hourly.

The other common antihistamine, promethazine, is described on page 49.

H_2 receptor antagonists

H_2 receptors are present on the gastric parietal cells. As discussed above, H_2 receptor antagonists inhibit gastric acid secretion.

Cimetidine (Tagamet) is given orally 300 mg three times a day followed by 400 mg at bedtime. It effectively decreases the volume and pH of gastric acid secretion.

It is used in the treatment of peptic ulcer, reflex oesophagitis and as a prophylactic anaesthetic premedication (see premedication).

Ranitidine (Zantac) is given either orally 150 mg twice a day or 50 mg IV or IM. It is used in the treatment of benign gastric and duodenal ulceration and reflex oesophagitis.

During emergency anaesthesia, ranitidine 50 mg IM can be used effectively to decrease the acid content and volume of gastric secretions.

Anticoagulants

Anticoagulants are those drugs which stop the formation of a further thrombus, i.e. of a new thrombus (prophylactically), or the extension of a pre-existing thrombus (therapy).

There are two types of anticoagulants: (a) direct acting and (b) indirect acting.

Direct acting

These include heparin, which is rapidly effective and only acts for a few hours; it should be given IV or IM.

Heparin is a highly acidic polysaccharide and is also found widely in the granules of mast cells of connective tissue surrounding blood vessels.

Heparin has a strong electronegative charge, and by its action with prothrombin and thrombin prolongs the clotting time.

Indications: in the theatre it is used as an anticoagulant during open heart surgery and vascular surgery (aortic). Pre- and postoperatively it is also given in a low dose subcutaneously to prevent deep vein thrombosis.

Dosage: heparin is available as units and the dose for open heart surgery is 3 mg per kg body weight (1 mg heparin is equal to 100 units). For prophylaxis, subcutaneous heparin is given in a dose of 5000 units in 0.2 ml 8 hourly.

Side-effects: occasional allergic reaction. It is incompatible with dextrose (which is highly acidic) and hydrocortisone.

Protamine sulphate is used as an antedote to heparin. Protamine is highly positive and can neutralize the negatively charged heparin molecule.

Indication: to reverse the effects of heparin.

Dosage: 1 mg of protamine is given IV for each 100 units of heparin injected. At the end of open heart surgery, residual heparin activity is checked with the prothrombin time and protamine is injected accordingly.

Indirect acting

These include the coumarin and inandione groups (Warfarin) and phenindione (Dindevan). These drugs take 72 hours to become effective and the action lasts for several days. Indirect-acting drugs are given orally.

These oral anticoagulants are stopped 72 hours prior to surgery, and the blood tested (prothrombin time). If necessary vitamin K is given to antagonize the effects and the patient is allowed to proceed to surgery.

DRUGS ACTING ON THE NEUROMUSCULAR SYSTEM

Local anaesthetic agents

Local anaesthetic agents are those agents which can produce a reversible depression of conduction of the nerve impulse.

Local anaesthetics can be injected into the subcutaneous tissue (infiltration), nearby to nerves (brachial plexus or individual nerve block), in the epidural space, the spinal cord or as an intravenous local analgesia.

General pharmacological actions and side-effects of local anaesthetics

They can penetrate the blood/brain barrier and stabilize neurones, thus some agents can control status epilepticus if given IV in adequate doses. If given in large doses, they can cause convulsions and coma. Local anaesthetics like lignocaine and procaine also have general analgesic properties. Some of the local anaesthetics such as procainamide and lignocaine have been used in the control of ventricular arrhythmias. All local anaesthetics except lignocaine and cocaine cause peripheral vasodilatation. Cocaine causes vasoconstriction. Some local analgesics have a mild antihistamine reaction which occurs when an excessive amount of the drug is given or when a normal dose is accidentally injected into a vein.

In a mild toxic reaction (or overdose) the patient becomes pale and restless and the symptoms pass off without treatment. In a severe reaction convulsions followed by cardiorespiratory arrest can occur. The management consists of injecting a small dose (100 mg) of thiopentone and supplying cardiorespiratory support if need be.

Use of adrenaline to prolong the action

The effect of a local anaesthetic wears off when it is removed from the site of absorption. Thus anything which delays its absorption into the circulation will prolong its local action and reduce toxicity. Adrenaline when used in a concentration of 1:200 000 will double the duration of action (e.g. 1–2 hours). Adrenaline should not be used with a local anaesthetic when performing blocks on finger, toe or penis, as those organs have their own blood supply cut off due to vasocontriction.

Some of the common local anaesthetic agents used are given below.

Lignocaine (Xylocaine) is a rapidly acting agent whose action is intense and lasts a long time.

Indications: lignocaine is widely used for a number of procedures by local infiltration, topical application (4% xylocaine for ET tubes and spray) and nerve, epidural and caudal blocks. It is also used to control dysrhythmias following myocardial infarction.

Dosage: lignocaine is used as follows with or without the use of adrenaline:

— For a nerve block 1% solution with adrenaline (10 ml for single nerves).
— For infiltration analgesia 0.5% solution 100 ml (500 mg) with adrenaline and 40 ml (200 mg) without adrenaline.
— For spinal analgesia 1–1.5 ml of 5% heavy xylocaine (plain) is used.
— For epidural and caudal blocks 15–50 ml of a 1.5% solution with adrenaline.
— For a topical spray of pharynx and larynx 4 ml of 4% solution is used.
— For intravenous regional analgesia (Bier's block) 25–40 ml of 0.5% lignocaine is used.

For the treatment of arrhythmias see page 62.

Bupivacaine (Marcain) has a longer duration of action (3–6 hours).

Indications: for nerve blocks and epidural analgesia in labour and for surgery. Nowadays heavy bupivacaine (0.5%) is used for spinal analgesia.

Dosage: Bupivacaine is available as 0.25%, 0.5% and 0.75% solutions, the first two being available either plain or with adrenaline. Heavy bupivacaine (0.5% with dextrose) is available for spinal analgesia.

The maximum dose is 2–3 mg/kg with or without adrenaline in a 4-hour period. For spinal analgesia, 3–4 ml of heavy marcain is used.

Prilocaine (Citanest) has a longer duration of action than lignocaine and is less toxic.

Indications: nowadays it is used regularly for IV regional analgesia (Bier's block) and for epidural and nerve blocks.

Dosage: for IV regional analgesia 30–40 ml of 0.5% plain solution is used. The maximum recommended dose is 400 mg with plain solution and 600 mg with adrenaline.

Side-effects: it can cause methaemoglobinaemia.

Cinchocaine (Nupercaine) has a slower onset with a long duration of action (2–3 hours).

Indications: cinchocaine was extensively used for nerve blocks in the past, but nowadays it is only used for spinal analgesia.

Dosage: for spinal analgesia (1:200 solution in 6% dextrose = heavy nupercaine) 0.5–2 ml is used. For epidural and caudal blocks 15–50 ml of a 1:600 solution and for nerve blocks 10 ml of 1:1000 solution are used.

Cocaine. In addition to its local anaesthetic effects, it causes cerebral excitement, tachycardia, hypertension and a rise in respiratory rate due to sympathetic stimulation.

Indications: it is used only as a surface analgesic and a vasoconstrictor in nose (SMR, polypectomy) and eye (dacryocystorhinostomy) surgery.

Dosage: because cocaine causes vasoconstriction, adrenaline is not used. A dose of 1.5 mg/kg should not be exceeded. In eye surgery a 4% solution is used and for operations on the nose 10 and 20% solutions are employed.

Side-effects: it is a drug of addiction. An over-dose causes headache, nausea and convulsions. The treatment consists of sedation and use of alpha and beta blockers to decrease the sympathetic over-activity of cocaine.

Muscle relaxants

As described in the section on physiology, at the junction between nerve and muscle there is a specialized portion of muscle membrane called a 'neuromuscular junction' (NMJ). At rest, the Na^+ ions are high extracellularly and the K^+ ions are high intracellularly, thus maintaining an electrical potential across the membrane of the cell; usually this potential inside is about −90 mV. At this NMJ, acetylcholine (ACh), a neurotransmitter, is stored in synaptic vessels. On arrival of a nerve impulse ACh is released and reacts with the receptors at the NMJ which facilitates the movement of Na^+ inside and K^+ outside the membrane. The NMJ loses its polarization and is called 'depolarized' when the membrane potential is reduced from −90 mV to −45mV.

This potential is moved (propagated) along the muscle fibre and causes it to contract.

After a few milliseconds, acetylcholine which was released earlier, now becomes completely hydrolysed to inactive choline and acetic acid in the presence of an enzyme, cholinesterase. The cell membrane becomes once again impermeable to Na^+ (being extruded out) and K^+ (being pushed back into the cell). Thus the muscle fibre becomes 'repolarized'.

At this point, a few terms will be introduced which will have a bearing on how and where the muscle relaxants work.

If the mechanism described above, i.e. release of ACh etc., is blocked then the nerve impulses reaching the muscle will be blocked (leading to relaxation).

There are two main types of blockers which are described below; two other terms used with muscle relaxants are also defined.

Depolarization block. Drugs in this category imitate the action of ACh at the NMJ (see above), but their action persists for up to three to four minutes. The initial depolarization these drugs cause (e.g. suxamethonium) produces a short period of muscle contraction (seen as fasciculation).

These drugs do not produce contraction (as expected) but relaxation, as they are not powerful enough to sustain contraction. The muscles recover contractibility as soon as the drug breaks down (see suxamethonium).

Non-depolarizing or competitive block. These drugs compete with acetylcholine for receptors at the NMJ. They do not cause depolarization themselves but protect the NMJ from depolarization by ACh. This results in paralysis of the muscles.

The action of these drugs can be reversed with anticholinesterase drugs (see p. 75) which will prevent the destruction of ACh by cholinesterases, thus allowing the concentration of ACh to build up and thus decreasing the concentration of the blocking agent.

Mixed block. This can be seen when a competitive muscle relaxant is administered before the action of a depolarizing agent wears off; e.g. before the action of suxamethonium wears off, a long-acting relaxant such as a tubocurare is given.

Dual block is seen when depolarizing relaxants are used in high doses or over a long period of time. This type of block can be reversed using anticholinesterase.

Monitoring of neuromuscular block. The neuromuscular block can be monitored using a peripheral nerve stimulator.

A single twitch stimulus is used for the diagnosis of a depolarizing block. A train of four stimuli is used for the diagnosis of a non-depolarizing block (see p. 73).

A. Competitive or non-depolarizing muscle relaxants

These muscle relaxants are further divided into those with a short to medium duration of activity and those of long duration. Examples of those of short to medium duration are given below.

Atracurium (Tracrium) is a potent non-depolarizing relaxant of medium duration. It has no cumulative effects (i.e. repeated doses last the same length of time). It undergoes spontaneous non-enzymatic degradation under normal body pH (7.4) and temperature (37°C) by the Hofmann elimination reaction. The drug is broken down irrespective of liver or renal damage. The action of a single dose lasts for 20–25 minutes.

Dosage: 0.6 mg per kg for intubation and maintenance of relaxation; 25% of the initial dose as 'top ups'. For continuous infusion, the rate is 0.4 mg per kg body weight per hour.

In large doses atracurium can cause histamine release. It is presented as 25 mg in 2.5 ml ampoules or 50 mg in 5 ml or 250 mg in 25 ml ampoules.

Vecuronium (Norcuron) is one of the cleaner muscle relaxants with no effect on the heart (the opposite of pancuronium which causes tachycardia due to a vagolytic effect). Its action lasts for 20–30 minutes. The drug is excreted in the bile, hence it should be used with caution in patients with liver failure.

Dosage: 0.1–0.15 mg per kg body weight.

Alcuronium (Alloferin) causes a slight tachycardia and a fall in blood pressure and peripheral resistance. Its onset of action is 90 seconds and it lasts for 20–30 minutes. It is effectively antagonized by neostigmine (see Anticholinesterases). It is partly excreted by the kidneys.

Indications: muscle relaxation for surgery of short to medium duration.

Dosage: 0.3 mg per kg body weight.

Precautions: alcuronium should be used with caution in patients with renal impairment.

Gallamine (Flaxedil). Its onset of action is 90–120 seconds lasting for 20–30 minutes. It causes tachycardia with a slight fall in blood pressure. It is excreted by the kidneys.

Indications: muscle relaxation of medium duration.

Dosage: 1.5–2 mg per kg body weight.

Side-effects: it crosses from the mother to the fetus via the placenta, hence gallamine is not used during caesarean section. Nowadays it is used very rarely.

Examples of muscle relaxants of long-duration are as follows.

Tubocurarine (Tubarine) takes 180 seconds to begin to act, the effect lasting for 30–40 minutes. Curare produces a fall in blood pressure with a rise in heart rate due to blocking of the sympathetic ganglia. It does not cross the placenta from mother to child. It is metabolized in the liver. Patients with liver disease require large amounts of this drug.

Indications: it is useful for long abdominal and thoracic operations.

Dosage: 0.45 mg per kg body weight and is safely reversed with neostigmine in normal conditions.

Side-effects and contraindications: its action is potentiated by hypercarbia and metabolic acidosis. It has a tendency to release histamine and can thus aggravate bronchospasm in patients with bronchial asthma.

Pancuronium (Pavulon). On IV injection the patient is adequately paralysed within 90–120 seconds, the action lasting for 35–40 minutes. Pancuronium causes a rise in heart rate, blood pressure and cardiac output (vagolytic effect). It is broken down in the liver and excreted in bile.

Indications: these are the same as for curare.

Dosage: 0.1 mg per kg body weight.

Side-effects and precautions: its action is potentiated by respiratory acidosis.

Mivacurium is a synthetic diester with non-depolarizing properties. It is rapidly hydrolysed by plasma cholinesterase. The action lasts for approximately twice that of suxamethonium and half that of atracurium. Its action can be reversed by anticholinesterase.

Doxacurium is a long-acting non-depolarizing blocker. It is very potent, the duration of action lasting for 60 minutes. It is highly cardiostable.

Pipecuronium is a long-acting non-depolarizing muscle relaxant with action similar to pancuronium. It is highly cardiostable.

Drugs such as mivacurium, doxacurium and pipecuronium are not available in the UK and will be shortly introduced.

B. Depolarizing muscle relaxants

Suxamethonium (Scoline, Anectine) is a short-acting relaxant. When it is injected IV it acts within 30 seconds, the action lasting up to 5 minutes. On IV injection, suxamethonium causes profound paralysis preceded by muscle fasciculations. It does not cross the placenta. When large and repeated doses of suxamethonium are used, it causes bradycardia and sometimes cardiac arrest (if inadequately monitored). In such cases either atropine is given beforehand or added to the suxamethonium infusion (see below). Suxamethonium causes an acute rise in serum K in patients with burns and major injury.

Suxamethonium causes an abrupt rise in intraocular pressure, hence it is contraindicated in patients with perforating eye injury (to avoid prolapse of the eye contents during this rise).

Suxamethonium is broken down by an enzyme, plasma cholinesterase, in the liver. If the plasma cholinesterase enzymes are low as in liver disease, malnutrition or due to genetic factors, suxamethonium will not be broken down for a longer period and hence will be long-acting.

Neonates and patients with myasthenia gravis are resistant to the action of suxamethonium.

Indications: it is used to facilitate rapid and easy intubation; Suxamethonium is used for endoscopies and electroconvulsive therapy (ECT). It can also be used for longer operations by a continuous infusion.

Dosage: 1–1.5 mg per kg body weight. For a continuous infusion 500 mg of suxamethonium is added to 500 ml of 5% dextrose and 600 micrograms of atropine. The drip rate is run according to the requirement of the patient.

Side-effects and precautions: following the use of suxamethonium young, fit patients experience muscle pains for several days. It is not given to patients with myotonia (a congenital muscle disorder), a history of malignant hyperpyrexia, liver disease or patients with a genetic disorder with plasma cholinesterase enzymes.

If suxamethonium is given to those patients (pseudocholinesterase deficient) unknowingly, a prolonged apnoea occurs. This is treated with IPPV and fresh frozen plasma.

Anticholinesterases

Anticholinesterases are those agents which inhibit or inactivate cholinesterases (which normally break down acetylcholine, see p. 72), thus raising the concentration and duration of acetylcholine at all sites at which it is being released. Anticholinesterases, when they are restoring transmission at the NMJs, produce salivation, bradycardia, bronchospasm and abdominal colic (called muscarinic effects). To counteract these atropine is given which produces a nicotinic effect and a rise in heart rate and blood pressure due to sympathetic stimulation.

Neostigmine is a synthetic anticholinesterase and has prominent action on the NMJ and gastrointestinal tract. Its other actions are as mentioned in the introduction.

Indications: neostigmine is used to antagonize the effects of competitive muscle relaxants and in the treatment of paralytic ileus (of the gastrointestinal tract) and myasthenia gravis.

Dosage: it is given orally for paralytic ileus and myasthenia gravis 15–30 mg three to four times a day. To antagonize the muscle relaxant neostigmine is given 0.05–0.08 mg per kg body weight with atropine 0.02 mg per kg body weight (ratio of neostigmine to atropine nearly 2:1).

Side-effects and precautions: it is used with caution in patients with heart disease and asthma. Atropine should always be given with neostigmine to avoid bradycardia, salivation etc.

Physostigmine (Eserine) is more potent than neostigmine and has the ability to penetrate the blood–brain barrier (unlike neostigmine which cannot).

Indications: in myasthenia gravis, to reverse the central nervous depressant effects of atropine, hyoscine and benzodiazepines. Physostigmine is also used in the treatment of glaucoma.

Dosage: 0.5–1 mg IV.

Pyridostigmine (Mestinon) is 50% less potent than neostigmine.

Indications: the same indications as for neostigmine.

Parasympathetic antagonists and anticholinergic agents

The neurotransmitter at all preganglionic and postganglionic nerve endings is acetylcholine (except sympathetic postganglionic nerve endings which are adrenergic).

Its action on the ganglion is nicotinic and on the effector cells muscarinic. Antagonists of the nicotinic action are ganglion blockers such as trimetaphan and at the effector cells (muscarinic action) atropine and its derivatives.

Interestingly, curare which blocks the release of acetylcholine is also used as an anticholinergic.

Atropine is an alkaloid from the plant *Atropa belladona*. It stimulates the cerebral and medullary centres initially, followed by depression at high dosage. By blocking the muscarinic actions of acetylcholine, atropine prevents sweating, increases body temperature and causes the blood vessels in the skin to dilate. Atropine increases the heart rate by blocking the cardiac vagus nerve. It causes a decrease in bronchial secretions and bronchial musculature is relaxed.

Indications: atropine is used to antagonize the muscarinic actions of neostigmine. It is also used as a premedication to decrease salivary and bronchial secretions. Atropine is used to correct hypotension with bradycardia following spinal anaesthesia. It is also used to dilate the pupils in the eye (mydriatic).

Dosage: it is given as 0.02 mg per kg body weight IV along with neostigmine (0.05–0.08 mg per kg) during the reversal of residual muscular paralysis.

For premedication 0.3–0.6 mg is given IM one hour before surgery, and in the treatment of hypotension with bradycardia 0.3–0.6 mg is given IV.

Side-effects and precautions: atropine overdose causes dilatation of the pupils, blurred vision, dry mouth, delusion and sometimes convulsions. The treatment consists of physostigmine 0.5–1 mg IV. Atropine is contraindicated in patients with glaucoma, and should be avoided in patients with marked tachycardia (e.g. thyrotoxicosis, cardiac disease).

Hyoscine is similar to atropine in a number of actions. In small doses it causes bradycardia and in large doses tachycardia. It causes amnesia, and in elderly patients induces excitement and restlessness. Hyoscine dries up salivary and bronchial secretions effectively (antisialagogue effect) and is a powerful antiemetic agent.

Indications: it is used as an antisialagogue, antiemetic and amnesic (during caesarean section) during general anaesthesia.

Dosage: 5–6 micrograms per kg body weight (approximately 0.2–0.4 mg) IV.

Side-effects and precautions: it can cause drowsiness and all the side-effects of atropine. It should be avoided in patients above the age of 65 years.

DRUGS ACTING ON THE GASTROINTESTINAL SYSTEM

Antiemetics

The vomiting centre is situated in the hypothalamus and the chemoreceptor trigger zone near the fourth ventricle. Vomiting occurs due to stimulation of the emetic centre by various causes. The emetic substances could be narcotic analgesics such as morphine, pethidine or digoxin which act on the chemoreceptor trigger zone (CTZ). Certain drugs such as digitalis act on the gastrointestinal tract as well as on the CTZ.

Post-anaesthetic vomiting is due to a combination of factors such as type of surgery (upper abdominal surgery, termination of pregnancy using prostaglandins), use of nitrous oxide and narcotics, and early mobilization in the postoperative period.

Vomiting can also occur during pregnancy, flying and following exposure to radiation.

The antiemetic effect of drugs on the vomiting centre is due to anticholinergic action and that on the CTZ is due to dopaminergic action. The important antiemetic agents available in the operating theatre are promethazine (see tranquillizers), dimenhydrinate (see antihistamines), prochlorperazine (see tranqullizers), hyoscine (see anticholinergics, parasympatholytics), droperidol (see major tranquillizers).

Metoclopramide (Maxolon, Primperan) has a central action on the CTZ and peripheral action on the upper gastrointestinal tract. It increases peristalsis and emptying of the stomach. If opiate analgesics are given, metoclopramide fails to empty the gastric contents.

Indications: to empty the gastric contents during labour and emergency anaesthesia and also to act as an antiemetic.

Dosage: 10 mg IV or IM every 8 hours.

Side-effects: it causes extrapyramidal dystonia (see phenothiazines).

Domperidone (Motilium) is used in the treatment of nausea and vomiting, the dose being 10–20 mg every 4 to 8 hours.

MULTIPLE CHOICE QUESTIONS

The answers to these questions can be found on page 253.

1. **A drug used for muscle relaxation is:**
   A buprenorphine (Temgesic)
   B prilocaine (Citanest)
   C cinchocaine (Nupercaine)
   D atracurium (Tracrium).

2. **One of the following drugs is used to treat bronchospasm:**
   A aminophylline
   B sodium cromoglycate (Intal)
   C digoxin
   D frusemide (Lasix).

3. **An IV injection of atropine causes:**
   A hypertension
   B salivation
   C tachycardia
   D nausea.

4. **One of the following drugs is a diuretic:**
   A adrenaline
   B digoxin
   C frusemide
   D ranitidine.

5. **Insulin is not given orally because:**
   A the blood flow through the stomach is insufficient
   B it is irritant to the stomach mucosa
   C it may cause peptic ulcer
   D the gastric juice inactivates or destroys the insulin.

6. **One of the following is not an antibiotic:**
   A Chloromycetin
   B gentamicin
   C prednisolone
   D penicillin.

7. **One of the following is not used as a premedicant:**
   A lorazepam
   B papaveretum
   C vecuronium
   D atropine.

8. **Adrenaline is mixed with a local anaesthetic agent to:**
   A increase the heart rate
   B decrease the blood pressure
   C increase the rate of absorption of local anaesthetic from the site
   D decrease the rate of absorption of local anaesthetic from the site.

9. **Suxamethonium is supplied in ampoules of:**
   A 100 mg in 2 ml
   B 100 mg in 5 ml
   C 100 micrograms in 2 ml
   D 25 mg in 2 ml.

10. **Diprivan (propofol) is supplied in 20 ml ampoules containing 200 mg. What dose, in millilitres, should be given to a 70 kg patient, if the dose is 2 mg per kg.**
    A 10 ml
    B 14 ml
    C 16 ml
    D 18 ml.

11. **One of the relaxants mentioned below is safe in patients with renal failure:**
    A alcuronium
    B atracurium
    C pancuronium
    D gallamine.

12. **One of the following drugs is a specific antidote for morphine:**
    A doxapram
    B nikethamide
    C naloxone
    D neostigmine.

13. **The last sensation to leave and the first to come back during general anaesthesia is:**
    A touch
    B pain
    C smell
    D hearing.

14. **Atropine causes:**
    A dry secretions
    B constriction of pupil
    C dilatation of pupil
    D bradycardia.

15. **One of the following is not an anaesthetic agent:**
    A carbon dioxide
    B halothane
    C cyclopropane
    D methoxyflurane.

3. Microbiology

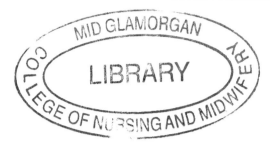

History

Since antiquity it has been known that diseases such as leprosy and gonorrhoea were contagious. In 1665, a haberdasher from Holland, Antony van Leeuwenhoek (1632–1723), known as the 'father of microbiology', examined water from a tub using his home-made lenses and found little animals, which in fact were protozoa (tiny organisms).

A French chemist, Louis Pasteur (1822–1895), proved that the conversion of sugar to alcohol in the production of wine was caused by the activity of living microorganisms. He also pointed out that specific microorganisms cause specific diseases in man and animals.

Robert Koch (1843–1910) from Germany proved in 1876 that *Bacillus anthracis* caused anthrax. In 1882 he also isolated *Mycobacterium tuberculosis*, the causative organism of human tuberculosis.

Alexander Ogston, a Scottish surgeon, showed in 1880 that cocci (round bacteria) produced inflammation and were the main cause of acute abscesses. He isolated Staphylococci and Streptococci.

Ivanowsky (1892) and Beijernick (1898) became aware that there were some organisms even smaller than bacteria; they showed that mosaic disease of the tobacco plant could be transmitted to healthy plants by means of tissue juices freed from bacteria by filtration. Thus a new group of minute organisms called viruses came to be recognized.

In 1940, Chain and Florey opened the antibiotic era by showing that penicillin was an effective chemotherapeutic agent.

Immunology, a subject which deals with the defence mechanisms of the body against bacteria and viruses, has grown with the knowledge of microbes and effective vaccines for preventing infectious diseases.

Classification of bacteria

Bacteria are classified on the basis of their morphology, staining reactions and metabolism, and have been divided and subdivided into orders, families, genera and species.

Higher bacteria are thin filamentous organisms which are sheathed and show simple branching e.g. the Actinomycetacea family comprising Actinomyces and Nocardia.

Lower bacteria are simple unicellular structures. The following terms are used:

— **Cocci cells** are spherical e.g. Staphylococci, Streptococci, Diplococci, Sarcinae.
— **Bacilli cells** are straight and cylindrical (rod-shaped). They are subdivided primarily according to their reactions when stained by Gram and Ziehl-Nielson techniques.
— **Vibrios** are curved and comma-shaped.
— **Spirilla** are spiral, non flexuous rods.
— **Spirochaetes.** These organisms are differentiated from Spirilla as they show active flexion of the cell. They do not possess flagella (tails) but are still mobile. There are three genera of pathogenic spirochaetes:
  • *Borreliae* are larger and more refractile; they can be identified by ordinary staining methods: they have large coils with a wavelength of 2–3 μm.
  • *Treponemata* are slimmer with a coil

wavelength of 1–15 μm. Silver impregnation techniques and dark ground microscopy can identify them.

- *Leptospirae* are very fine, with a coil wavelength of 0.5 μm or less. One or both poles of the organism are hooked. They are identified under dark ground illumination.

— *Mycoplasmas.* These are very small organisms (50–300 nanometres in diameter) and behave like bacteria with no rigid cell wall. Thus they assume various shapes and are very delicate. They were originally known as 'pleuro pneumonia-like organisms' (PPLO).

— *Chlamydiae.* These are spherical bodies of about 300 nanometres in diameter and are intracellular parasites.

— *Rickettsiae and coxiellae.* These organisms are intermediate between bacteria and viruses. They range from being spherical (300–500 nanometres in diameter) to thin rods (up to 2 μm in length). They can be seen by the light microscope but do not pass through filters.

Methods of identification

Gram's method

This is the most important staining procedure used in medical bacteriology. Based on staining properties, bacteria can be divided into two classes:

Gram-positive organisms retain the violet stain following treatment with acetone or ethanol.

Gram-negative organisms lose the violet stain in the decolorization process, but take up the counterstain and are pink.

All cocci are Gram-positive except for the genus Neisseria. All rod-shaped bacteria are Gram-negative except for the genera Bacillus, Clostridium, Corynebacterium and Mycobacterium.

Growth of bacteria

A standard method of obtaining organisms in pure culture is by plating out on a solid medium.

A small quantity of material (pus, sputum) is streaked on to a surface of the medium in a culture plate (petri dish) using a sterile wire loop.

Periodically, initially inoculated material is streaked with a sterile wire loop and reinoculated into different areas of the medium. When the plate is incubated, a crop of colonies appears. Isolated colonies can be picked off and the characteristics of the pure cultures can be studied in fresh media.

The common media used are:

(i) For general purposes—nutrient agar, blood agar, heated blood agar (chocolate agar), cooked meat medium, MacConkey's agar

(ii) For intestinal organisms—MacConkey's agar, deoxycholate citrate agar (DCA), selenite F broth

(iii) For mycobacteria—Dorset's egg medium, Lowenstein-Jensen medium, Dubos medium

(iv) For *Corynebacterium diphtheriae*—Loeffler's medium, tellurite medium

The important pathogens and commensals seen in clinical practice are summarized below:

I. RODS

A. Non-spore forming

1. *Gram-negative*
a. Enteric bacteria e.g. *Escherichia coli, Klebsiella pneumoniae, Pseudomonas aeruginosa, Vibrio cholerae*
b. Respiratory pathogens e.g. *Haemophilus influenzae, Bordetella pertussis*
c. Genitourinary pathogens e.g. *Haemophilus ducreyi*
d. Blood and tissue pathogens, e.g. Brucella, Bacteriodes.

2. *Gram-positive*
a. Gastrointestinal pathogens e.g. Bovine tuberculosis.
b. Respiratory pathogens e.g. *Corynebacterium diphtheriae, Mycobacterium tuberculosis*
c. *Mycobacterium leprae*
d. Blood and tissue pathogens e.g. *Listeria monocytogenes.*

B. Endospore forming

1. *Gram-negative*
The bacteria included in this class are of no medical importance.

Table 3.1 Principle diseases and their causative pathogens.

Genus	Species	Mode of transmission	Disease
Gram-positive bacteria			
Actinomyces	*A. israelii*	Endogenous	Actinomycosis: abscess in facial region, abdomen
Mycobacterium	*M. tuberculosis*	Airborne	Pulmonary tuberculosis
Corynebacterium	*C. diphtheriae*	Airborne and close contact	Diphtheria
Bacillus	*B. anthracis*	Skin contact with contaminated hides, bone meal	Anthrax
Clostridium	*Cl. welchii*	Wounds contaminated with soil	Gas gangrene
	Cl. tetani	Wounds contaminated with soil	Tetanus
Streptococcus	*S. viridans*	Endogenous bacteraemia	Dental abscess; endocarditis
	S. pyogenes	Airborne, contact with a carrier	Acute tonsillitis
	S. faecalis	Endogenous	Urinary tract, wound infection, cholecystitis
	S. pneumoniae	Endogenous or airborne	Lobar pneumonia
Staphylococcus	*S. aureus*	Endogenous or carrier by direct or indirect routes	Boils, styes, osteomyelitis, septicaemia
Gram-negative bacteria			
Neisseria	*N. meningitidis*	Endogenous or airborne spread from carrier	Meningococcal meningitis
	N. gonorrhoeae	Acquired during sexual intercourse or birth	Gonorrhoea, ophthalmia neonatorum
Haemophilus	*H. influenzae*	Endogenous or from carriers	Bronchopneumonia, meningitis, epiglottitis
Bordetella	*Bord. pertussis*	Airborne, close contact	Whooping cough
Vibrio	*V. cholerae*	Water and food borne. Close contact with carrriers	Cholera
Pseudomonas	*Ps. aeruginosa*	Endogenous or contact with contaminated areas or instruments	Infected wounds, chronic otitis media, septicaemia
Escherichia	*E. coli*	Endogenous or exogenous	Wound infections, peritonitis, septicaemia, gastroenteritis
Klebsiella	*K. aerogenes*	Endogenous or exogenous	Urinary tract infections
Proteus	*P. mirabilis*	Endogenous, sometimes exogenous	Urinary tract and wound infections
Salmonella	*S. typhi*	Water or food borne by ingestion	Typhoid fever
	S. paratyphi a,b,c,	Water or food borne	Paratyphoid
Shigella	*Sh. dysenteriae*	Ingestion or by hand-to-mouth routes involving faecal contamination	Bacillary dysentery
Bacteroides	*Bact. fragilis*	Endogenous	Appendicitis and peritonitis, brain abscess
Mycoplasma	*M. pneumoniae*	Airborne	Mycoplasma pneumonia

2. *Gram-positive*
a. Aerobic or facultative (produce spores only in contact with free oxygen) e.g. *Bacillus anthracis*
b. Anaerobic or microaerophilic (produce spores and germinate only in an atmosphere without oxygen) e.g. Clostridium species such as *Clostridium tetani, Clostridium perfringens, Clostridium botulinum.*

II. COCCI

A. Diplococci

1. *Gram-negative*
Neisseria species e.g. *Neisseria gonorrhoeae, Neisseria meningitidis.*

2. *Gram-positive*
a. Streptococcal species e.g. *Streptococcus pneumoniae, Streptococcus pyogenes* Enterococcus group (*Streptococcus faecalis*)
b. Staphylococcal species e.g. *Staphyloccus aureus.*

III. HELICAL, FLEXIBLE BACTERIA

Treponema species e.g. *Treponema pallidum.*

IV. BACTERIA WITHOUT CELL WALLS

Mycoplasma.

V. MINUTE BACTERIA

Two orders:
Order I Rickettsiales: genus Rickettsia
Order II Chlamydiales: *Chlamydia trachomatis.*

'Carrier state'—its implications

In a number of infectious diseases the causative organisms are not eliminated completely at the time of recovery of the patient.

Following diphtheria or streptococcal sore throat, the organisms may still persist in the throat; similarly, following typhoid fever, dysentery or poliomyelitis patients continue to excrete the organisms in the faeces. These types of patients are *convalescent excreters* or *carriers.*

The number of people who continue to harbour and excrete these organisms after two months can be up to 5–10%. Sometimes the carrier state remains indefinitely. *Temporary carriers* or *excreters* excrete the organisms for more than a year. Chronic carriers, e.g. patients with typhoid fever, excrete the organisms for a long period.

Contact carriers

Some people who come into contact with a patient suffering from an infectious disease may acquire the organisms and harbour them without suffering from the disease. Such persons are called *contact carriers* or *Symptomless excreters.* This state may be temporary or chronic.

Over half the population, and an even higher proportion of hospital workers, carry *Staphylococcus aureus* in the nose and skin; they are an important source of disease.

The diseases often found in contact carriers are: diphtheria, streptococcal sore throat, meningococcal meningitis and hepatitis B. As these contact carriers go unrecognized, they constitute a special hazard for the rest of the uninfected population.

INFECTION

Sources of infection

The organisms causing disease in man are derived from three sources: human beings, animals, and other sources.

1. Human source

Some organisms such as Bacteroides and *Escherichia coli* live harmlessly in the bowel, but acting together they can cause peritonitis if the bowel wall is mechanically damaged. *E. coli* is also the commonest cause of urinary tract infection. *Haemophilus influenzae, Streptococcus pneumoniae* and *Streptococcus viridans* live harmlessly in the upper respiratory tract, but can cause bronchitis, sinusitis, bronchopneumonia and otitis media.

Sometimes *S. viridans* may enter the bloodstream and settle on a damaged heart valve causing subacute bacterial endocarditis.

2. Animals

Diseases primarily affecting animals which are transmitted to man are called zoonoses. Cows may excrete *Mycobacterium bovis* (tuberculosis) or *Brucella abortus* (brucellosis) in their milk.

3. Other sources

Pseudomonas aeruginosa, Proteus and clostridial species live freely in the soil and as commensals in the intestines of man and animals.

They may infect burns, wounds and the urinary tract. *Clostridium tetani* and *Clostridium perfringens* can gain access to deep wounds contaminated with soil, causing tetanus and gas gangrene.

Legionella pneumophila which grows in soil and water may contaminate the water in air conditioners and humidifiers.

Sepsis, asepsis, antisepsis

Sepsis means the presence of pathogenic organisms growing in tissues or blood.

An *antiseptic* is a substance that combats sepsis. It can be applied to exposed living tissues without damage to the tissues: examples are dilute alcohol and tincture of iodine.

Asepsis means absence of any living organisms.

Aseptic technique is a procedure aimed at eliminating live organisms; modern surgical and microbiological procedures are based on an aseptic technique.

Local infection control policies

In any hospital, infection control policies are based on:

1. Eradicating the source of infection
2. Interrupting the mode of transmission
3. Increasing the individual's resistance.

Surveillance of infection

A microbiologist (Infection Control Officer) assisted by an Infection Control Nurse is usually responsible for maintaining up-to-date records of all hospital infections. The main sources of these records are:

1. Laboratory records of pathogenic organisms isolated
2. Data collected from:

(i) Doctors, nurses, occupational health departments
(ii) Routine visits to all wards and departments
(iii) General practitioners.

Infection control policies relating to specific infections

A. Infection caused by Gram-negative bacilli

Gram-negative bacilli contribute to 40–50% of all cases of sepsis in surgical wounds. Some infections due to coliform bacteria are due to contamination rather than true infection. The infection is usually due to *Pseudomonas aeruginosa*, Klebsiella, Proteus and Escherichia.

Burns become infected with Pseudomonas resulting in delayed healing, failure of grafts and septicaemia, possibly causing death.

Sources of infection. Most of the Gram-negative bacilli are usually normal intestinal flora and sometimes free-living organisms.

Mode of infection. Coliform infections are common following operations on the intestinal tract e.g. appendicectomy. Sometimes they infect clean operation wounds due to cross infection.

Some patients acquire new strains of coliforms on admission to hospital, which account for urinary tract and wound infections.

Some outbreaks of coliform infections have been traced to infected suction apparatus, endotracheal tubes, anaesthetic machines and hand creams.

Control of infection. This depends on appropriate ward and theatre hygiene. It usually involves using sterilizing methods, rather than disinfecting, and regular checks on the sterility of moist equipment such as humidifiers in which coliforms can multiply.

B. Infections caused by staphylococci

Staphylococcus aureus is responsible for 30–40% of all cases of sepsis occurring in surgical wounds. *Staphylococcus aureus* is widely distributed among patients and hospital staff and is a major source of cross infection.

Source of infection. Deep-seated infection within a few days of an operation and before the wound has been dressed indicates a theatre infection.

Ward infections are superficial and follow the dressing of wounds and burns in the ward.

Control of infection

(i) *Isolation*. All patients with *Staphylococcus aureus* infection should be isolated and barrier nursed. Infected members of staff should not be allowed into operating theatres and wards until they are cured.

(ii) *Search of carriers*. Swabs are taken from the nose, throat, skin, minor septic spots and pimples of individuals who are suspected as a possible source of infection.

(iii) *Treatment of carriers*. If they are patients, they should be isolated; if working personnel they should be taken off work and prescribed local treatment with an antibacterial preparation such as a cream containing chlorhexidine and neomycin (for nose) and hexachlorophane soap (for skin).

C. Infections caused by streptococci

Group A haemolytic streptococci are the source of infection in burns, plastic surgery operations and wound sepsis.

Sources of infection are nasal and throat carriers.

Control of infection. Systemic penicillin is used to treat carriers.

D. Viral hepatitis

Source of infection. Viral hepatitis is caused by hepatitis A virus* and hepatitis B virus.

Hepatitis A causes small outbreaks of infection;

---

*Viruses are small infective agents which grow and reproduce only in living cells. They have the power to enter specific living cells within which they multiply and give rise to signs of disease.

the virus is excreted in the faeces and infection is acquired by mouth.

Hepatitis B virus reaches people through contaminated injection needles (e.g. heroin addicts); haemophiliacs and patients requiring haemodialysis are also vulnerable to injection.

Control of infection. Control of the hepatitis A virus depends upon preventing the contamination of food or water by faeces, and hygienic measures to prevent faecal spread of the disease.

Serum hepatitis (hepatitis B virus) can be prevented by: (i) avoiding the use of infected blood, (ii) the use of separate needles for each patient, and (iii) screening blood for transfusion to exclude the hepatitis virus.

PHYSIOLOGY OF BODY DEFENCE MECHANISMS

The body's defence mechanisms against infection can be divided into two types: non-acquired and acquired.

1. Non-acquired mechanisms

A. Outer defences

Mechanical barriers. An intact skin is a highly effective barrier against bacteria as compared to mucous membranes which are permeable.

Mechanical removal. Mucous membranes of the respiratory tract trap bacteria in a layer of mucus and carry them towards the oesophagus by ciliary action; coughing, sneezing, blinking, tears, sweat, saliva, urine and gastrointestinal secretions remove many bacteria.

Bactericidal activity (cidal = destroying)
Skin acts as a bactericidal for *Streptococcus pyogenes*, *Escherichia coli*, Salmonella and Pseudomonas.
Gastric juice, because of its acidity, kills all bacteria except *Mycobacterium tuberculosis*.
Prostatic secretions which enter the bladder at the end of micturition contain an antibacterial agent.
Breast milk contains various antibacterial substances and an antiviral agent.

Lysozyme, an enzyme, is present in high concentration in tears and has the ability to destroy bacteria.

Normal flora or commensals. They act as defensive organisms and can also cause disease. The mechanism by which they fight disease-causing organisms is by competition for space and food.

B. Inner defences

Body fluids. Serum from a normal person, if incubated for a few hours with certain species of bacteria, will kill them (bactericidal action) and may dissolve some Gram-negative non-pathogenic organisms such as *E. coli*, *Haemophilus influenzae* and *Salmonellae* (bacteriolysis action).

Body fluids also have the property of neutralizing bacterial endotoxins, enzymes and viruses. The substances responsible for these actions are lysozymes, complement, properdin and natural antibodies.

Phagocytosis. Phagocytes are body cells (polymorphs, macrophages) which are specialized in the capture, ingestion and destruction of invading bacteria.

2. Acquired defences

These defence mechanisms depend on the previous contact of the body with microorganisms or their products. They are divided into two types:

a. Antibody-relayed immunity (humoral immunity) which depends on the production of specific antibodies*
b. Cell-relayed immunity (cellular immunity) which depends on the development of specifically sensitized cells (T-lymphocytes)†.

---

*An antibody is an immunoglobulin produced as a result of the introduction of an antigen into the tissues of an animal. An antigen is a substance which, when introduced into the tissues of an animal, can provoke an immune response.

†T-lymphocytes are derived from lymphoid tissues such as the spleen and lymph nodes. They circulate in the blood and extravascular fluids and encounter antigens anywhere in the body.

The acquired defence mechanisms differ from the non-acquired in the following respects:

(i) They take time to develop because of the late arrival of antibodies and sensitized lymphocytes.
(ii) They are more powerful because of the strengthened action of antibodies and lymphocytes against bacteria and their products.
(iii) Because of a prolonged production of antibodies or sensitized lymphocytes, they leave a varying degree of acquired immunity.

CHEMOTHERAPEUTIC AGENTS AND ANTIBIOTICS

Chemotherapeutic agents are drugs which are lethal or inhibitory to the organisms which cause infectious diseases.

An antibiotic is an antimicrobial substance produced synthetically or from living microorganisms.

Alexander Fleming in 1929 found that the products of a mould, *Penicillium notatum*, were strongly active against a wide range of bacteria, but attempts to concentrate the active agent (penicillin) were unsuccessful.

In 1940 Chain and Florey at Oxford isolated penicillin preparations of high antibacterial activity.

Type of action

Antibacterial agents are divided into two types, based on their action:

1. *Bactericidal drugs* destroy all bacteria; examples are penicillins, cephalosporins, aminoglycosides and polymyxin.
2. *Bacteriostatic drugs* are those which merely inhibit the growth of organisms; examples are sulphonamides, tetracylines and chloramphenicol.

Mode of action

Sulphonamides act by competitive inhibition of a bacterial enzyme which has as its substrate the structurally similar substance para-aminobenzoic acid, an essential metabolite for many bacteria.

Trimethoprim inhibits the bacterial enzyme, dihydrofolate reductase.

Pencillins, cephalosporins, bacitracin, vancomycin and cycloserine interfere with cell wall synthesis and secondarily cause cell fragility and bacteriolysis.

Tetracyclines and chloramphenicol act as a specific inhibitor of protein synthesis.

Streptomycin and other aminoglycosides inhibit protein synthesis.

Polymyxin becomes firmly bound to the cytoplasmic membrane and acts by damaging this structure.

Range of action

1. Antibiotics active against Gram-positive organisms include penicillins and erythromycin.
2. Antibiotics active against Gram-negative organisms include polymyxin and nalidixic acid.
3. Antibiotics active against both Gram-positive and Gram-negative organisms (broad-spectrum) include tetracylines, chloramphenicol, ampicillin and sulphonamides.

Antibiotics in regular use

Penicillins and related compounds such as the cephalosporins contain a beta-lactum ring in their chemical structure and hence are called β-lactum antibiotics. They are divided into four groups:

Group 1 Benzylpenicillin (Penicillin G) and penicillins with similar activity e.g. phenoxymethylpenicillin (Penicillin V)

Group 2 Penicillins with broad-spectrum activity e.g. ampicillin, amoxycillin and carbenicillin

Group 3 Penicillins resistant to staphylococcal penicillinase (β-lactamase) e.g. cloxacillin and flucloxacillin

Group 4 Penicillins more active against Gram-negative bacilli than against

Gram-positive organisms e.g. mecillinam.

Group I penicillins. Benzyl penicillin (Crystapen) is the antibiotic of choice in infections caused by *Staphylococcus aureus*, *Streptococcus pyogenes*, *Streptococcus pneumoniae*, Clostridium and other gas gangrene organisms, and syphilis. Similarly, *Corynebacterium diphtheria*, *Neisseria meningitidis* and *Neisseria gonorrhoea* are sensitive to penicillins.

Benzyl penicillin is destroyed by gastric hydrochloric acid, hence it is given by intramuscular (IM) injection. Penicillin V (Crystapen) and phenethicillin (Broxil), which are acid resistant, can be given by mouth.

Dosage. Benzyl penicillin (Crystapen) 300–600 mg is given four times daily by IM route or up to 24 g by intravenous (IV) injection. Penicillin V (Crystapen V) 250–500 mg is given every 6 hours.

Group II penicillins. Ampicillin (Penbritin) is less active than benzyl penicillin against Gram-positive organisms except *Streptococcus faecalis*. It is active against many Gram-negative bacilli, such as salmonella, shigella, *Escherichia coli*, *Proteus vulgaris* and *Haemophilus influenzae*.

It is inactivated by β-lactamase and is normally given by mouth.

Amoxycillin (Amoxil) resembles ampicillin in its activity.

Dosage

Drug (Trade name)	Dose	Route	Interval (hours)
Ampicillin (Penbritin)	250 mg to 1 g	Oral	6
	500 mg	IM or IV	6
Amoxycillin (Amoxil)	250 mg	Oral	8
	500 mg	IM or IV	6
Carbenicillin	5 g	IV slowly	6
Ticarcillin (Ticar)	15–20 g	IV	Divided doses
Mezlocillin (Baypen)	2 g	IV	6–8
	500 mg to 2 g	IM	6
Piperacillin (Pipril)	100–300 mg per kg body weight	IM or IV	8–12

Group III penicillins. Cloxacillin (Orbenin) and flucloxacillin (Floxapen) are unaffected by the β-lactamase enzyme produced by penicillin-resistant *Staphylococcus aureus*. Both of them are absorbed when administered orally.

Dosage

Drug (Trade name)	Dose	Route	Interval (hours)
Flucloxacillin (Floxapen)	250 mg	Oral	6
	500 mg	IV	6
Cloxacillin (Orbenin)	500 mg	Oral	6
	250 mg/500 mg	IM or IV	6

Group IV penicillins. Mecillinam (Selexidin) is highly active against *Escherichia coli* and other Gram-negative intestinal bacteria.

Dosage. 5 to 15 mg per kg body weight is given 6 hourly IM or IV.

Side-effects of penicillin are hypersensitivity and urticarial rash.

Cephalosporins resemble penicillins in being bactericidal and of low toxicity. They have a broad spectrum of activity and can be used against streptococci, staphylococci (including penicillin-resistant strains) and a wide range of Gram-negative bacteria.

Cephalexin (Keflex, Ceporex), cephradine (Velosef), cefaclor (Distaclor) are active when given by mouth. Cefuroxime (Zinacef), cefoxitin (Mefoxin), cefotaxime (Claforan) and ceftazidime (Fortum) are often effective against strains of

Dosage

Drug (Trade name)	Dose	Route	Interval (hours)
Cephalexin (Keflex)	250 mg	Oral	6
Cephradine (Velosef)	250 mg	Oral	6
	500 mg	IM or IV	6
Cefaclor (Distaclor)	250 mg	Oral	8
Cefuroxime (Zinacef)	750 mg	IM	8
	1.5 g	IV	8
Cefoxitin (Mefoxin)	1–2 g	IM or IV	6–8
Cefotaxime (Claforan)	1 g	IM or IV	12
Ceftazidime (Fortum)	1–6 g	IM or IV	Divided doses

Gram-negative bacilli resistant to other cephalosporins. They are given either IM or IV.

Side-effects. The principal side-effect of the cephalosporins is hypersensitivity. Haemorrhage due to interference with blood clotting factors has been reported.

Aminoglycosides. This group of antibiotics includes neomycin, kanamycin (Kantrex), gentamicin (Genticin, Cidomycin), amikacin (Amikin), framycetin (Soframycin). They are similar in chemical structure, antibacterial activity, pharmacological properties and toxicity.

They are bactericidal and active against some Gram-positive and many Gram-negative organisms.

Streptomycin and kanamycin are also active against *Mycobacterium tuberculosis*, while amikacin and gentamicin have activity against *Streptococci faecalis* and Pseudomonas.

Dosage

Drug (Trade name)	Dose	Route	Interval (hours)
Neomycin	1 g	Oral	4
Kanamycin (Kantrex)	250 mg	IM	6
Gentamicin (Genticin)	2–5 mg/kg body weight	IM or IV	8
Amikacin (Amikin)	15 mg/kg body weight	IM or IV	12
Framycetin (Soframycin)	2–4 g	Oral	Divided doses

Side-effects are ototoxicity (impaired hearing) and nephrotoxicity (damage to the kidneys) which occur commonly in adults and patients with renal failure.

Plasma concentrations are measured approximately one hour after an IM dose or 20 minutes after an IV dose. One hour concentrations of gentamicin should not exceed 10 μg/ml and the pre-dose concentration should be less than 2 μg/ml.

Tetracyclines. This group includes tetracycline (Achromycin), oxytetracycline (Terramycin), chlortetracycline (Aureomycin), demeclocycline (Ledermycin), doxycycline (Vibramycin) and minocycline (Minocin).

They are normally given by mouth and are broad spectrum antibiotics active against Gram-positive and Gram-negative bacteria as well as *rickettsiae*, *chlamydiae* and *mycoplasmas*. They are also effective against many Gram-negative bacilli which are resistant to penicillin, including *Escherichia coli*, Salmonellae, Shigellae, Coliform organisms, and the haemophilus and brucella groups.

Dosage

Drug (Trade name)	Dose	Route	Interval (hours)
Tetracycline (Achromycin)	250–500 mg 100 mg	Oral IM	6 12
Oxytetracycline (Terramycin)	250–500 mg	Oral	6
Chlortetracycline (Aureomycin)	250–500 mg	Oral	6
Demeclocycline (Ledermycin)	300 mg	Oral	12
Clomocycline (Megaclor)	170–340 mg	Oral	6–8
Doxycycline (Vibramycin)	200 mg initially then 100 mg	Oral	Daily

Side-effects. Large intravenous doses can cause severe liver damage. Tetracyclines should not be given to a patient with renal failure as they aggravate biochemical abnormalities. They inhibit growth and the development of bones and teeth in the developing fetus and infant. Children up to the age of 8 years who receive tetracycline develop permanent unsightly staining of teeth.

Chloramphenicol (Chloromycetin) has a range of activity similar to that of the tetracyclines; it is normally given by mouth. It is the drug of choice in typhoid fever, meningitis and acute epiglottitis caused by *Haemophilus influenzae*.

Dosage. 500 mg is given orally, 6 hourly or 50 mg per kilogram daily in divided doses IM or IV.

Side-effects. Depression of bone marrow function is a rare but potentially fatal complication. It also causes severe shock and death in premature infants (grey baby syndrome).

The use of chloramphenicol should be restricted to short courses of treatment.

Erythromycin (Erythrocin) is a member of the macrolide group of antibiotics. It is effective against *Mycoplasma pneumoniae*, Legionella and Campylobacter. It is reserved for patients who are hypersensitive to penicillin or are infected with penicillin-resistant organisms.

Dosage. 250–500 mg is given orally 6 hourly or 2 g daily in divided doses IV.

Side-effects are minor gastrointestinal upsets; erythromycin estolate may cause jaundice and impaired liver function if treatment is prolonged.

Sulphonamides. As bacterial resistance has increased against sulphonamides they are being replaced by antibiotics. Folic acid antagonist co-trimoxazole (Bactrim) is indicated in urinary tract infections, prostatitis, exacerbations of chronic bronchitis, salmonella infections, brucellosis and *Pneumocystis carinii* infections.

Sulphonamides are of value in the prophylaxis of meningococcal infections caused by sensitive strains.

Dosage

Drug (Trade name)	Dose	Route	Interval (hours)
Co-trimoxazole (Bactrim)	960 mg 960 mg	Oral IM or IV	12 12
Sulphadiazine (Sulphatriad)	1–1.5 g	IM or IV	4
Sulphafurazole (Gantrisin)	1 g	Oral	4–6
Sulphamethizole (Urolucosil)	200 mg	Oral	6
Trimethoprim (Monotrim)	200 mg	Oral	12

Anti-tuberculous drugs. The drugs used in the treatment of tuberculosis are listed below:

Side-effects. Rifampicin causes severe hypersensitivity reactions and thrombocytopenic purpura.

Isoniazid can cause peripheral neuropathy when a high dosage is used. Pyridoxine (vitamin B6) 10 mg daily should be given prophylactically to prevent this.

Ethambutol causes visual disturbances, such as colour blindness and restriction of visual fields.

Dosage

Drug (Trade name)	Dose	Route	Interval (hours)
Isoniazid (Rimifon)	300 mg 1 g	Oral Oral	Daily Twice a week
Rifampicin (Rifadin)	450–600 mg	Oral	Daily
Ethambutol (Myambutol)	15 mg per kg body weight	Oral	Daily
Streptomycin	1 g	IM	Daily
Pyrazinamide (Zinamide)	20–30 mg per kg body weight	Oral	Daily

Other antibiotics

Polymyxin B (Aerosporin) is reserved for severe infections caused by *Pseudomonas aeruginosa*.

Spectinomycin (Trobicin) is active against a wide range of organisms including gonorrhoea.

Metronidazole (Flagyl) is active against strict anaerobes, trichomonal urethritis, vaginitis amoebic dysentery and giardiasis, and in the prevention and treatment of anaerobic infections associated with bowel surgery.
Dosage. 400 mg is given 8 hourly by mouth or 500 mg 8 hourly for 7 days by intravenous infusion.

Amphotericin B (Fungilin, Fungizone) is used for the systemic treatment of severe generalized infections by yeasts and fungi e.g. cryptococcosis and blastomycosis.
Dosage. 200 mg is given every 6 hours by mouth; it can also be given as an intravenous infusion.

Antiviral chemotherapeutic agents

Acyclovir (Zovirax) is highly active against herpes virus. It is valuable in the treatment of life-threatening infections with herpes simplex and the varicella zoster virus (smallpox virus), particularly in patients having immunosuppressive therapy.
Dosage. 200 mg is given five times daily orally or 5 mg per kg body weight 8 hourly IV.

Idoxuridine (Iododeoxyuridine) inhibits DNA viruses. It is highly toxic for systemic use but can be used in the form of eye drops for the treatment of herpetic keratitis.

Amantadine (Symmetrel) inhibits certain myxoviruses. When given orally it is effective in preventing infection with type A influenza virus.
Dosage. 100 mg is given 12 hourly orally.

METHODS OF STERILIZATION AND DISINFECTION

Sterilization is defined as the destruction or removal of all living microorganisms in or on an object.

Disinfection is defined as the destruction or removal of pathogenic microorganisms so as to make the object non-infective.

A summary of the various methods of sterilization and disinfection is given below:

A. Physical methods
I. Heat
a. Dry heat
b. Autoclaving
c. Steam/formaldehyde
d. Pasteurization
e. Boiling.

II. Cold
a. Gamma irradiation
b. Ethylene oxide
c. Ultraviolet light.

B. Chemical methods
a. Salts
b. Halogens
c. Oxidizing agents
d. Alcohols
e. Soaps and detergents
f. Phenols
g. Diguanide compounds

A. PHYSICAL METHODS

I. Heat

a. Dry heat

Contaminated swabs, dressings and human tissue are collected in disposable bags and burnt.

b. *Autoclaving* (steam under pressure)

This is the usual method of sterilizing surgical instruments, dressings, gowns, towels and culture media.

An autoclave is a closed chamber in which objects are subjected to steam at high pressures and temperatures above 100°C. Steam is a more efficient method of sterilization than air at the same temperature. If air is present in the sterilizing chamber, a satisfactory temperature will not be achieved and pockets of air may prevent penetration of the load of articles by the steam. The air must therefore be removed.

Types of autoclaves. There are two types in frequent use:

Downward-displacement autoclaves. Air is removed in two stages and sterilization is effected by an atmosphere of pure steam. The minimum exposure time required for sterilizing instruments is 15 minutes at 121°C or 10 minutes at 126°C. Bulky dressings and surgical packs require exposures two or three times as long.

High vacuum/high pressure autoclaves. Air is removed by a powerful pump. Steam penetrates the load instantaneously and very rapid sterilization of dressings and packs is possible in 3 minutes at 134°C.

The causes of failure to produce a sterile load are:

— Faults in the autoclave and the way it is operated e.g. poor quality steam, failure to remove air and condensate, faulty gauges and timings, leaking door seals
— Errors in loading e.g. large packs, excessive layers of wrapping material, overpacking
— Recontamination after sterilization due to an inadequate air filter, leakage into the chamber, wet or torn packs, incorrect storage.

Methods of testing the effectiveness of autoclaves are as follows:

(i) Automatic dial recording of temperatures and times of each sterilizing cycle.
(ii) Heat-sensitive tape fixed to the outside of each pack.
(iii) A chemical indicator placed in the most inaccessible part of each load e.g. routine use of Browne's TST strips or Browne's tubes.
(iv) For high vacuum/high pressure autoclaves, daily tests in an empty chamber using a heat-sensitive tape fixed as a cross in the middle of 24–36 towels. If all the air has been removed there will be a uniform colour change; if air remains, the colour change is incomplete at the centre (Bowie-Dick test).
(v) Daily checks for leaks by evacuating the chamber and confirming that the leak rate does not exceed 1.3 kPa over a 10 minute period.

c. *Steam/formaldehyde*

Autoclaving and dry heat are not practical for heat-sensitive articles such as plastics and optical devices.

In a modified autoclave, steam under sub-atmospheric pressure at temperatures below 90°C will rapidly kill non-sporing organisms after the air in the chamber has been removed by a high-vacuum pump. All but a few resistant spores are killed; if formaldehyde vapour is added to the steam it can destroy all spores and effect sterilization.

d. *Pasteurization*

This involves the immersion of instruments, such as endoscopes, for 10 minutes in water at a temperature of between 75°C and 85°C. It is effective in destroying vegetative bacteria.

e. *Boiling*

At 100°C for 5 minutes boiling kills all vegetative organisms, but a few spores may survive. Boiling is satisfactory for disinfecting contaminated cups, plates and cutlery, but is not safe for instruments used in surgery.

II. Cold

a. *Gamma irradiation*

This method involves the use of gamma radiation from a cobalt 60 source and is used commercially.

b. Ethylene oxide

This is a well-established technique for sterilizing heat labile articles. The essential part of this sterilizing process consists of using a 15% ethylene oxide, 85% carbon dioxide mixture and controlled humidity.

It can be used for sterilizing artery and bone grafts, heart-lung machines, plastic articles such as disposable syringes, surgical instruments such as cystoscopes, catheters, bacteriological media and vaccines.

It is toxic to man; when it contaminates the skin it can cause vesicles and is also known to produce cancer.

c. Ulraviolet light

This is a form of surface radiation. As its penetrating capacity is poor, it is used for sterilizing surfaces, bone chips, grafts and blades.

B. CHEMICAL METHODS

a. Salts
Simple salts in high concentration inhibit bacteria, though they may not kill them.

b. Halogens

Chlorine is used to disinfect water. A very strong solution of hypochlorite (which liberates chlorine) is used to disinfect articles and surfaces contaminated with blood. It is effective against hepatitis B virus.

Iodine as a 2–5% aqueous or ethanolic solution in potassium· is used effectively to disinfect intact skin before surgical operations.

Povidone-iodine (Betadine) is a non-staining, non-irritant, water soluble iodine complex. It is a topical disinfective, killing all spores with a prolonged action. Betadine is used undiluted for skin preparation preoperatively and as a surgical scrub.

c. Oxidizing agents

These are effective against bacteria and viruses. *Hydrogen peroxide* is used for cleaning and disin-

fecting wounds. *Potassium permanganate* is used for disinfecting drinking water, fruit and vegetables.

d. Alcohols

Pure alcohol has no antibacterial activity. 70% alcohol kills vegetative bacteria and some viruses rapidly and is also active against *Mycobacterium tuberculosis*. It is used for preparing the skin prior to injections and for disinfecting trolley tops and other clean surfaces in high risk areas.

e. Soaps and detergents

Soaps have minimal germicidal activity, killing streptococcus, *Haemophilus influenzae* and the influenza virus. Anionic detergents, such as sulphated long-chain fatty alcohols, are excellent cleansing agents for floors, walls, ledges, furniture and trolleys.

Cationic detergents include the quarternary ammonium compound cetrimide (Cetavlon). Their surface-active properties make them excellent cleansing agents for intact skin, wounds and burns. They are active against most Gram-positive bacteria. Non-ionic detergents, such as ethylene oxide condensates, are excellent cleansing agents but have no germicidal activity.

f. Phenols

Clearsol contains 40% of phenols and is used as a general disinfectant in a dilution of 1%. It is used effectively against Gram-positive and Gram-negative organisms, including *Pseudomonas aeruginosa*.

Chloroxylenol (Dettol) is used at a dilution of 5% for general disinfection purposes, and is used effectively against most organisms, excluding certain Gram-negative organisms.

g. Diguanide compounds

Chlorhexidine (Hibitane) is an established antibacterial agent. Hibitane Hospital concentrate 5% is a solution of 5% chlorhexidine gluconate; an aqueous dilution of 0.5% of this concentrate is used for the surface disinfection of towels, tables, etc.

Hibitane concentration	Use
1% Hibitane in water (0.05%)	Prophylactic treatment of wounds
10% in 70% methylated spirit (0.5%)	Pre-surgical skin disinfection
10% Hibitane in 70% industrial methylated spirit (0.5%)	For emergency pre-surgical disinfection of heat labile instruments
1% Hibitane in 70% industrial methylated spirit (0.5%)	Pre-surgical rinse of hands

(Dilutions in brackets are the effective concentration of the antibacterial agent.)

Hibitane concentrate is effective against a wide range of Gram-positive and Gram-negative organisms.

Hexachlorophane is an antibacterial agent and can be combined with soap in a 2% proportion. It is more effective against Gram-positive than Gram-negative bacteria.

SUMMARY OF METHODS OF STERILIZATION OF VARIOUS EQUIPMENT

Anaesthetic apparatus	Methods
Rubber face masks, rebreathing bags, corrugated tubes, airways, endotracheal tubes	Immerse in 0.5% aqueous Hibitane or Savlon or Cidex for 10 minutes
Corrugated tubes, Y pieces, Heidbrink valves, rubber airways, endotracheal tubes	Autoclave
Electrical apparatus: electrical leads and illuminators, diathermy cautery electrodes, electric bone saws, drills, electrical lamps	Read manufacturer's instructions. Autoclave or immerse in 10% Hibitane for 30 minutes. Ethylene oxide
Metal ware	Autoclave at 134°C for 6 minutes

Anaesthetic apparatus	Methods
Linen (gowns, caps, operation drapes packed into packets)	Sterilize at 126°C for 30 minutes
Endoscopes such as cystoscopes, bronchoscopes, oesophagoscopes	Sub-atmospheric steam formaldehyde
Glassware	Autoclave after careful packing
Metal instruments. a. scissors, dissecting and artery forceps, metal bougies and catheters	Autoclave in open trays for 6 minutes
b. Carbon steel instruments such as solid scalpels, twist drills, osteotomes	Dry heat or ethylene oxide
Nail brushes	Autoclave at 130°C for 6 minutes
Rubber goods such as non-disposable tubing, drainage, sheeting, catheters	Autoclave
Plastics, polyvinyl chloride, polythene tubing, nylon tubing	Wet heat. Ethylene oxide or sub-atmospheric steam/formaldehyde steam sterilization
Suture material: unopened inner sachets	Immersion in a fluid recommended by the manufacturer for 30 minutes before use
Monafilament nylon and silkwork gut	Autoclave
Metal wire, mesh, suture clips	Autoclave
Braided, twisted, plated and floss silk	Autoclave

ACQUIRED IMMUNE DEFICIENCY SYNDROME (AIDS)

The acquired immune deficiency syndrome (AIDS) is the terminal result, in a certain number of people, of infection with a virus earlier known as HTLV III and now known as human immunodeficiency virus (HIV).

It was reported for the first time in the USA in 1979; the first case was reported in the UK in 1981. Since then it has been reported from various parts of the world.

In the western world the disease is found in high-risk groups such as:

(i) Homosexuals
(ii) Intravenous drug abusers
(iii) Children born to HIV infected women
(iv) Heterosexual partners of HIV carriers.

Before donor bloods were screened for the HIV virus, some patients became infected after receiving a contaminated blood transfusion.

The vast majority of cases in the USA and UK are homosexual and bisexual males, with a fair number of drug abusers (mainly in Scotland) as positive carriers.

In central Africa, AIDS is present in both sexes with predominant spread in heterosexuals.

Aetiology

The causative agent—human immunodeficiency virus (HIV)—is a member of a group of retroviruses. This virus destroys the defences that protect humans against infection by many different agents.

Human beings can normally resist infection due to the activities of a variety of specialized cells (e.g. phagocytes, lymphocytes) which are present in the lymph nodes and spleen.

The phagocytes destroy invading bacteria; the lymphocytes, which are of two types, produce antibodies (B-lymphocytes) and attack virus-infected cells (T-lymphocytes). Some lymphocytes control the activity of other cells of the immune system. One sub-population of these promotes the immune response to infection and these cells are called T-helpers (Th). Another sub-population regulates the response, thus exerting control; these cells are known as T-suppressor cells (Ts).

Before the HIV can infect cells it attaches onto the surface of the T-helper lymphocytes. As a result of infection the Th cells may be irreversibly damaged and lost from the blood; this can be detected as a reduced cell count or a change in the ratio of Th to Ts cells. It is this decrease in the cells responsible for activating the immune response that reduces the individual's ability to resist infection. Despite this immunodeficiency, an infected person can remain healthy.

However, some patients develop a secondary 'opportunistic' infection, particularly with organisms against which T-lymphocytes normally afford protection.

Acquired immune deficiency can be suspected when a previously healthy individual develops pneumonia due to a normally harmless parasite, *Pneumocystis carinii*, or the uncommon tumour known as Kaposi's sarcoma.

Clinical features

1. Patients can be asymptomatic with a detectable anti-HIV in the serum.
2. They may also present with symptoms such as fever, malaise, pharyngitis, arthralgia (acute glandular fever-like syndrome) within one to eight weeks of exposure.
3. Patients may develop a chronic illness called AIDS-related complex (ARC) or 'pre-AIDS'. The symptoms range from generalized lymphadenopathy to fever, weight loss, diarrhoea and thrombocytopenia, but without opportunistic infections.
4. AIDS is characterized by 'opportunistic infections' such as *Pneumocystis carinii* pneumonia, candidiasis, toxoplasmosis, *Herpes simplex* stomatitis, gingivitis and Kaposi's sarcoma.

The incubation period for AIDS is variable, ranging from six months to five years or longer. In a majority of infected individuals, HIV infection is unaccompanied by signs or symptoms and can be identified only by the presence of virus antibodies in the serum.

Mode of transmission

a. Sexual contact. HIV is present in semen and can be transmitted by vaginal or rectal intercourse. The incidence of heterosexual transmission in Africa is much higher, with females and males equally infected by HIV infection.

b. Blood-borne. HIV is present in the blood of infected individuals, hence transfusion of blood and blood products can cause transmission of the virus to the person receiving them.

The individuals who are at risk are haemophiliacs receiving Factor VIII and intravenous drug abusers who share needles and syringes contaminated with HIV infected blood.

c. Mother to fetus. Infected mothers can transmit HIV infection to the fetus via the placenta during pregnancy, by infected blood during delivery, and to the neonate via breast milk.

d. Needlestick injuries. Accidental 'needlestick' injury whilst handling the blood of an AIDS patient could result in the transmission of HIV infection. There are only two cases of infection reported in this manner (one in the UK). These cases are asymptomatic, although the serum is positive.

Preventative measures

These include the following:

1. Prevention of puncture wounds, abrasions, and cuts in the presence of body fluids and blood, and protection of existing wounds
2. Control of surface contamination with blood and body fluids by the use of disinfectants and taking proper care
3. Application of simple protective measures to prevent contamination of personnel or clothing, and practice of good basic hygiene such as regular hand washing
4. Safe disposal of contaminated waste.

It is essential to realize that operating theatre personnel will be handling patients or specimens which have not been identified as presenting a risk of infection. Hence, extra care should be taken in handling patients who are homosexual or bisexual males, intravenous drug addicts and haemophiliacs.

Testing of health staff

Staff exposed to specimens or patients infected with HIV should be aware that laboratory tests are available to detect antibodies to the virus. The occupational health department in each hospital should make local arrangements for these tests. Staff who have an accident handling infected material should be offered the chance of having their serum tested or stored for future testing. In such circumstances, an 'immediate' specimen should be tested followed by further specimens at regular intervals.

Care of the patient

The infected patient should be looked after by staff trained in the precautions appropriate for HIV infection. Staff looking after patients who require isolation should be properly trained in isolation techniques and the use of gloves, gowns, aprons and eye protection.

Blood, body fluids and tissue specimens for diagnosis must be taken by experienced staff who must wear gloves, gowns, aprons, eye and face protection. Resheathing of the needle must not be done. All disposable sharps must be placed in a puncture-proof bin which is suitable for incineration. Non-disposable items should be placed in a suitably secure enclosure for sterilization or disinfection. After closing securely, the specimens must be labelled by whatever system is recognized locally to indicate a danger of infection.

Labelled specimens should be sealed in plastic bags without using staples, metal clips or pins. The request form accompanying them should clearly mention the suspicion or knowledge of HIV infection and must be kept separate from the specimen container to avoid contamination.

The physician/surgeon is responsible for making the laboratory staff aware of the risk and specimens should not be sent to the laboratory without an agreement between the doctor and senior laboratory staff.

Precautions for body handling and disposal

If a person known or suspected to be infected with HIV dies, either in hospital or elsewhere, it is essential that funeral personnel involved in handling the body are informed that there is a risk of infection.

Sometimes powered devices implanted in the body during life (i.e. a cardiac pacemaker) may present a risk of injury to staff if the body is cremated. These should be removed before cremation in a hospital using a 'no touch' technique through a tiny incision. The skin should be stitched and the wound sealed with waterproof adhesive tape. The body should be replaced in a plastic body bag after local skin disinfection.

Waste disposal

Material which comes in contact with HIV-infected patients should be either autoclaved or incinerated as necessary.

Disinfection and sterilization

As the HIV retrovirus is stable at room temperature in both the wet and dry state it is essential to establish thorough disinfection and sterilization practices whenever contamination occurs.

Chemical disinfectants. The retrovirus is inactivated by alcohols, hydrogen peroxide, hypochlorite, formalin, Lysol and glutaraldehyde. Of these, hypochlorite, glutaraldehyde and isopropyl or ethyl alcohol are the most useful.

If HIV-positive blood, body fluid and excreta are spilled onto surfaces, either 2% glutaraldehyde or hypochlorite solution containing 10 000 ppm (parts per million) chlorine should be used.

For general good hygiene or treatment of minor surface contamination, 1% phenolic disinfectant or a lower concentration of hypochlorite (1000 ppm available chlorine) should be used.

Physical treatment: Ultraviolet light and gamma rays do not eliminate HIV retrovirus.

Sterilization: HIV is destroyed by conventional sterilizing regimes using moist or dry heat treatment.

Maintenance and cleaning

It is the responsibility of the head of the department or a designated deputy to implement written codes of practice which should specify the procedures to be adopted for the protection of maintenance and service staff working in patient facilities and laboratories.

MULTIPLE CHOICE QUESTIONS

The answers to these questions can be found on page 253.

1. **Penicillin was discovered by:**
   A Koch
   B Pasteur
   C Fleming
   D Penn.

2. **Diplococci are found:**
   A in pairs
   B in clusters
   C in chains
   D singly.

3. **The organism *Pseudomonas pyocyanea* is often found to be resistant to:**
   A chlorhexidine
   B proflavine
   C glutaraldehyde
   D iodine.

4. **The following bacteria form spores:**
   A *Clostridium tetani*
   B *Pseudomonas aeruginosa*
   C Pneumococci
   D Meningococci.

5. **Gas gangrene is caused by:**
   A *Staphylococcus aureus*
   B *Streptococcus viridans*
   C *Clostridium welchii*
   D *Proteus vulgaris.*

6. **Aerobic bacteria multiply in the presence of:**
   A carbon dioxide
   B oxygen
   C hydrogen peroxide
   D hydrogen.

7. **Which of the following organisms does not cause food poisoning?**
   A Staphylococcus
   B Salmonella
   C Neisseria
   D Clostridium.

8. **Streptococci are usually seen in stained smears (Gram stain) as:**
   A clusters
   B chains
   C arranged in straight rows
   D single organisms.

9. **Urinary tract infection is caused by:**
   A Klebsiella
   B *Treponema pallidum*
   C Staphylococcus
   D Pseudomonas.

10. **The organism which commonly causes tonsillitis in children is:**
    A adenovirus
    B haemolytic streptococci
    C *Candida albicans*
    D *Staphylococcus aureus.*

11. **The process time for a high vacuum autoclave is:**
    A 20 minutes
    B 3 minutes
    C 10 minutes
    D 30 minutes.

12. **Browne's tubes are used for:**
    A lumbar puncture
    B blood sampling
    C testing autoclaves
    D abdominal paracentesis.

13. **The most reliable test of sterility following high vacuum temperature autoclaving is:**
    A thermistor
    B spore test
    C Bowie-Dick test
    D Browne's tubes.

14. **In the high vacuum, high pressure autoclave, the temperature probe is found in the:**
    A door
    B jacket
    C steam inlet
    D drain.

15. **The temperature in an autoclave is accurately measured by:**
    A a bimetallic strip
    B a clinical thermometer
    C temperature-sensitive tape
    D a thermistor.

16. **Microorganisms can be destroyed at:**
    A $4°C$ for 24 hours
    B $-20°C$ for 24 hours
    C $160°C$ for 1 hour
    D $40°C$ for 10 minutes.

17. **Disinfection is:**
    A sterilization with chemicals
    B destruction of vegetative forms of bacteria
    C destruction of bacterial spores
    D the same as sterilization.

18. **Stewart's medium is used as a transport medium for:**
    A biochemistry
    B bacteriology
    C blood cross-match
    D histology.

19. **Which one of the following organisms is used for testing an autoclave?**
    A *Bacillus steartothermophilus*
    B *Clostridium perfringens*
    C *Bacillus anthracis*
    D *Bacillus subtilis.*

20. **Which of the following is not a micro-organism:**
    A virus
    B protozoa
    C fomite
    D bacteria.

4. Physics and electronics

UNITS OF MEASUREMENT

Initially, measurements were made using commonly available objects. During Anglo-Saxon times standards were adopted; for example there was a standard yard in the form of an iron bar kept at Winchester. At the end of the 18th century metric standards were developed in France, measuring length in metres and weight in kilograms.

Until 1960 there were two main systems of measurement in the UK: the imperial system which was used for most purposes and the metric system used in certain branches of science.

In 1960, the organization responsible for maintaining standards of measurements formally approved and introduced the Systéme International d'Unités (SI units).

SI units

This a refinement of the traditional metric system: there are six basic SI units (Table 4.1).

Table 4.1 Basic SI units

Physical quantity	Name of unit	Symbol
Length	Metre	m
Mass	Kilogram	kg
Time	Second	s
Electric current	Ampere	A
Thermodynamic temperature	°Kelvin	°K
Luminous intensity	Candela	cd

There are 15 supplementary units and derived units which are mentioned in the Appendix.

Physical state of matter

Matter is made up of gases, liquids and solids and they are all composed of molecules.

A molecule is the smallest part of an element or compound which can exist by itself. It is made up of individual parts called atoms.

An atom is the smallest part of a molecule which can take part in a chemical change.

Atoms and molecules have a weight. These weights are not 'real' but factors by which they are heavier than hydrogen. The original reference of hydrogen with an atomic weight of 1 was replaced by carbon with an atomic weight of 12.

An atom contains a large nucleus surrounded by a cloud of electrons. The nucleus contains protons which are positively charged and neutrons without any charge.

The electrons are negatively charged. At any period the total number of electrons is equal to the total number of protons in an atom which is electrically neutral.

For some atoms, one or more of the outermost electrons can become separated from the atom if sufficient energy is supplied. The proton/electron balance is destroyed and the atom is said to be ionized; the two parts produced are a positive ion and a negative ion.

An ion, therefore, is a charged particle, either an electron or an atom, which has lost or gained one or more electrons.

Speed is the rate of change of distance.

Velocity is the distance travelled in unit time in a given direction.

Force is that which changes or tends to change the state of rest or uniform motion of a body.

Force = Mass × Acceleration

The unit of force is the newton (N), which produces an acceleration of one metre per second in a mass of one kilogram.

Friction is the resistance which must be overcome when one surface moves over another.

The friction between two surfaces depends on how tightly they are pressed together. It is useful because if there was no friction between our feet and the ground, we would not be able to walk.

Work in science has a definite meaning. Mechanical work is done whenever anything is moved against a force or resistance.

The unit of work energy is the joule (J). One joule of work is done when a force of one newton moves through a distance of 1 metre measured in the direction of force.

Energy is the capacity for doing work. There are two kinds of energy (Fig. 4.1):

a The kinetic energy of a body is the energy it possesses by virtue of its velocity or movement (swinging pendulum in Fig. 4.1A).
b The potential energy of a body is the energy it possesses because of its position or state (poised weight in Fig. 4.1B).

Power is the rate of doing work. When we speak of power we mean how quickly work is done.

The unit of power is the watt (W). One Watt is used when one joule of work is done in one second.

The mass of a body is the amount of material it contains.

Weight: the pull of the earth or the force of gravity on a body is called the weight of that body.

Density is the mass of unit volume of a substance.

$$\text{Density} = \frac{\text{Mass of object}}{\text{Volume of object}}$$

It is measured in kilograms per cubic metre.

Pressure

Pressure is the distribution of force over an area.

$$\text{Pressure} = \frac{\text{Force}}{\text{Area}}$$

The unit of pressure is the newton per square metre (N/m^2), also called the pascal (Pa).

A gas will always flow from a high pressure region to one of lower pressure if it is free to do so. An instrument called a manometer can measure these pressures; it consists of U-tubes made of glass or plastic and half-filled with some liquid (oil, water or mercury depending on the pressure to be measured) (Fig. 4.2). One side of the tube is connected to the pressure source to be tested. With both sides at the same pressure, both liquid columns are at the same level. A difference in pressure is shown by a difference in the levels of the columns of fluid.

The manometer measures pressure in terms of a head of liquid, but it is useful in medical practice

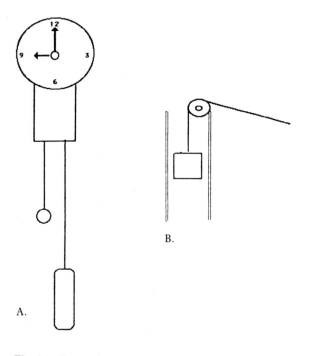

Fig. 4.1 Types of energy: A, kinetic and B, potential.

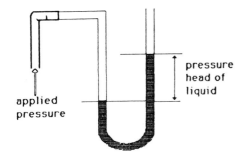

Fig. 4.2 A manometer.

to have a direct reading pointer instrument to measure pressure. A bourdon gauge is an instrument made up of a curved metal tube of oval cross-section, which tends to straighten out when the pressure inside it is increased.

As the tube straightens out the toothed quadrant rotates and turns the pointer round the seal.

The scale is calibrated in the first place using a series of known pressures measured by a manometer. (Fig. 4.3).

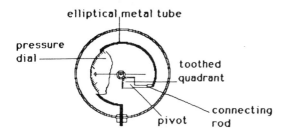

Fig. 4.3 A bourdon pressure gauge.

Atmospheric pressure is the pressure exerted by the atmosphere on all objects. At sea level this pressure is 760 mmHg; this decreases at high altitudes. The air is made of three main components: oxygen, nitrogen and water vapour.

In air the percentage of oxygen is 21%, nitrogen 78% and water vapour 0.8%. The remainder is made up of other gases. These three components contribute to a total atmospheric pressure of 760 mmHg; each constituent is said to exert a partial pressure.

Composition of air at sea level:

	Pressure (mmHg)	Percentage
Oxygen	149	20.9
Carbon dioxide	0.3	0.04
Nitrogen	564	74
Water vapour	47	6

If we climb a mountain to 14 000 feet and measure the atmospheric pressure it will be found to be around 450 mmHg. At this height the percentage of gases remains the same as at the sea level, i.e. the percentage of oxygen would be 20–21% but the partial pressure of oxygen would decrease to:

	Pressure (mmHg)	Percentage
Oxygen	95	21
Nitrogen	351	78
Water vapour	3.6	0.8

At this point, a few definitions which will be related later to anaesthetic gases (Ch. 6) are introduced.

Vapour pressure (Fig. 4.4)

In a closed space when evaporation takes place from a liquid, the volume above the liquid contains air molecules and vapour molecules. All the molecules will be bombarding the walls of the container and exerting a pressure. The pressure exerted by the vapour molecules is called vapour pressure.

Saturated vapour pressure. If a liquid is heated, at some stage the number of molecules of vapour re-entering the liquid is exactly the same as the number of molecules leaving it. The pressure exerted at this point is called the saturated vapour pressure. This principle is used in anaesthetic vaporizers.

Boiling point. The words boiling and evaporation are used to describe the change from liquid to vapour. Evaporation is a slow process which occurs at all temperatures; it occurs from the surface of the liquid. Boiling takes place when bubbles of vapour are formed inside the bulk of the liquid. The constant temperature at which boiling takes

EVAPORATION

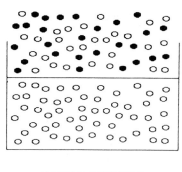

VAPOUR PRESSURE

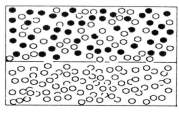

● = air molecules
○ = liquid vapour
    pressure

Fig. 4.4 Saturated vapour pressure.

place is the boiling point. The boiling point of water is 100°C.

The specific latent heat of vaporization is the heat required to change 1 kg of liquid into vapour at boiling point without change of temperature. The unit of specific latent heat is the joule per kilogram (J/kg).

THE GAS LAWS

Dalton's law of partial pressures

In a mixture of gases, each gas exerts the same pressure which it would if it alone occupied the container.

For example if two gases, carbon dioxide and oxygen, were inside a cylinder and carbon dioxide (CO_2) exerts a pressure of 3 and oxygen (O_2) exerts a pressure of 5, then the total pressure in the cylinder would be 8. If oxygen is removed from the cylinder, the molecules of carbon dioxide spread out and the pressure in the cylinder remains at 3.

There are three other gas laws which show an inter-relationship between pressure (P), volume (V) and the temperature of gases.

Boyle's law (Fig. 4.5)

Boyle's law states that at constant temperature, the pressure of a gas is inversely proportional to its volume.

$$P \propto \frac{1}{V} \text{(at constant temperature)}$$

Boyle's law holds accurately for real gases such as oxygen and nitrogen over a wide range of pressures.

Charles' law

Charles' law states that, at constant pressure, a given quantity of a gas expands by a constant proportion of its volume for each degree rise in temperature.

$$T \propto V \text{ (at constant pressure)}$$

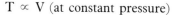

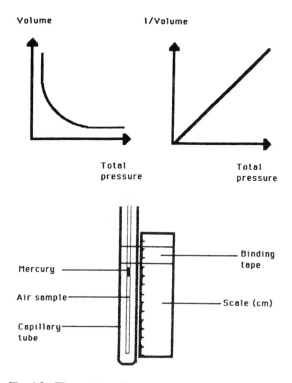

Fig. 4.5 The gas laws: Boyle's law and Charles' law.

Gay-Lussac's law

At constant volume, the pressure of a gas is directly proportional to its temperature.

$$P \propto T \text{ (at constant volume)}$$

A general equation for the three laws is:

$$P \propto \frac{T}{V}$$

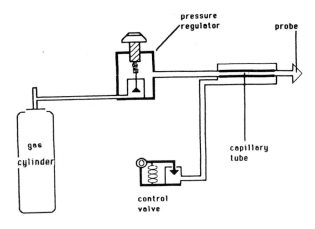

Fig. 4.6 A cryoprobe.

Ideal or perfect gas

An 'ideal' or 'perfect' gas is one in which the attraction between molecules can be regarded as negligible and the volume of molecules small compared to the space in which they are enclosed.

A 'perfect gas' obeys the laws of Boyle and Charles always. These laws can be combined to give the equation of state of a perfect gas, thus PV/T is a constant.

Adiabatic changes in a gas

The gas laws mentioned above are a description of the behaviour of a gas when one of the three variables, i.e. pressure, temperature or volume, is maintained at a constant value. For these conditions to apply, heat energy is required to be added to or taken from a gas as the change occurs.

The state of a gas can be altered without allowing the gas to exchange heat energy with its surroundings. This change of state is called an adiabatic change. A typical example of adiabatic change is when a gas cylinder connected to an anaesthetic machine or regulator is turned on quickly—the pressure of the gas in the connecting pipes and gauges rises rapidly. As the gas is compressed adiabatically there is a considerable risk of fire, because of large temperature rises. Alternatively, if a compressed gas is made to expand adiabatically, cooling occurs. This principle is made use of in the working of a cryoprobe.

Cryoprobe (Fig. 4.6)

Principle. The cooling effect of a cryoprobe is due to an adiabatic process. A gas such as nitrous oxide or carbon dioxide flows from a cylinder

through an adjustable pressure regulator which is used to set the cooling rate.

The gas flows through a capillary tube in the cryoprobe and expands in the probe tip where a temperature as low as $-7°C$ can be produced. The cooling effect is controlled by a hand or foot-operated valve which turns off the flow of gas through the probe. The gas is allowed to expand rapidly out of a capillary tube and the temperature falls due to this expansion.

Uses. It is used in eye surgery to weld detached retinas and in neurosurgery to remove single lesions (i.e. cysts in the brain or isolated cerebral tumours). It is also used in the management of chronic pain. Its application to nerves causes local degeneration resulting in long-term analgesia (3–6 months).

Critical temperature

The critical temperature of a gas is that temperature above which a gas cannot exist as a liquid no matter how much pressure is applied. Oxygen has a critical temperature of $-118°C$ and in all practical situations it is a gas within the cylinder. As it is used, the pressure drop in the cylinder over a period is constant.

Nitrous oxide has a critical temperature of $36.5°C$. In the UK and countries with a cold climate it always exists as a liquid in the cylinder, whereas in very hot countries it exists in gaseous form.

When nitrous oxide is used the liquid vaporizes and produces more and more nitrous oxide gas at the top of the liquid. At the same pressure, gas is continuously produced until all the liquid is used, and only then does it behave like a true gas such as oxygen.

In anaesthetic practice it is not possible to find out how much nitrous oxide is left in the cylinder by measuring the pressure: the amount of nitrous oxide left in the cylinder can be found by weighing it.

'Tare weight' is the weight of an empty nitrous oxide cylinder, and when subtracted from the total weight of the cylinder gives the weight of nitrous oxide in the cylinder.

Filling ratio is the weight of a substance (e.g. nitrous oxide) in a cylinder divided by the weight of the same cylinder filled with water.

$$\frac{\text{Weight of substance (liquid + gas) in a cylinder}}{\text{Weight of water required to fill the cylinder completely}}$$

Cylinders of nitrous oxide have a filling ratio of 0.75—a 'full' cylinder, then, contains about 9/10 liquid, the rest being gas. The means of keeping a check on the contents of carbon dioxide and nitrous oxide cylinders is by weighing them.

Property	N$_2$O	CO$_2$	O$_2$
Boiling point	−88.6°C	—	−183.1°C
Critical temperature	36.4°C	31.04°C	−118.4°C
Molecular weight*	44.01	44.00	32.00

*Molecular weight is the sum of the atomic weights of the atoms of which an element is composed.

HEAT

Heat is another form of energy; it can be transferred from a hotter substance to a colder substance. Temperature is the thermal state of a substance which determines whether it will give heat to another substance or receive heat from it.

Transmission of heat

Heat is transmitted from a higher to a lower temperature by different mechanisms.

Conduction is the transfer of heat through a material which is not at uniform temperature, from points of high to points of low temperature.

Conduction is the method of heat transfer in solids. Heat can be transferred in this manner by a heating mattress for temperature control during surgery.

Convection is the transfer of heat energy by circulation of the material due to differences in temperature.

Convection, by its very nature, can occur in fluids and gases. During anaesthesia, the process of breathing causes heat loss as the inspired gases will be at room temperature and the temperature of the expired gases will be from 34° to 36°C.

Radiation is the transfer of heat by means of electromagnetic waves. Radiant heat travels through empty space and is the method by which heat energy reaches the earth from the sun. In intensive care units, infra-red heaters are employed to maintain the temperature of infants by radiant heating.

Temperature scales

A thermometer is an instrument for measuring temperature. It is calibrated by choosing two temperatures (called fixed points) and dividing the interval between them into a number of equal spaces called degrees. In this way temperature scales are derived.

The lower fixed point, the ice point, is the temperature of pure melting ice at standard atmospheric pressure. The upper fixed point, the steam point, is the temperature of steam from pure boiling water at standard atmospheric pressure.

(i) On the Celsius (or centigrade) temperature scale, the interval between the fixed points of 0°C and 100°C is divided into one hundred degrees.
(ii) On the Fahrenheit scale, the ice point is 32°F and the steam point 212°F.

The relationship between the two scales is as follows:

$$°F = 9/5°C + 32$$

Techniques of temperature measurement

Temperature is measured by either a non-electrical or an electrical technique.

1. Non-electrical techniques

Any property which changes with temperature can be used in a thermometer to measure a temperature change. The most commonly used property is that of the expansion of a liquid in a glass tube.

The liquid commonly used is mercury or alcohol. Mercury is used because of its low freezing point (−39°C) and high boiling point (357°C); the thread can be seen easily; it expands regularly and gives readings consistent with other methods of measuring temperature.

Clinical thermometer (Fig. 4.7). The normal body temperature for human beings is 36°–37°C (97°–99°F). When someone is ill, his body temperature often rises and a clinical thermometer is used to take his temperature. It is placed in the mouth under the tongue. As the mercury rises it can force its way past the kink in the thermometer tube. When the thermometer is removed from the patient and the mercury begins to contract the thread breaks at the kink and the reading can be taken.

To set the thermometer ready for a second reading it is given a sharp shake. In order to read the correct temperature, the thermometer must be left for a certain time (usually one or two minutes) in the patient's mouth. The time is marked on each thermometer.

The two main disadvantages of a mercury thermometer are: firstly, a period of one to two minutes is required to achieve a uniformity between the mercury and its surroundings; secondly, it may be difficult to introduce the thermometer into some orifices because of its rigidity and the risk of breaking the thermometer with consequent injury to the patient.

Sometimes alcohol is used instead of mercury in thermometers. It is suitable for measuring low temperatures because mercury solidifies at −39°C. But alcohol thermometers are unsuitable for high temperatures because alcohol boils at 78°C.

The other non-electrical method of temperature measurement is the Dial thermometer. Dial thermometers use either a bimetallic strip or a bourdon gauge principle.

Bimetallic thermometer (Fig. 4.8). The sensing element of this device consists of two different types of metal which are fixed together. When heated they bend: the longer the element is the more movement there will be at the end of the bar. A long strip is coiled into a spiral to make the instrument compact and sensitive. One end is fixed while the other is attached to a pointer which moves over a circular scale graduated in degrees. This instrument is robust but has the disadvantage of not responding quickly to rapidly changing temperatures.

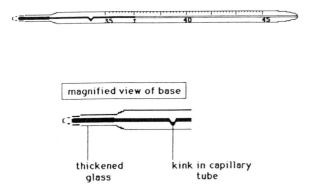

Fig. 4.7 A clinical thermometer.

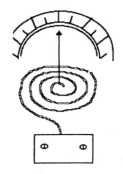

Fig. 4.8 A bimetallic thermometer

The bourdon gauge thermometer is in fact a device for measuring pressure and is attached to a sensing element containing a small tube of mercury. Slight variations in temperature lead to changes in volume or pressure in the sensing fluid. The bourdon gauge, which is calibrated for temperature, picks up these changes.

2. Electrical techniques

There are three main electrical techniques for measuring temperature: a thermocouple, a thermistor and a resistance thermometer.

(i) **Thermocouple** (Fig. 4.9). When the junction between two different metals is heated an electromotive force (EMF) is produced. Heat energy is converted to electrical energy. This is the thermoelectric or Seebeck effect and the arrangement of metals is called a thermocouple. The metals often used are copper and constantan— constantan being an alloy of copper and nickel.

In order to measure temperature it is necessary to maintain the temperature of one junction at a constant value so that the other can be used to determine the required temperature, provided the EMF of the thermocouple is measured.

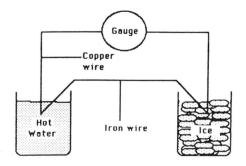

Fig. 4.9 A thermocouple.

(ii) **A thermistor** is a semiconducting element consisting of a small bead made of either manganese, nickel or cobalt oxides. Thermistors have a very small thermal capacity and can respond to a change of temperature in as little as 0.2 seconds.

As thermistors are highly sensitive, they are well suited for measuring small changes e.g. within the

pulmonary artery during thermal dilution procedures for measuring cardiac output (see Ch. 6).

The disadvantage of thermistors is that they age by increasing their resistance with time over a period of months.

(iii) **Platinum resistance thermometer.** The working of this thermometer is based on the electrical resistance of a metal increasing linearly with a rise in temperature. It consists of a temperature-sensitive platinum wire resistor, a Wheatstone bridge circuit (Fig. 4.10) containing a number of coils, and an ammeter to measure current which can be calibrated to indicate temperature.

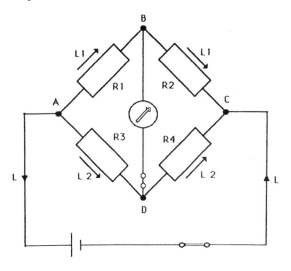

Fig. 4.10 The Wheatstone bridge circuit.

For medical use, the chief disadvantage of these resistance thermometers has been the physical size of the coil in the Wheatstone bridge circuit and a slow response time.

Although rectal and oesophageal thermometers have been produced commercially, smaller probes are not readily available.

See Chapter 6 for the clinical application of measurement of body temperature.

HUMIDITY

The mass of water vapour present in a given volume of air is called the humidity. Humidity is expressed in two ways:

a. Absolute humidity—which is the mass of water vapour present in a given volume of air
b. Relative humidity—the ratio of the mass of water vapour in a given volume of air to the mass required to saturate the same volume at the same temperature.

The values of absolute humidity are mg/l (milligrams per litre). The amount of water vapour that is present in a given volume of air is limited by temperature.

Measurement of humidity

All the instruments available measure relative humidity: they are called hygrometers. There are two types of instrument:

(i) **Wet and dry bulb hygrometers** consist of two thermometers. Around the bulb of one is a muslin bag constantly supplied with water by a wick and reservoir. As the water evaporates, it cools the bulb down and a lower temperature is recorded. When the air is dry, evaporation takes place more quickly and the temperature drop is greater. When the air is saturated, no evaporation takes place and both thermometers read the same. Tables are supplied with this instrument, and the relative humidity can be determined from the dry-bulb temperature and the difference between the wet-bulb and dry-bulb readings.

(ii) **Hair hygrometers** (Fig. 4.11) give a direct reading of relative humidity. They work on the principle that a hair gets longer as humidity rises and the hair length controls a pointer moving over a scale. This instrument is simple to use and can be accurate if its working is restricted to humidities between 15% and 85%.

Another instrument called Regnault's hygrometer is available which measures humidity accurately. It consists of a silver tube containing ether. Air is blown down the ether to cool it, thus initiating condensation on the shiny outside surface of the tube. The temperature at which condensation occurs is noted and called the dew point. This dew point represents the temperature at which the ambient air is fully saturated.

Relative humidity is calculated from the dew point as follows:

$$\text{Relative humidity} = \frac{\text{Actual vapour pressure}}{\text{Saturated vapour pressure at that temperature}}$$

$$= \frac{\text{Saturated vapour pressure at dew point}}{\text{Saturated vapour pressure at ambient temperature}}$$

From the dew point noted, and saturated vapour pressure which can be derived from tables, both relative and absolute humidities can be calculated at the temperature required.

Importance of humidity

1. Normally when a patient breathes through his nose the inspired air is warmed to body temperature and saturated with water vapour before entering the trachea i.e. to a level of 34 g/m^3 at 34°C.

During anaesthesia, when the nose is bypassed by an endotracheal tube or a tracheostomy tube, dry air enters the trachea. The secretions present in the trachea may become dry and their mucous plugs tend to block the respiratory tract. At the completion of surgery, it may become difficult for the patient to cough up these secretions, and the anaesthetist has to aspirate them via an endotracheal tube.

Similarly in the intensive care unit, if a patient is ventilated for prolonged periods he receives dry inspired gases which inhibit the cilia lining the tracheal mucous membranes. Eventually these cilia

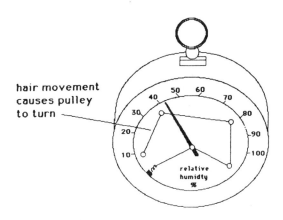

hair movement causes pulley to turn

Fig. 4.11 A hair hygrometer.

disappear and the lining of trachea becomes keratinized.

For these reasons humidification of inspired gases using various devices is recommended (see Ch. 6).

2. The atmosphere of the operating theatre, for which there is usually air conditioning, should be kept at a suitable level of relative humidity. This should be between 50% and 70%. A high humidity results in a most uncomfortable and tiring atmosphere for the theatre staff, and a very low humidity can increase the risk of explosion due to a build up of static electricity.

MAGNETISM

The study of magnetism is one of the oldest in physics. A magnet has the property of attracting iron and steel (and special alloys of iron), and to a lesser degree cobalt and nickel. These substances are know as magnetic or ferromagnetic materials and all other substances are non-magnetic. When a magnet is dipped in a pile of iron filings and removed, it is seen that most filings cling to the ends of the magnet and very few to the middle. These ends are called the poles of the magnet. When these magnets are suspended in a paper stirrup, after rotating freely they settle down pointing in a northerly and southerly direction.

The law of magnetism is that:

Unlike poles attract, like poles repel.

This can be demonstrated by bringing two different poles together.

Repulsion is a definite test for a magnet. The method of identifying a magnet from an unmagnetized bar of iron is by bringing the pole of a known magnet to each end in turn of the iron bar. With an unmagnetized bar there will be attraction at both ends, but with the magnet there will be attraction at one end (unlike poles) and repulsion at the other (like poles).

ELECTROSTATICS

It has been known since ancient times that certain substances when rubbed with fur or cloth attract light objects to them. Amber, which is a yellow glass-like solid, showed this property in early years. Nowadays plastics behave in a similar way.

After a piece of plastic is rubbed against an arm sleeve it will pick up small pieces of paper. The Greek word for amber is elektron.

Substances like the above, when rubbed, were said to be charged or electrified with electricity. As the charge stays on these amber rods or plastic and does not move, this kind of electricity is called static electricity. The study of this field in physics is called electrostatics.

Just as there is a magnetic field round a magnet, so there is an electric field round a charged body or between two charges.

The electric field between two metal plates is uniform except at the edges. A field like that is used in the cathode-ray oscilloscope to deflect electrons. This instrument is used to display an electrocardiogram trace which can be photographed directly with a time exposure.

The ability to store a charge is not limited to amber rods or plastics and capacitors. It can build up on the surface of any object insulated from its surroundings. In the case of a bobbin in a variable orifice flowmeter of an anaesthetic machine (see Ch. 6), friction can result in electrons being removed from the bobbin surface when it moves up rotating against the wall of the flowmeter. Thus the opposite electric charges on the wall and bobbing can exert a force of attraction leading to the bobbin sticking. A temporary solution to this is to coat the inside of the tube with stannic oxide; a permanent solution is to use some other conductive material in the manufacture of flowmeters.

Similarly, insulators may develop static charge on their surface with risks of sparks which can be dangerous in the presence of an inflammable anaesthetic agent (see Hazards p. 118).

ELECTRICITY

The word current means a movement or flow. An electric current is a flow of electrically charged particles. There needs to be a source of electricity to light a lamp. The source could be either a dynamo or a battery. The method whereby the lamp is connected to a battery via a switch is called a simple circuit. For an electric current to flow there must be a complete path for its movement without any gaps.

There are two types of electric current:

a. Direct current (dc) in which a steady flow of electrons occurs in only one direction along a wire. A common example is a battery or a thermocouple.
b. Alternating current (ac) in which electrons flow first in one direction and then in the opposite direction along a wire.

Conductors and insulators

Substances which allow electricity to flow through them are called conductors. Materials which do not allow a current to flow through them are called insulators. Most wires used for making electrical connections are covered with a layer of insulating material so that if two wires touch they will not cause a short circuit. Metals are good conductors while non-metallic substances such as rubber and plastic are good insulators.

Conduction of electricity in metals. The atoms of metals are in a regular sequence, being held together by electrical forces. The electrons are loosely held in the outer layer and shared between the atoms. As the ends of a metallic conductor are connected to a battery, the negatively-charged electrons move towards the positive end; the movement of electrons is called an electric current.

As each electron carries a negative charge, an electric current is a movement of charge.

In addition to conductors and insulators there are certain substances which contain fewer free electrons than conductors. These are called semiconductors.

Measurement of current

The ampere (A) is the unit of current in the SI system. The instrument used to measure the amount of electric current is the ammeter. The ammeter is connected to the circuit in such a way that current to be measured flows through it.

Whenever an electric current flows in a wire, a magnetic field exists around the wire. Thus when a wire carrying an electric current is placed in a magnetic field there is a force on the wire which tends to move the wire in a direction perpendicular to both the electric current and the magnetic field.

The galvanometer is an instrument which works on the principle of interaction between an electric current and a magnetic field. In a galvanometer a coil of wire is suspended on a jewelled bearing in a magnetic field. The current which is being measured passes through this coil and the interaction between the magnetic field and electric current causes the coil to rotate. The rotating force on the coil is balanced by a hair spring. The deflection of the coil is proportional to the electric current passing through the coil, which is indicated by a pointer moving over a scale.

In operating theatres, many recorders and display devices are based on the principle of the galvanometer.

Effects of an electric current

When an electric current flows in a conductor it produces certain changes in the space around the conductor and in the conductor itself. An electric current has a heating effect, a chemical effect and a magnetic effect.

Heating effect

As electricity is a form of energy, it has the capacity to change into other forms of energy, such as heat energy.

When the current supplying a domestic electric radiator is switched on, the coil of wire called the element in the radiator becomes red hot. In the element electric energy is being converted into heat energy.

Fuses are a safety device for ensuring that the current in any particular circuit does not rise above a certain value and either cause the element to overheat and start a fire or damage the equipment. A fuse consists of a thin piece of tinned copper wire. It is carried in a three-pin plug which connects appliances to the main supply of electricity.

A fused three-pin plug (Fig. 4.12) consists of a live wire (brown wire) which carries the current, an earth (green and yellow wire) and a neutral (blue wire) with a fuse.

It is important that the correct value of fuse should be used, so that when a safe value of the

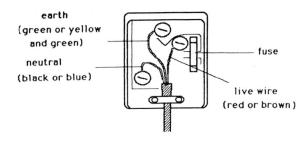

earth
(green or yellow
and green)

neutral
(black or blue)

fuse

live wire
(red or brown)

Fig. 4.12 A fused three-pin plug.

current is exceeded the fuse wire melts and breaks the circuit.

Chemical effect

Certain solutions of acids, alkalis (like caustic soda) and salts (like common salt) conduct electricity. Water is a poor conductor of electricity. Liquids which conduct electricity are called electrolytes.

When an electric current is passed through an electrolyte, a chemical change takes place which is termed electrolysis. The apparatus in which electrolysis occurs is called a voltameter.

The electrode at which current enters the liquid is called the anode, and the electrode at which current leaves the liquid is called the cathode.

Magnetic effect

As electric current flows it produces a magnetic field. The path of the current sets the pattern of the magnetic field, which in turn depends on the shape of the conductor which carried the current.

The magnetic field produced by a current flowing in a straight wire is different from that produced by a flat coil or a solenoid.

Any source of electricity which converts one form of energy into electric energy has an electromotive force (EMF). EMF measures the ability to drive a current through a circuit. It is measured by a voltmeter. The unit of electromotive force is the volt (V).

Charge. A current is the rate of flow of charge. The unit of charge is the coulomb (C), which is the quantity of charge involved when a current of one ampere flows for one second.

Current is the flow of electrons carrying a charge. The unit of current is the ampere (A). It represents a flow of 6.24×10^{18} electrons per second past a fixed point.

The potential difference determines whether or not a current will flow, and if so in which direction. The unit of potential difference between two points is the volt (V), when one joule of energy is required to transfer one coulomb of charge from one point to another.

Resistance is the opposition offered by a conductor to the flow of current. The unit of resistance is the ohm (Ω). A conductor has a resistance of one ohm when a potential difference of one volt across its ends produces a current of one ampere.

Ohm's law states that 'the current (I) flowing through a conductor is directly proportional to the potential difference (V) across its ends provided the temperature is constant.'

$$I \propto V \text{ or } \frac{V}{I} = \text{constant}$$

The constant quantity V/I is the resistance of the conductor. A conductor has a high resistance if the ratio V/I is large; only a small current can pass through it. If the V/I ratio is small, a large current can flow through and so the resistance of that conductor must be small.

Properties of common electrical components

The following illustrations (Fig. 4.13) are standard symbols for some common electrical components which are used in the daily routine.

Alternating current (AC) is a current which changes its direction and magnitude at regular intervals. The current grows to a peak volume, diminishes to zero, grows to a maximum in the opposite direction and then decreases to zero again.

Alternating current produces a heating effect, thus it can be used for heating and lighting. It can

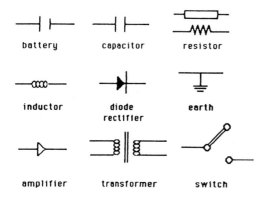

Fig. 4.13 Standard electrical symbols.

also be used to make an electromagnet, although the polarity is constantly changing. One of the advantages of AC is that it can be 'transformed' i.e. the voltage can be altered using a transformer.

Capacitance measures the ability of an object to hold electric charge, the charge being a measure of the amount of electricity. The unit of charge is the coulomb (C). The coulomb is the quantity of electric charge which passes one point when a current of one ampere flows for one second.

Coulomb (C) = amperes (A) × seconds (s)

If two conductors are separated by an insulator, the resulting capacitor develops the property of storing electrons when a potential difference is applied to its terminals.

A transformer consists of an iron core with two coils of wire wound round it. The coil connected to the AC input is called the primary coil and the coil connected to the galvanometer is the secondary coil. When the primary current is switched on and off, a current is induced in the secondary coil; but the current only flows in the secondary coil when the primary current is changing. If a primary coil is connected to a source of alternating current (which is changing all the time) there will be an induced current in the secondary coil. This current in the secondary coil will be changing in the same way and at the same rate as the primary alternating current. The transformer is used to change voltage; thus low voltages are supplied to

laboratories and high voltages are used for television sets and radios.

ELECTRICAL COMPONENTS USED IN MEDICAL EQUIPMENT

A potential difference exists between the surface of a cell and the underlying cytoplasm. A nerve fibre is a part of a cell and an impulse travels along it when a wave of depolarization occurs (see Ch. 1). Similarly a wave of depolarization occurs in muscle fibres before they contract. These waves of electrical changes are also transmitted through the tissues overlying the nerve fibres and muscles, and these signals can be detected by appropriate electrodes placed on the skin and displayed as an electrocardiogram (ECG), electromyogram (EMG) or electroencephalogram (EEG).

The graphs which are derived from these recordings consist of complex wave patterns which are plotted as voltage against time. These complex wave patterns can be analysed and grouped using Fourier analysis.

Fourier analysis. In the 19th century Fourier showed that however complex a waveform is, it can be analysed as the composite of a number of simple waveforms. These simple waveforms have a similar shape to the alternating current mains voltage and are called sinusoids or simple harmonic waveforms.

Electrocardiogram (ECG). As the sine waves of different frequencies are added, they result in a complex ECG waveform. As described earlier, the potentials from the heart are transmitted through the tissues and can be detected by electrodes, thus giving rise to an ECG trace. The appearance of an ECG depends on the positioning of the electrodes on the surface of the body—the recordings being the difference in potential between two electrodes.

The frequency range for an ECG is about 0.5 to 80 Hz.

Electromyogram (EMG). The potentials from muscular contraction are picked up by surface electrodes. The potentials generated are large with sharp spikes, thus indicating that analysis of this wave will result in a large frequency distribution of sine waves.

Electroencephalogram (EEG). The changes in potential which occur in the cerebrum and brain stem can be picked up by electrodes placed over the patient's scalp.

The EEG tracing consists of various waves i.e. β, B, S, δ. The frequency distribution of these waves is small i.e. in the range of 1–60 Hz.

All the above signals generated (i.e. ECG, EMG and EEG) should be displayed on a screen and if possible recorded on a device. To record these biological signals three devices, i.e. an input transducer, amplifier and a display device, are required. These devices are regarded as a series of black boxes. It is important that electrical signals such as voltage, current, frequency from the output of one black box matches the input of the next black box in the system. If these three black boxes are well matched, then they can be connected together to give a good monitoring device (Fig. 4.14).

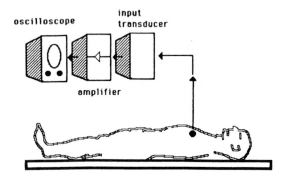

Fig. 4.14   The black box concept.

The amplifier available should have a high input impedance which is the total resistance to alternating circuits (see below).

Impedance

Circuits consisting of resistors, inductors and capacitors possess a resistance to the flow of electric current, which in turn depends on the frequency of current flowing. The term used for this resistance is impedance. Its unit of measurement is the ohm.

For picking up EEG signals, whose voltage and electrode impedance are small, amplifiers should be provided with an input impedance of around 10 000 000 ohms (10 mega ohms). For ECG and EMG amplification, although input impedances required are small they are still in the mega ohm range.

Band width

To produce a perfect reproduction of an input signal all the frequencies contained in it should be equally amplified. There is always a range of frequencies within which the degree of amplification is reasonably constant, but outside which there is attenuation of the output signal. The acceptable band width of an amplifier is the range of frequencies in which there is less than 50% relative loss. The band width of an amplifier should cover the range of frequencies that are important to pick up a signal. For an ECG machine, a flat band width from 0.14 to 50 Hz is required, whereas for an EEG machine the band width extends from 0.5 to 100 Hz. An EMG recorder requires a flat response from 20 Hz to 10 kHz (kiloHertz) which will enable it to record high frequencies contained in the signal.

Amplifiers which pick up ECG signals should have long time constants.

Time constant

This is the length of time that 100% change should take if the initial rate of change is maintained. In one time constant 63% of the final value is completed. In two time constants 63% of the remaining difference is completed: 63% + 63/100 × 37% = 86%. In three time constants 86 + 63/100 × 14 = 94%.

The time constant of an ECG amplifier is fixed, and is usually 3 seconds, which means if the trace is displaced it will return to baseline position in 9 seconds.

EEG recorders have short time constants of 0.03, 0.1, 0.3 and 1 seconds.

The gain of amplifiers can be correctly adjusted with the aid of calibration voltages. An ECG machine when calibrated will produce a 1 cm deflection of the trace with a 1 mVolt input; similarly an EEG machine produces a 1 cm deflection of the trace with 0.1 mV input.

Display of signals

The biological potentials (ECG, EEG, EMG) can be displayed in two forms, i.e. as analogue or digital recordings.

Analogue. This display allows a lever to move over a scale which can provide a clear visual indication of the size of a signal.

The recorders based on the analogue principle are:

(*i*) *Galvanometers* (see p. 107). These recorders have certain disadvantages, for example there is no permanent record or tracing, and the inertia of the coil and needle prevents the display of rapidly changing signals. Thus monitors based on the principle of galvanometers are used for displaying slowly changing signals such as patients' pulse rate or temperature.

These recorders can be modified to provide a continuous record: one method uses a galvanometer needle with a heated tip, so that a record may be produced on heat-sensitive paper. Another method conducts ink through a capillary to a writing point at the end of the galvanometer needle.

(*ii*) *Potentiometric recorders*. A potentiometer, as the name suggests, compares potential differences (pd). It consists of a length of uniform resistance wire to the end of which a difference of potential is applied so that a steady current flows.

These recorders have a limited frequency response. They are used for longer term recordings such as patients' temperature. They can also provide overlapping tracings.

Digital. A digital meter displays values as a set of figures. These types of meters are used to record pulse rates.

Oscilloscope. When this instrument is used to display signals the trace can be photographed directly with a time exposure. Note that:

Cathode = negative charge

Anode = positive charge.

The cathode ray oscilloscope (CRO) as it is called consists of:

a. an electron gun which produces a beam of electrons from a heated cathode.
b. a deflecting plate which can deflect the beam side to side and upwards and downwards.
c. a fluorescent screen on which the electrons produce a line or spot of light.

All these components are present in a highly evacuated glass tube. The electrons are produced by an indirectly heated cathode.

The outside controls of a cathode ray oscilloscope typically consist of:

a. an off/on switch
b. X-shift and Y-shift controls to centre the spot on the screen
c. a focus control
d. X-gain and Y-gain controls connected to the amplifiers between the input terminals and the deflector plates
e. a time-base control which applies a steadily changing voltage to the X-plates
f. an ac/dc switch to use with alternating and direct current.

The electron beam produced by the hot cathode passes between the deflecting devices, one of which deflects the beam on the Y-axis and the other on the X-axis. The beam then strikes a fluorescent screen thus producing a tracing. A signal such as arterial blood pressure from a transducer of ECG deflects the beam in the Y-axis direction.

The oscillating circuit supplying the time-base produces a sawtooth voltage. For an ECG signal the sensitivity control of the CRO is adjusted to a 1 millivolt calibration signal which thus gives a 1 cm vertical displacement of the trace.

The CRO is essentially a voltage-measuring apparatus and whenever there is a potential difference between the deflecting plates a deflection occurs. Its great advantage is the electron beam, which is the only moving part, with minimal inertia. The beam responds instantly to any deflecting force and returns instantly to a zero position when the force is removed, thus making the CRO an apparatus with a very high frequency response.

Other electromedical equipment

a. Defibrillator

This instrument is used for the treatment of ventricular fibrillation. In the defibrillator electric charge is stored in a capacitor and then released in a controlled fashion. Defibrillators are set according to the amount of energy stored, this energy depending on both the charge and the potential.

For treating a patient with ventricular fibrillation, electrodes are applied across the patient's chest and, by means of switches, 400 joules of energy are released as a current passes across the patient's chest and heart. This current gives a simultaneous contraction of the myocardium.

Defibrillators are also provided with lower energy settings suitable for use with internal cardiac electrodes in a patient with an open chest. Some makes of defibrillators are designed for a synchronized mode, the principle being that the energy must be supplied at the correct time in the cardiac cycle i.e. simultaneously with the R wave in the electrocardiogram. If the delivery of energy is mistimed it can cause ventricular fibrillation. This type of defibrillator is used in the treatment of certain dysrhythmias.

b. Pacemaker

Patients with heart block and fainting attacks (syncope) due to slow ventricular rates are prescribed cardiac pacemakers.

Placement of electrodes when using a pacemaker. The myocardium can be stimulated by placing two electrodes on the heart (bipolar leads) or a single electrode on the heart and a second electrode on another part of the body (unipolar leads).

A typical theatre or bedside pacemaker with a catheter electrode provides a rate ranging from 30 to 150 beats per minute. These cardiac pacemakers can be either a demand type or a fixed type.

Demand type. The output from the pacemaker is inhibited if a spontaneous R-wave is detected. If this expected beat is not found then the pacemaker delivers a pacing pulse. Similarly if the spontaneous heart rate drops below a pre-set limit then the pacemaker will pace continuously at this rate.

The operating theatre personnel usually encounter this type inserted in patients following cardiac surgery.

Fixed type. As the name suggests the pacemaker delivers a fixed pacing pulse to the heart.

Pacemakers can be inserted for short term as an emergency procedure either via a transvenous or oesophageal route.

Long-term pacing is carried out using:

(i) External pacemakers which consist of wire running from the pacemaker to an electrode situated on the surface of the heart. These are not used regularly nowadays.
(ii) An internal or implanted pacemaker, consisting of an electrode passed via a subclavian vein into the heart and the pacemaker implanted in the abdomen below the breast or in the infra-clavicular region. The connecting wire between the wire and the electrode runs subcutaneously.

Diathermy (Fig. 4.15)

Diathermy is the passage of a high frequency electric current through the tissues whereby heat is produced. It is used in surgery to coagulate blood and to cut through body tissues.

'*Current density*' is the amount of current passed per unit area. It is necessary to be familiar with this term in order to understand the principles of diathermy.

Diathermy equipment consists of an active part which is the electrode used by the surgeon and a plate which is kept below the patient's shoulder or thigh (patient plate). When a current is passed the same current flows through the electrode and the patient plate.

The degree of burning produced by diathermy depends on the current density. When the current flows through the electrode used by the surgeon it is focused on a very small area, thus leading to local heating and burning due to a high current density. The same circuit flowing through the patient plate should not cause any burning as it passes through a large area. If the area of contact is reduced due to movement the current density is considerably increased with a risk of burning to the patient. If the patient plate falls off the patient,

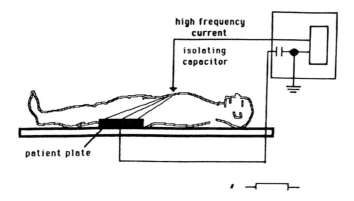

Fig. 4.15 Diathermy

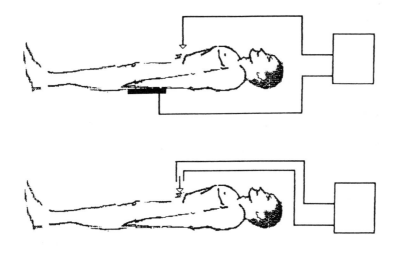

Fig. 4.16 Bipolar and unipolar diathermy.

the diathermy current flows to earth through any point at which the patient is touching an earth metal source. This is the principle of a unipolar lead arrangement.

Bipolar leads (Fig. 4.16). In certain diathermy sets there are facilities for a bipolar system in which the current passes from one blade of forceps to another. The current does not pass through any part of the patient's body other than that grasped by the forceps, and the circuit is earth-free.

This type of bipolar lead is used for coagulation of tiny blood vessels and small pieces of tissue and thus finds a suitable place in neurosurgical and ophthalmic procedures.

Current strength used in diathermy. Normally, if an alternating current from the mains electrical supply (60 Hz) passes through a patient, complications such as muscle contraction, cardiac dysrhythmias or cardiac arrest occur.

However, if alternating currents of frequency above 10 kHz pass through the body the above-mentioned effects are not seen. This principle is used in the manufacture of a diathermy machine.

Diathermy units are basically of three types:

a. Spark-gap generators which employ a current frequency of 0.4 MHz (megaHertz). This generator produces a damped wave which is used for coagulating tissues.

b. Valve oscillators employ a current frequency of between 1 and 1.5 MHz. This oscillator produces a sine waveform which is used for cutting tissues.

c. Transistorized diathermy sets produce both a cutting and a coagulation current, although the latter effect is not as satisfactory as that produced by spark-gap generators.

Modern diathermy apparatus used in operating theatres is designed to produce both a coagulating and a cutting effect.

Accidents due to faulty use of diathermy sets

These can be either electrical burns to the patient, or fires or explosions caused by the use of diathermy in the presence of inflammable vapours.

Electrical burns can be due to the following:

a. If the foot switch of the diathermy is accidentally pressed when the forceps are in contact with part of the patient's body which is not to be operated on, burns can occur. This hazard is usually prevented by keeping the forceps in an insulated container when not in use. Many diathermy sets are equipped with a buzzer which sounds when the foot switch is depressed.

b. A poor contact between the plate and the patient can cause burns.

Modern diathermy sets are equipped with an audible warning system if the plate is not making a good contact or is not plugged in, or if the electrical continuity is broken.

Fire and explosions can occur in the presence of an inflammable liquid or vapour. In addition to anaesthetic vapours (i.e. ether, trichlorethylene), agents used to clean skin prior to an operation, such as ethyl alcohol and isopropyl alcohol, can be dangerous. They are usually soaked up and remain in the drapes and can cause a fire by contact with an active electrode or a faulty mains lead or floor switch.

Caution. Surgical diathermy should not be used on patients using a cardiac pacemaker as unwanted signals from the diathermy can cause false triggering of the pacemaker.

Interference with electromedical equipment

All the equipment necessary for measuring biological potentials (i.e. ECG, EMG, EEG) have a major problem with interference or noise. This could be due to noise originating in the patient or his surroundings or in the instrument itself.

Ideally all instruments should have a high signal to noise ratio. This means that noise should be reduced to a minimum by eliminating its source or by the use of a differential amplifier.

A differential amplifier is an amplifier which measures the potential difference between two sources and eliminates interference from the mains supply.

The noise originating from an instrument is reduced by good design, adequate screening and the use of high quality components.

The major sources of noise are the patient or his surroundings.

Noises from the patient. The EEG signal detected from the scalp has a potential difference of 50 V whereas the ECG signal has a potential difference of 0.5 to 2 mVolts. The EMG has a much larger potential than the EEG and ECG signals. Thus it can submerge the other two signals. This is avoided by the use of differential amplifiers.

Noises from the patient's surroundings. These could be due to electromagnetic induction or electrostatic induction.

Electromagnetic induction. When a current flows it generates a magnetic field around and through the patient and any apparatus connected to him. This form of interference is seen in the vicinity of wires carrying alternating currents from the mains supply.

The magnetic field is developed in the loops of wire with their own voltage, thus causing interference. This type of interference can be minimized by keeping the wires together and twisted around one another.

Electrostatic induction. If a cable from the mains supply lies close to the input lead of an amplifier or a patient it will induce an electrostatic charge in the lead or the patient.

An interference will be seen because the mains cable or the lead act as one plate of a capacitor which superimposes on the signal from the patient.

This interference can be decreased by increasing the distance between the leads of an amplifier and the mains supply cable, or decreasing the resistance of the patient-lead combination.

Safety precautions with monitoring apparatus

When a number of monitoring instruments with mains supply are connected, it is essential to make sure that the patient does not receive a dangerous shock. The operating rooms should be supplied with earth-free mains supply.

The isolated mains supply should not come into contact with an earthed object, because if it does a small leakage current will flow. The minimum leakage current allowed is 5 mA $\sqrt{}$R.M.S. (R.M.S. = root mean square) which can be detected by an earth leakage current detector. If this leakage current exceeds the minimum, the faulty condition should be detected as soon as the warning is given.

RADIOACTIVE SUBSTANCES

Atoms and isotopes

An atom consists of a nucleus containing positively-charged protons and uncharged neutrons; this nucleus is surrounded by negatively-charged electrons in an orbit.

An element consists of atoms containing the same number of protons (the atomic number). For example, carbon has six protons, hydrogen has one proton. The neutrons contribute towards the stability of the nucleus.

Atoms containing the same number of protons but with different numbers of neutrons are called isotopes. A number of elements have stable isotopes which do not disintegrate spontaneously. However, there are other isotopes which are unstable and their nuclei break down in a number of ways and are said to be radioactive.

Types of radiation following atomic disintegration. When an atom disintegrates it may be accompanied by the emission of energy or particles or both. There are three types of radiation:

1. Alpha radiation: its emission results in the formation of an element with an atomic number two less and an atomic weight of four less than the original element.

The alpha particles are easily absorbed and as they are doubly charged can be extremely harmful biologically if retained in a tissue.

2. Beta radiation: in this type of nuclear disintegration a neutron breaks down into a proton and an electron, the electron being ejected as a beta particle.

Beta particles emerge with a wide range of energies and are slowed down by collision with electrons of any atom which they encounter. The electrons are absorbed easily and they transfer their energy if administered internally.

3. Gamma radiation is a shortwave type of electromagnetic radiation, similar to light waves and X-radiation.

Methods of detecting radiation

There are two main methods of detecting radiation: scintillation detectors and Geiger-Müller counters.

Scintillation detectors: when radiation reacts with certain materials it produces small flashes of light. These materials are called scintillators or phosphors.

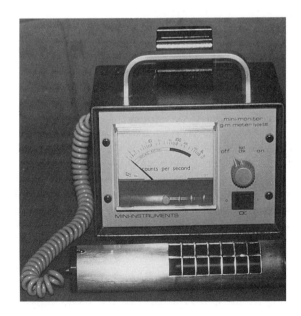

Fig. 4.17 A Geiger-Müller counter.

Gamma radiation can be detected by using a detector made up of a crystal of sodium iodide which produces a small flash of light when in contact with the rays.

Beta rays can be detected by these methods, but as the penetrating power of these rays is less, this technique is ineffective.

Geiger-Müller counters (Fig. 4.17). The principle of this equipment is that radiation causes inert gases to ionize. When a voltage is applied to the gas contained between two electrodes, ionization of gas occurs producing free electrons and positively-charged gas ions which tend to migrate under the influence of an electric field to produce an electrical signal. Geiger counters are sensitive to beta radiation but relatively insensitive to gamma radiation.

Units of measurement — the becquerel (Bq)

A given quantity of radioactive substance is presumed to have an activity of 1 becquerel if one disintegration of a nucleus takes place on average every second.

Formerly, the basic unit was the curie (Ci) which was defined in terms of the absolute rate of disintegration. A substance which underwent 3.7×10^{10} disintegrations per second contained 1 curie of activity.

Half-Life. The rate of decay of radioactive material is measured by the half-life. This is the time required for half the radioactive atoms present to disintegrate.

Uses of radioactive isotopes

Isotopes are used for diagnostic and therapeutic purposes.

Diagnostic. Radioactive isotopes can be used for diagnostic purposes in two forms — imaging and non-imaging.

Imaging. This technique uses gamma rays emitted from an isotope, and the distribution of these rays in the body can be detected using a gamma camera.

A commonly used isotope is technetium-99 m, thus technetium-99 m labelled red blood cells or albumin are used for vascular imaging and assess-

ing cardiac activity. Technetium-99 m pertechnetate is used in brain and thyroid scans.

Non-imaging techniques. Fibrinogen labelled with radioactive iodine-125 is used to detect deep vein thrombosis. This labelled fibrinogen is injected intravenously and should a clot begin to form, fibrinogen (from the normal clotting factors) begins to concentrate with the clot. A part of this fibrinogen in the clot is the injected radioactive fibrinogen which emits gamma rays. A scintillation counter detects a high level of radioactivity just above the formed blood clot.

Blood flow into and/or out of a body organ such as the liver or kidney can be measured if a radioisotope is used as an indicator.

Therapeutic. Radiation may be given either by means of an internal or external source in the treatment of tumours. For example a sealed caesium-137 capsule is implanted in the uterus for uterine tumours. As an external source the commonest radioactive material used is a sealed capsule of cobalt-60.

Radiation hazards and safety

All radioactive substances and X-rays can cause tissue damage and abnormalities in chromosomes. Hence it is essential to limit exposure to a minimum. An individual can be exposed to radiation from either outside (i.e. from the surroundings outside the body) or from radioactive elements within the body.

Exposure to external radiation can be minimized by keeping radioactive sources in containers that absorb radiation.

As alpha particles travel only a few centimetres in air, it is essential to contain them in specialized containers. Beta particles travel a distance of a few metres in air before they are absorbed. As beta particles also produce X-rays it is safer to provide a protective shield for staff, made of Perspex, a material with a low density.

A dense material such as lead is used as a shield against gamma rays which travel long distances. Lead also tends to absorb X-rays, hence it is added to aprons (during manufacture) which are worn by staff exposed to radiation.

The dose of radiation received is directly proportional to the square of the distance, hence

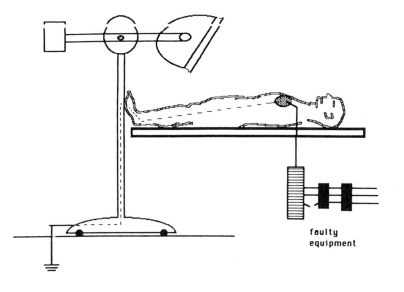

Fig. 4.18 The safety of electromedical equipment.

the risk of exposure can be considerably reduced by moving away from the source of radiation.

As a fetus is at specific risk from radiation, women of child-bearing age should be X-rayed only in the first 10 days of their menstrual cycle (i.e. before ovulation and to exclude conception).

Personnel who are constantly exposed to X-rays should wear a photographic film badge to monitor the total radiation dose received. The badge consists of a small piece of photographic film behind several filters through which passes the dose of radiation received.

Each hospital has a radiation control officer who is consulted before radioactive compounds are used.

HAZARDS IN THE OPERATING THEATRE

The source of power for most anaesthetic apparatus and monitoring equipment is an alternating electric current. In the UK electrical power is supplied at a frequency of 50 Hz.

It is essential to be aware of the principles behind the mains supply to the hospital and the operating theatre.

The hospital site receives electrical power as a three-phase 11 000 volts supply. A local transformer transforms this power in to three 240 volts supplies. Each 240 V supply is 120° out of phase with the other two, so it is obvious that interconnected electrical devices should not receive power from different phases. Hence all the wiring outlets of the operating theatre should be connected to the same phase supply. The current used in electromedical equipment passes between a live 240 V wire and the neutral.

Electromedical equipment connected to the mains consists of a live component called 'load' which is covered by an insulated 'earthed' metal casing. This earth is important for the safety of the equipment (Fig. 4.18).

If the insulation tends to deteriorate a connection is established between the load and the earthed metal casing, and current produced due to this connection is called 'leakage current'. If this is high the line current will exceed the rating of the fuse, making it blow and thus breaking the circuit.

The fuse protects the equipment from the effects of large leakage currents. But if the earth connection becomes faulty a dangerous situation develops. The current does not flow because of loss of the earth connection, the fusing does not blow and the metal casing (Fig. 4.18) remains at the same potential as the leakage source. At this point if a person standing on an antistatic floor

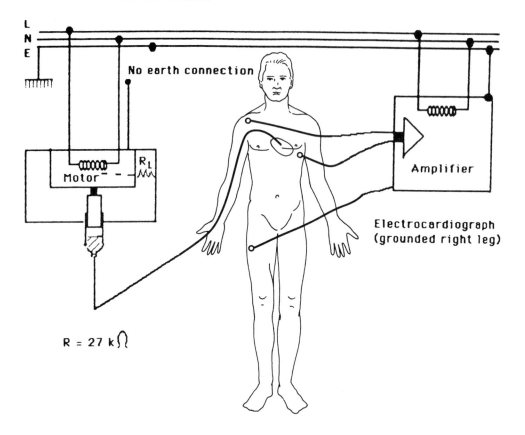

Fig. 4.19   Microshock.

touches the case, current passes through him to the earth and mains, giving him a painful shock.

However if he touches this case with a wet hand, he will receive a dangerous electrocuting current.

Protection against electric shock

Electromedical equipment can be divided into three classes by the degree of protection needed to protect against the risk of electric shock.

Class I equipment. In this type of equipment, any conducting part that can touch a user, such as the metal case of an instrument, is connected to an earth wire which becomes the third wire connected via the plug to the mains supply socket.

Class II equipment. In this type of equipment (also called double-insulated equipment), parts that can be touched easily are protected by two layers of insulation. An earth wire is not required.

Class III equipment. In this type of equipment, there are no potentials exceeding 24 V ac, so it does not produce an electric shock, but it can still produce a microshock.

Risks of shock with earthed equipment

If the patient is allowed to get in contact with Class I type equipment in the theatre, there is a risk that he will be electrocuted. In older diathermy machines, the patient's plate acted as a possible connection between earth and the patient, increasing the risk of electrocution in the event of an electrical fault occurring in any equipment to which he was attached.

Microshock. If an electric current passes through the myocardium, it can cause ventricular fibrillation due to electric shock. If an electric current passes from a hand to the feet, the current flows not only through the heart but also through a part of the body, so that the total current flow through the heart is a fraction of 24 mA which may pass from the hand to the feet. It is that fraction of the current passing through the myocardium, or the current density in the region of the myocardium, which determines whether ventricular fibrillation will occur.

If there is a faulty intracardiac catheter passing from the monitoring equipment into the heart (Fig. 4.19) and if this catheter touches the wall of the heart, an electric current flowing along the catheter will pass through a very small area of the heart. In such a case a current of 150 μA (micro amp) can produce the same current density in a portion of the myocardium as that produced by 24 mA flowing from a hand to the feet, and ventricular fibrillation can occur. This phenomenon is known as a microshock.

Microshock can occur in patients who have an intracardiac pacemaker with an external head.

ULTRASOUND

This is used as a diagnostic tool when X-rays are contraindicated as in pregnancy or when they give poor images such as those of soft tissues. Ultrasound instruments using the Doppler principle were introduced in 1958. The Doppler technique allows repeated measurements of the same patient without causing any harm. It is used to measure the blood flow (eg. limb blood flow) and differentiate between a solid or cystic swelling.

Principles of ultrasound

The human ear can detect sound waves between 20 and 20 000 Hz. Any sound waves generated above this level (i.e. above 20 000 Hz.) which are inaudible to the human ear are called ultrasound. In diagnostic instruments the frequency of ultrasound employed is between 1 and 10 MHz (megahertz).

In some instruments ultrasound can be produced as a narrow continuous beam with a set direction at the target organ, whereas in others it can be produced as a series of short bursts.

Ultrasound is generated and detected by transducers made up of crystals with a piezo-electric effect.

The piezo-electric effect. When crystals made up of quartz or rochelle salt (potassium, sodium tartarate) are pressurized an electric charge appears on their surface (both positive and negative). This effect is called the piezo-electric effect.

Display of ultrasound signals

As ultrasound signals have a short duration they are continuously displayed on a cathode ray oscilloscope. The types of scanning techniques available are:

— A-scan (A-mode or amplitude scan). This is simple although expensive. It is used to differentiate between solid and cystic lesions (e.g. in the kidney) and for obtaining accurate measurements such as identifying the midline of the brain when there is a suspected mass in the cranium.

— B-scan (B-mode or brightness scan). B-scan is used in obstetrics to detect multiple pregnancies, fetal size and abnormality, and the size of the placenta. In cardiology it is used to detect the mobility of cardiac muscle and heart valves.

Clinical uses of ultrasound and the Doppler technique

Ultrasound and the Doppler technique are used in the following situations:

1. In the indirect measurement of systolic and diastolic blood pressure in operating theatres, using arteriosonde
2. To detect air embolism during neurosurgery
3. To detect fetal heart movement during labour
4. To detect the patency of a peripheral blood vessel after a suspected embolism.

MULTIPLE CHOICE QUESTIONS

The answers to these questions can be found on page 253.

1. **The Joule is a unit of:**
   A energy
   B temperature
   C power
   D resistance.

2. **Temperature is normally measured in medical practice in one of the following units:**
   A kelvin
   B kilogram
   C centigrade
   D celsius.

3. **An ion consists of:**
   A a neutron
   B an element
   C an atom or molecule carrying an electrical charge
   D a mixture of elements.

4. **An atom of hydrogen contains**
   A one electron and one proton
   B one electron and one neutron
   C one neutron and one proton
   D two electrons and two protons.

5. **Mass and weight are:**
   A different in that the latter varies with gravity
   B always proportional to each other
   C identical
   D different in that mass varies with gravity.

6. **Boyle's law applies to which one of the following?**
   A the relationship between the pressure and volume of a gas
   B the temperature of a gas
   C the pressure within an autoclave
   D the difference between a gas and a vapour.

7. **One of the following components allows the passage of alternating current, but not direct current:**
   A inductor
   B resistor
   C capacitor
   D solenoid.

8. **Latent heat is:**
   A produced by the sun
   B necessary for boiling
   C the extra heat necessary to change a physical state
   D necessary to increase pressure.

9. **Water boils at 100°C due to:**
   A decreased pressure
   B atmospheric pressure
   C type of container it is in
   D increased pressure.

10. **Static electricity can be reduced by:**
    A wearing dark clothes
    B having humid surroundings
    C wearing nylon clothes
    D wearing rubber boots.

11. **The colour of the neutral wire in a 13 amp plug is:**
    A black
    B blue
    C green and yellow
    D brown.

12. **Ohm's law relates to:**
    A voltage produced by a cell
    B current flowing through a resistor
    C light produced by a laser
    D number of ions in 100 ml of a solution.

13. **Before handling faulty mains-operated equipment, it is essential that the:**
    A equipment is earthed
    B fuse be removed
    C mains should be switched off
    D plug be removed from the mains.

14. **Radioactive isotopes emitting gamma rays should be stored in:**
    A water
    B a glass bottle
    C a lead container
    D a thick plastic container.

15. **The term ferrous metal means it:**
    A is magnetic
    B contains iron
    C rusts easily
    D conducts electricity.

16. **Low dose radiation is hazardous to the:**
    A nervous system
    B skin
    C respiratory system
    D reproductive system.

17. **Ionization is produced by:**
    A sound waves
    B X-rays
    C alpha particles
    D neutrons.

18. **A device that converts electrical energy into mechanical energy is a:**
    A transformer
    B motor
    C dynamo
    D rectifier.

19. **Mains electrical frequency is:**
    A 120 Hertz
    B 50 Hertz
    C 240 Hertz
    D 100 Hertz.

20. **Diathermy is not recommended in:**
    A a child
    B an adult with a pacemaker fitted
    C an adult with hyperthermia
    D an elderly patient.

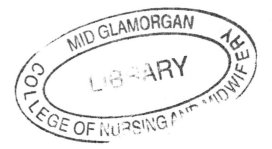

5. Patient care and theatre technique

In every hospital, from the simplest operation to the most complicated, nurses and technicians should understand their roles within the organizational structure of the operating theatre to be effective members of the surgical team. The role and relationships of each member of the team should be clarified in order to achieve a safe environment for the care of the patient.

In addition to the medical profession (i.e. surgeons and anaesthetists), charge nurses/nursing officers, theatre sisters, staff nurses, technicians and ancillary staff form part of the theatre team.

The time spent by patients in the operating theatre is relatively short (but important) compared to their overall stay in hospital. The responsibility of theatre personnel lies in maintaining safety, comfort and the welfare of the patient from the time he arrives in the operating theatre until the time he departs. Many patients are anxious about surgery, its outcome and the new environment when they arrive in the operating theatre. The role of theatre personnel is to allay the patient's apprehension, explain adequately what he will be undergoing, and assure him that his welfare will be looked after when he is unable to do so himself.

In the present hospital set-up, because of the number of patients being treated, sometimes scant attention is paid to patients' needs. Theatre personnel play a vital role in ensuring that every patient arriving in the theatre is treated as an 'individual' and not identified by his 'operation'. This will enable the patient to adjust to a strange environment while trying to retain his dignity in the process.

In some operating theatres, patients' aids or prostheses are not allowed, which can cause discomfort, embarrassment and confusion. For example, an edentulous patient (patient without teeth) may not be able to speak without his prosthesis; patients with hearing aids may not be able to understand pre- and postoperative commands; some patients may be wearing wigs due to premature baldness; ethnic minority patients (Sikhs) do not like having their turbans removed because of their religious beliefs. Hence, concessions need to be made regarding these factors, to maintain patients' dignity and safety, and to respect their religious beliefs.

In the operating theatre the nurse who receives the patient from the ward explains the entire operation to him; hence kind, friendly attention to the patient is of great importance. In addition to caring for their physical needs, attending to patients' emotional needs will help many of them to remember their time in theatre more pleasantly. On arrival in theatre, the patient should be transferred to quiet surroundings. Many patients will have received a premedication 45 minutes to one hour prior to arrival and they may appear sleepy, awake but relaxed; they should not be disturbed either by the environment or personnel, and loud laughter, friendly chats and joking amongst theatre personnel should not be permitted within their hearing.

PREOPERATIVE PREPARATION OF THE PATIENT

Elective

Normally patients scheduled for elective surgery are admitted at least the day before the operation and in some cases even earlier. This allows patients to undergo haematological, biochemical, radiological or any other appropriate investigation. If the patient is anaemic he may receive a blood transfusion to bring his haemoglobin to an adequate level. If a diabetic patient (receiving long-acting insulin treatment) is admitted, his blood sugar is controlled by changing the regime to short-acting insulin and repeated blood sugar estimation (see p. 183).

A patient who is adequately prepared for surgery can be assessed the day before the operation by the anaesthetist, and prescribed a premedication drug (see p. 140). Some adults and children undergoing minor surgery are admitted on the same day of the operation (day case surgery). They are usually fit, and are investigated when seen in the outpatient clinic.

Starvation. Adult patients coming for surgery in the morning are starved from 10 p.m. overnight and children for four hours before surgery. Diabetic patients usually receive a 5% dextrose infusion at 6 a.m. on the day of the operation (with or without soluble insulin added to the dextrose infusion).

In many hospitals, patients scheduled for afternoon surgery receive a light breakfast (toast and tea) at 6 a.m. and are then starved.

Emergency

Patients are presented for emergency surgery at short notice. Some of them are very sick, not adequately starved, dehydrated and hypovolaemic due to bleeding (e.g. ruptured ectopic pregnancy or ruptured aortic aneurysm).

The aim of doctors in these situations is to rehydrate the patient, make sure blood and blood products are available (see p. 170), and transport the patient immediately to theatre so that appropriate surgical procedures can be carried out.

If the patient is being resuscitated in the anaesthetic room, the role of the nurse is to closely observe the patient. The theatre technician's role is to help the anaesthetists in resuscitating the patient and in administering the anaesthetic.

Starvation. Patients who have eaten within four hours of injury, pregnant women and patients with intestinal obstruction are potentially in danger because their gastric emptying time is delayed. A patient with a full stomach can soil his lungs by aspiration if he vomits during the induction of anaesthesia or in the immediate postoperative period because his swallowing reflexes are either absent or inadequate. The methods used to empty the stomach are described on page 193.

Safety period for anaesthesia

There is no definite safety period for the induction of anaesthesia with regards to gastric contents, regurgitation, etc. Hence, in spite of a minimum four-hour interval after eating, if the patient arrives for an anaesthetic the role of a theatre technician is to apply cricoid pressure during the induction of anaesthesia and intubation (see p. 194 for details on application of cricoid pressure).

Reception of the patient

All patients arriving in theatre should have someone in constant attendance; they should never be left alone on a trolley. The patient should be welcomed by the operating room nurse with a relaxed, well-modulated tone of voice. A short period of conversation, including an introduction to the operating theatre, is reassuring to the patient.

Identification of the patient

Patient identification is absolutely essential in order to avoid the possibility of operating on the wrong person. The nurse in the reception area of the operating theatre should ask the patient's name. The patient is correctly identified and his identification band should correspond with the case notes and operating list regarding his registration number and name, etc. The site of the operation (e.g. amputation of the right leg) should be checked and identified with a marker by the surgeon before the patient arrives in theatre.

The patient should not be transferred into the anaesthetic room until the nurse is certain that he has been correctly identified. The nurse should also make sure that relevant X-rays and laboratory reports have accompanied the patient, and blood (if need be) is cross-matched and readily available in theatre.

Protecting the patient's possessions

Prostheses, such as contact lenses and dentures, should be removed before the patient leaves the ward. As discussed earlier, hearing aids, and occasionally dentures, should be allowed into theatre until the patient is anaesthetized. If the dentures or prostheses are removed after the induction of anaesthesia, they should be looked after by the anaesthetic nurse until the patient recovers from his anaesthetic. If the patient has crowned or loose teeth, they should be mentioned in the notes and to the anaesthetist once again before the induction of anaesthesia.

Transfer of the patient

In many hospitals in the UK patients are transferred from the reception area to the anaesthetic room, but certain hospitals in this country, and many hospitals around the world, lack this facility; hence the patient is brought directly into the operating room on a trolley and then transferred to the table.

For elective surgery the patient is usually anaesthetized on a theatre trolley, but in some emergency cases (e.g. aneurysms, ectopic pregnancies, intestinal obstruction, Caesarean sections), despite the availability of the anaesthetic room, the patients are anaesthetized on the table in the operation room. This allows the patient's abdomen to be explored immediately if the patient becomes hypotensive during induction of anaesthesia (e.g. aneurysms, ectopic pregnancy), or the table can be tilted, head down, if the patient tends to regurgitate.

Regardless of where the patients are anaesthetized or transferred, they should be encouraged to move by their own effort, provided they are not heavily sedated. It is safer if one person stabilizes the trolley while another person stands on the opposite side of the table to receive the patient.

If the patient is too drowsy due to premedication, he must be lifted correctly by at least four people—one supporting his head and shoulders, one lifting his feet and legs, and one on each side to lift his trunk.

For the protection of the patient and personnel, it is advisable to have enough people to lift the patient to the table, otherwise accidents and strained backs can result. In many hospitals, rollers and lifter sheets are used. Once the patient is placed on the table, to prevent him from falling he should be carefully observed until he is anaesthetized.

Anaesthetic management

The patient, after being identified and made comfortable, is anaesthetized using either a general or regional anaesthetic technique (see p. 152).

Positioning of the patient

After administration of the anaesthetic, the patient is positioned as required for the surgical procedure. The ideal position allows good access to the operating site, does not hinder respiration and circulation, does not cause injury to nerves and blood vessels (see p. 189) and allows adequate monitoring of the patient.

Operating table. All the operating theatre personnel should be accustomed to the working conditions of the operating table. They should be able to manipulate the controls, make and break, and lock and unlock the table.

Measures before positioning

The patient should be moved gently after administration of the anaesthetic; rapid turning or moving the extremities can cause dislocations and fractures. The head and neck of the patient are usually supported by the anaesthetist to prevent injury and accidental extubation.

The patient's clothing is removed before positioning, and afterwards parts of the body, other than the surgical site, are covered with aluminium foil to prevent accidental hypothermia.

Usually one arm is secured to a padded armboard so that intravenous infusion can be given during the operation. The angle of abduction should not be more than 90 degrees, i.e. at right angles with the body. If the arm is severely abducted, the brachial plexus will be stretched causing paralysis of the nerves in that arm. The elbow should be protected with cotton wool to prevent friction of the ulnar nerve (which lies on the medial side of the elbow joint) against a hard surface.

If the patient is placed in a lithotomy position (see below) the knee joint should be protected on the lateral side from being rubbed against the stirrups to prevent injury to the lateral popliteal nerve. If this nerve is damaged it can lead to foot drop.

Supine (dorsal) (Fig. 5.1)

The patient lies flat on his back; both arms are secured at his sides with palms down or one arm extended on an armboard for intravenous therapy. The patient's heels are supported with either a pillow or a sandbag and the legs uncrossed.

Patients are anaesthetized in this position routinely for abdominal, some thoracic and thoracoabdominal operations and some operations on the hip and lower extremities. A few modifications are made to this position for good surgical access; e.g. for surgery on the face and neck the head is stabilized in a doughnut. For shoulder and thyroid operations a small sandbag or rolled sheet is placed under the shoulder.

For operations on an upper extremity, e.g. the breast, the arm on the affected side is placed on an armboard at right angles to the body. For operations on the groin or varicose veins the knees are slightly flexed over a pillow with the thighs externally rotated.

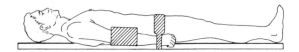

Fig. 5.1 The supine position.

Sitting (Fig. 5.2)

Initially the patient lies supine with the knees over the lower break of the table, a padded footboard

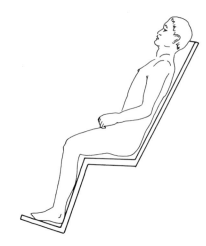

Fig. 5.2 The sitting position.

supporting the feet. The foot of the table is lowered with slight flexion of the knees. The upper section of the table is raised to a full sitting position, the head being supported on a headrest. The arms rest on a large pillow in the lap with shoulders and thighs strapped to the table.

This position is used for craniotomies and some facial operations.

Prone

The patient is turned onto his abdomen with rolled sheets or pillows placed under the chest and pelvis, thus facilitating free movement of the diaphragm during respiration. Arms are secured along the side of the body. The feet and the ankles rest on a pillow to prevent pressure on the toes, with a safety strap placed below the knees.

This position is used for operations on the posterior chest and legs. A slight modification, adjusting the mattress so that the patient's lumbar area is over the upper break in the table, is suitable for laminectomy.

Trendelenburg (Fig. 5.3)

The patient is placed on the table in a supine position with his knees directly over the lower break of the table. The foot of the table is lowered to flex the knees and the table tilted to lower the

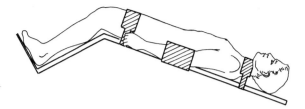

Fig. 5.3 The Trendelenburg position.

head. A knee strap helps to prevent the patient sliding towards the head of the table.

This position is used for operations on the pelvis or lower abdomen where it is essential to obtain better exposure by letting the abdominal viscera fall into the upper abdomen.

Reverse trendelenburg

With the patient in the supine position, the table is tilted upwards to raise the head and lower the feet. A padded footboard is used to prevent the patient from sliding.

This position is used for thyroidectomy to decrease the blood supply to the operative site, thus facilitating surgery.

Lithotomy

The patient is placed on the table in a supine position. A polyethylene pad is placed at the lower end of the table (to prevent the mattress being soaked with blood etc.) and the patient is moved onto the pad so that the buttocks extend slightly past the lower break in the table. The legs are put into stirrups. It is essential to lift and flex both legs simultaneously to prevent lower back strain for the patient when either leg is placed in the stirrups. Similarly, the legs should be removed from the stirrups simultaneously.

Strap stirrups are commonly used and preventive measures should be taken using paddings to prevent direct contact between metal and the patient's legs at any point.

After the foot section of the table is lowered, a footboard may be attached to provide a ledge for the surgeon. The arms are secured across the patient's abdomen by folding the gown over them

and tucking it under the body. During perineal operations a better surgical access can be achieved in male patients by gently pulling the genitalia onto the lower abdomen and strapping them with an adhesive plaster.

This position is used for cystoscopy, vaginal, perineal and rectal operations.

Lateral (Fig. 5.4)

The patient is turned onto the unaffected side with his back near the edge of the table. The arm on the affected side is placed on an armrest with slight flexion and minimal abduction. Cotton wool or padding below the elbow joint prevents compression on the ulnar nerve, and minimal abduction prevents stretching of the brachial plexus. The unaffected arm is placed on an armboard for venous access or folded across the chest with a folded sheet in between. A sandbag is placed below the chest to support and elevate it. The lower leg is flexed and the upper leg remains straight; a large pillow between the legs relieves the pressure of one leg on the other. Braces are attached to the table—the short one at the patient's back, the long one in front of him. A safety strap over the hip provides stability.

This basic position can be modified for operations on the chest, kidney and ureters. For operations on the kidney the mattress is adjusted so that the kidney area is over the kidney elevator. The table is flexed at the upper break and the kidney rest is raised to spread the space between the lower ribs and the iliac crest.

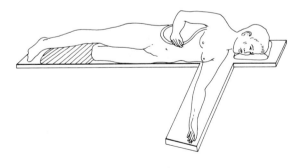

Fig. 5.4 The lateral position.

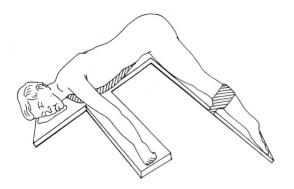

Fig. 5.5   The jack knife position.

Jack knife (Fig. 5.5)

The patient is placed in a prone position with the hips over the upper break in the table and the safety strap below the knees. The foot of the table is lowered, and the arms are placed on armboards at right angles to the body or placed on either side of the head with padded support under the elbows. The chest and pelvis are supported on sandbags and the entire table tilted head down so that the hips are elevated.

This position is used for haemorrhoidectomy and the excision of pilonidal sinuses.

OPERATING THEATRE ENVIRONMENT

The following points need to be considered: design, ventilation, and control of pollution and traffic.

A. Design

A proper design of the operating theatre allows a one-way flow of traffic and prevents the return flow of contaminants into the clean area. Separate rooms are allocated for the:

— Anaesthetic room
— Scrub-up area
— Sterile supply area
— Dirty utility area
— Sterilizing room
— Unsterile stock and heavy equipment
— Plaster room

— Recovery room
— Medical, nursing and technicians' lounge rooms
— Dark rooms for processing X-rays
— Staff changing rooms
— Cleaners' room.

Lighting and power. Fluorescent lighting is best for general lighting, with provision for emergency back-up. In the patient areas, white light is preferred as blue light can make the patient appear cyanosed.

Overhead lights. These are specially-designed, shadowless lights made up of tungsten lamps and incandescent bulbs with heat filters which act as heat reflectors to prevent overheating of patients and theatre staff. The lights can be dimmed or increased by turning a knob. They have handle covers which are autoclavable so that the surgeon can adjust the position of the light on the operating site.

Ventilation

The air movements and air conditioning in the operating theatre are regulated so that the patient and theatre staff are comfortable. Air flow in the operating room is directed from clean to less clean areas.

The method of ventilation used to remove bacteria (in the air) in the operating theatre is as follows:

Plenum ventilation. A positive pressure is applied to force a downward displacement of fine filtered air from ceiling level. The air is filtered, humidified and either warmed or cooled. Humidity prevents bacterial growth and build-up of static electricity. Relative humidity (see p. 105) is maintained at between 50 to 55%. Heat and water loss can occur in small babies during prolonged operations in cool air conditioning; hence the humidity needs to be adjusted.

Air change

a. *Pressurization.* Each operating room should have an air change rate of about 20 times an hour.

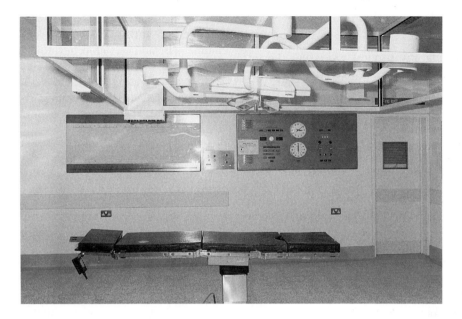

Fig. 5.6 The Charnley tent.

Air supply and exhausts are adjusted in such a way that the operating room and the adjacent clean areas are at positive pressure in relation to the surrounding areas.

b. *Doors*. The doors should be kept closed at all times to maintain the correct pressure in the operating room and surrounding rooms.

c. *Exhaust*. Exhaust vents are positioned in such a way that bacteria and dust particles do not get distributed into the atmosphere.

d. *Lamina flow ventilation*. This ventilation provides 100 changes of air per hour with bacteria-free air in the operating theatre. It is a highly efficient but expensive method of removing bacteria. Lamina flow is used in cardiac surgery and hip replacement surgery to control infection.

e. *Recirculation of air*. A certain amount of the exhaust air is filtered to remove bacteria and is then reintroduced. This is a less expensive means of ventilation.

f. *Charnley downflow clean-air enclosure (Fig. 5.6)*. This allows the patient and the operating team to be isolated in an enclosure from other people in the operating room. The flow of air produces a positive movement in a determined route, with 300 changes of air an hour. The air is taken from outside the hospital into the enclosure. The surgeon and the team inside the enclosure wear special gear using a 'body exhaust' system. A vacuum is used to remove bacteria, dust particles and expired air from the inside of the gown.

C. Control of pollution and traffic

Anaesthetic gases are scavenged from the expiratory valve of the anaesthetic apparatus to the atmosphere via tubing.

Traffic of personnel is restricted in the operating theatre. There should be a limited number of people in the operating room during surgery. The important factors which need to be considered whilst planning traffic controls are:

— movement of staff and patients
— removal of linen and contaminated waste
— delivery of supplies.

If visitors arrive in the theatre complex, they are taken to the changing rooms and shown how to wear appropriate clothes.

PREPARATION BY THE THEATRE PERSONNEL

Before beginning any surgical procedure the following points need to be followed strictly:

a. Personal hygiene. All theatre personnel should have a bath or shower and change underwear daily. Hands should be washed frequently and nails cut.

b. Operating theatre clothing. Theatre personnel change into theatre clothes and wear caps which cover all their hair. They wear antistatic rubber-sole shoes. No jewellery is worn in the operating room. A mask is tied securely around the nose and mouth to allow the air to filtrate through the mask and not escape around the sides. Masks should be thrown away after each use and not worn around the neck.

Aseptic technique

Staff in the operating theatre should make sure that they maintain asepsis to limit the risk of contamination of a surgical wound. The main principles of an aseptic technique are:

(i)   All instruments used in the theatre must be sterile.
(ii)   Sterile and non-sterile instruments must be kept apart.
(iii) Correct sterile scrubbing, gowning and gloving procedures must be followed.
(iv)   The patient's skin must be prepared properly.
(v)   The patient must be draped with an aseptic technique.
(vi)   An unsterile person should always face a sterile fluid, never lean over a sterile trolley and never walk between sterile trolleys and the operating table.

Surgical scrubbing

The surgical hand scrub is essential to remove bacteria and dirt from the hands and arms, and to provide an antiseptic cover on the skin to prevent the growth of bacteria.

A brush is used to remove visible soil from the fingernails and between the fingers. Brush dispensers are attached to the wall of a scrub-up area

from which sterile scrub-brushes are dispensed. A number of antiseptic agents, such as povidone iodine (Betadine), chlorhexidine (Hibitane) or hexachlorophane (pHisohex), are available.

In each operating area there is a separate 'scrub-up' zone outside the operating room. The first scrub of the day lasts for five minutes and is described below:

(i)   Hands and arms are rinsed under running water.
(ii)   Antiseptic agent is squeezed into the palm of the hand and the hands and arms are washed to the elbows for two minutes.
(iii)   The lather is rinsed off with running water.
(iv)   The fingers and finger nails are scrubbed with a brush for one minute.
(v)   The hands are rinsed.
(vi)   The procedure of washing hands and arms for two minutes is repeated.
(vii)   Following a rinse, the hands and arms are elevated away from the body.
(viii) The hands and arms are dried using a sterile towel before wearing the gown and gloves.

Wearing gown and gloves (Fig.5.7)

Each hospital has a different technique but a common procedure is:

(i)   The gown is lifted upwards, holding it at the neck end.
(ii)   The scrubbed person touches only the inside of the gown as the outside of the gown is sterile.
(iii) The gown is worn by sliding the arms into the armholes.
(iv)   The hands are left within the sleeves of the gown to allow gloves to be worn.
(v)   The hands and fingers are kept within the cuff of the gown and with the left hand the right glove is picked up.
(vi)   The palm of the glove is put against the palm of the right hand with the thumbs together and fingers of the glove pointing to the right elbow.
(vii) The folded edge or the cuff of the glove is grasped in the left hand and inverted over

Fig. 5.7   Gloving technique (from Kaczmarowski N 1982 Patient care in the operating room. Pitman).

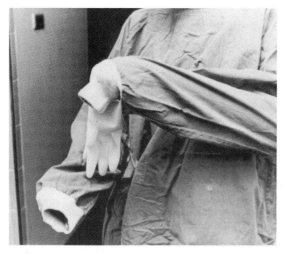

a. Unexposed left hand holds the right-hand glove, thumb faces upwards.

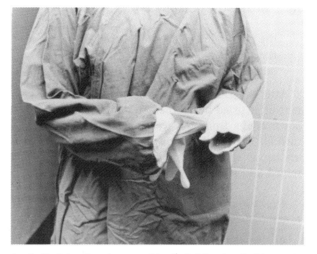

b. Cuff of the glove is grasped in the left hand and slid over the right hand.

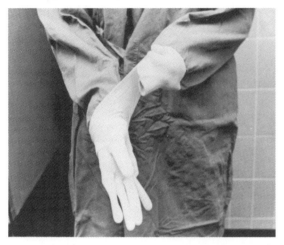

c. Cuff of the glove is stretched over the stockinette cuff of the sleeve.

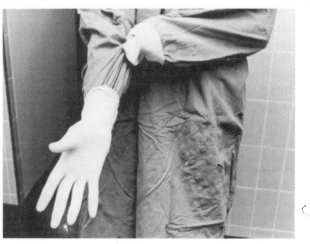

d. Stockinette cuff of the sleeve is positioned over the wrist.

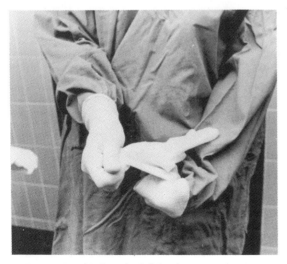

e. Repeat the technique for left hand.

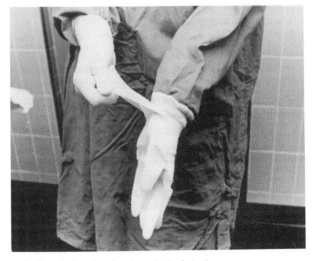

f. Completing the closed method of gloving.

the right hand. The glove is pulled on at the same time over the wrist area. The same procedure is repeated for the left hand.

After wearing gown and gloves, the scrubbed person, assisted by another 'sterile' person, ties the gown at the front. A sterile person should never turn his back to the sterile trolley and should keep his hands above waist level. The arms are never folded and sterile people pass back to back.

Discarding the gown and gloves. The gown is removed first, then the gloves.

Patient preparation

Skin preparation. Preoperative skin preparation removes bacteria and dirt from the skin and provides an antiseptic cover on the skin surface. On the ward, the skin area is shaved according to the type of surgery. The surgeon in the operating theatre prepares the patient's skin with a swab attached to sponge-holding forceps dipped into an antibacterial skin solution. The various antiseptic solutions used were mentioned earlier.

Draping (Fig. 5.8). Sterile drapes are used to provide a safe barrier between sterile and non-sterile parts of the body, thus preventing cross-infection and contamination of the surgical wound. Drapes may be disposable or re-usable, and their use depends upon the operating room policy and the surgeon's preference.

Draping is carried out by two 'sterile' people. The sterile drapes are placed over the patient, allowing only the operative site to be exposed. For an abdominal operation the patient is draped from the incision site to the foot of the operating table. The next drape is arranged from the incision site to the head of the operating table. The side drapes are then placed to provide a sterile surgical field. A split (fenestrated) sheet may be used to cover the initial drapes for added protection. An anaesthetic screen is used to separate the sterile surgical area from the non-sterile anaesthetic area. It is covered by extending the sterile drape over the skin.

Fig. 5.8 Sterile draping (from Kaczmarowski N 1982 Patient care in the operating room. Pitman).

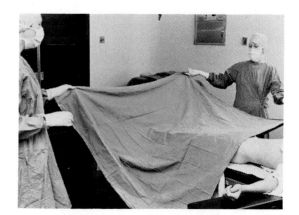

a Placing the first sterile drape over the lower part of the patient's body for an abdominal operation.

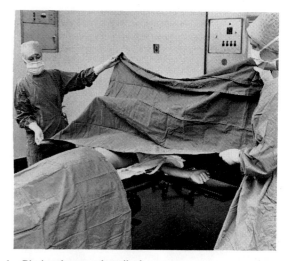

b Placing the second sterile drape.

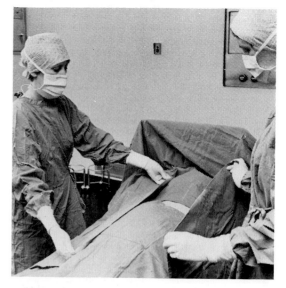

c Placing the sterile side drapes.

Swabs, sponges, instruments and needles

It is extremely important to count the various pieces of surgical equipment and inform the surgeon at the end of surgery that the count is correct. During each case a circulating nurse counts the swabs with the scrub nurse and writes the number correctly on the swab board. Before the closure of the peritoneum, the scrub nurse and the circulating nurse check the board to ascertain the total number of swabs in use along with the swabs on the instrument trolley and the ones which the surgeon is using. When the check is complete the scrub nurse informs the surgeon that the swabs are correct. If the count is not correct the surgeon is informed and a search made until the swabs are found. The wound is not closed until the swab count is correct. Before skin closure a third count is made. Where there is a discrepancy in the swab count and swabs are not found, even after X-ray of the patient, the senior nurse must be informed.

The red tags off each bundle of swabs must be kept and checked to ensure that the swabs recorded tally with the number of tags.

Instrument check. Each scrub nurse is responsible for checking all her instruments before, during and after every operation. Particular attention is paid to any loose blades and screws on retractors.

Special instrument set. Arterial clamps should be checked and recorded on a board. The time of application and removal of arterial clamps should be recorded. At the end of each operation the scrub nurse must sign the card which is in the instrument tray and check that the patient's name label is on the card; the circulating nurse witnesses her signature.

Needles and tapes must be counted before and after an operation.

Atraumatic sutures are placed on a discard-a-pad and the cut-off end of the suture packet placed on the pad with the used needle alongside.

Procedure for application of diathermy pad

Operating theatre personnel ensure that the diathermy pad is in satisfactory working order before the list begins. The scrub nurse checks the lead and forceps. After positioning the patient on the theatre table, operating theatre personnel check the thigh where the diathermy pad is to be placed to make sure that the skin is clear (with no abrasion or redness). The diathermy pad is placed on the thigh and bandaged firmly, but not tightly, in position. At the end of surgery, the diathermy pad is removed and the site checked for any signs of redness. If any redness is seen, the surgeon is informed immediately, an accident form is completed and the senior theatre nurse advised of the incident.

Tourniquet

A tourniquet is applied to make the operative site bloodless, e.g. for arthroscopy, upper limb surgery or toe surgery. The tourniquet consists of a cuff and a pressure gauge (Fig. 5.9). When a tourniquet is applied the time of application is recorded with the patient's name on the tourniquet board; the time is recorded again when the tourniquet is released. This is important as surgeons will put these times in the patient's notes after surgery. The surgeon should be reminded after each half-hour of tourniquet time during surgery. The sister-in-charge should check that the tourniquet has been removed before the patient leaves the theatre.

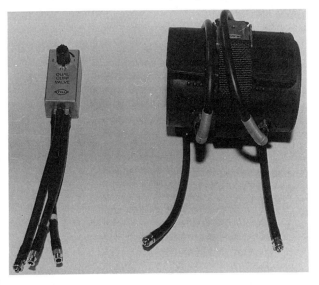

Fig. 5.9 Dual-cuff tourniquet.

Frozen section specimens

During surgery the surgeon takes a piece of suspected tissue (e.g. suspected breast cancer) and sends for a frozen section biopsy. The laboratory technician is informed by the medical staff before starting surgery with details of the patient who is to have a frozen section operation and the time the specimen will be available from theatre. A pathology form is completed in advance.

When the section is taken, the tissue is put in a dry sterile container and sent immediately to the pathology department. The result of the pathological examination is telephoned to theatre and the medical staff take the message.

Specimen collection for histology and bacteriology

The scrub nurse finds out from the surgeon if any tissue removed from the operative site is to be sent for laboratory examination.

Histology specimens. The specimen is put in a container and covered with formal saline. Two patient name labels are removed from the patient's notes by the circulating nurse who, after checking with the sister, puts one label on the container and one on the histology form. The medical staff complete the form. The specimen book is completed by the circulating nurse and the specimen sent to the laboratory.

Bacteriology specimens. The same procedure is carried out as for histology specimens but the specimen is not covered with formal saline; it is left dry in its sterile container.

Procedures for Australian antigen-positive patients undergoing surgery

a. Preparation of theatre. All unnecessary furniture and equipment are removed from the theatre and disposable equipment is used. The circulating staff wear plastic aprons/disposable gowns and gloves. The scrub team wear disposable plastic aprons under disposable gowns and all staff wear goggles.

b. During surgery. The used swabs are placed in bags labelled 'Infected material' and removed immediately for collection. All the used instruments and anaesthetic equipment are placed in a BIO-HAZARD bag and sent to HSSU for autoclaving. If linen is used it should be placed in special linen bags and removed for collection. All equipment and furniture are cleaned with hypochlorite solution and specimens are placed in adequate-sized containers with the lid fully secured. The specimen container is placed in a plastic bag, sealed and sent to the pathology laboratory with a form clearly marked that the specimen is from an Australian antigen patient.

Any injury to staff, no matter how trivial, is reported to the senior theatre nurse and the member of staff sent to the occupational health department.

The same procedure is followed for AIDS patients; further details can be read on page 92.

The procedures for harvesting donor organs vary from one hospital to another.

Death of a patient in theatre

In the event of the death of a patient in theatre, the sister-in-charge informs the senior theatre nurse, and the medical staff advise the ward sister. An oxygen mask and blankets are placed on the patient who is transferred to the ward for the last offices.

Accidents to staff

In the event of an accident occurring to a member of staff on duty, an accident form is completed by the sister-in-charge and the incident reported immediately to the senior nurse. Arrangements are made for the member of staff to go to the occupational health department for examination and treatment. All accident forms are forwarded to the senior theatre nurse.

Scheduled drugs

The recovery nurse, in liaison with the anaesthetic sister/charge nurse, maintains stocks of scheduled drugs and lotions. Stocks are checked weekly to avoid over- or under-stocking. A member of the trained staff on night duty checks the pharmacy in the emergency theatre each morning.

THEATRE SAFEGUARDS

The Medical Defence Societies and the Royal College of Nursing in association with the National Association of Theatre Nurses have formulated guidelines for working in theatre, a summary of which is as follows:

a. Label all patients admitted for surgery immediately on admission.
b. Place identity bracelets on unconscious patients in the A & E department.
c. Day-bed patients should be admitted in the same way as inpatients.
d. The nurse in charge of theatre sends for the patient in agreement with the anaesthetist.
e. The senior ward nurse is responsible for checking that all patients going for surgery are properly labelled.
f. The side and site of operation are marked with a skin marker.
g. The patient is identified in the anaesthetic room by full name and hospital number on the identity bracelet. An additional check is made against the theatre list. The consent form is also valuable in identifying the patient and the proposed operation.
h. The nurse who sends for the patient and the anaesthetist are responsible for making sure that the correct patient has been brought into the anaesthetic room.
i. The surgeon or his assistant should check that the patient's full name, hospital number, date of birth and nature of the operation, as set out on the operation list, correspond with the entries in the clinical notes and on the identity bracelet.
j. The operation list is drawn up by the surgical team indicating the nature and site of the proposed operation.
k. The procedures or site are written in full. Abbreviations such as 'l' for left and 'r' for right are avoided.
l. The site of the operation is marked by a member of the surgical team before the patient arrives in theatre.
m. All swabs and packs to be used should be in bundles of five and should be counted again before the start of the operation.

n. The swabs from previous operations are removed. The circulating nurse or operating department assistants should count all swabs and packs before any body cavity or joint space is closed.
o. The circulating nurse or operating department assistant counts the swabs during the operation (see page 133).
p. Swabs used in the theatre should be radio-opaque. Non-radio-opaque swabs should not be given to the surgeon until the wound is closed. The radio-opaque swabs should not be cut into pieces.
q. When using powered tools and other similar instruments it is important to check that attachments and fitments are neither faulty nor loose.
r. Patients' notes should be marked with warnings of allergies to plaster, to skin cleansing agents and to drugs.
s. Cross-matched blood should be checked and made available in the theatre before induction of anaesthesia.
t. Care is taken during lifting and transferring anaesthetized patients between theatre trolleys and the operating table.
u. In positioning the patient, nerves must be protected from pressure (see page 189), particularly in thin patients.
v. Eyelids should be closed with tape in an unconscious patient to prevent exposure and damage from falling foreign bodies.
w. All pneumatic cuff pressure gauges and monitors should be checked regularly by qualified engineers. When a tourniquet is applied, the operating department assistant should make a note of the time and inform the surgeon (see page 133).
x. The surgeon and the nurse in charge of theatre should make sure that instruments heated during sterilization are cooled before being used on the patient.
y. Staff should be familiar with the use of diathermy and other electrical equipment.
z. Regular checks are made to make sure that equipment has been maintained on the due dates.

MULTIPLE CHOICE QUESTIONS

The answers to these questions can be found on page 253.

1. **It is essential to remove make-up and nail varnish preoperatively because it:**
   A may obscure physical signs
   B can react with anaesthetic agents
   C can cause skin irritation following anaesthesia
   D can cause cross-infection.

2. **If a patient arrives in theatre with his dentures still in, the theatre personnel should:**
   A consult the anaesthetist
   B leave them in his mouth
   C place the dentures in a labelled pot and return them to the ward
   D wrap them in paper and place them under the pillow.

3. **Which of the following is the most suitable for wiping the scrub trolley during preparation?**
   A Dettol
   B detergent hypochlorite
   C Cidex
   D Hibitane in spirit.

4. **The site and side of operation in a small child should be marked:**
   A by the ward sister
   B just before the premedication is given
   C in the presence of the parent or guardian
   D just before leaving for theatre.

5. **False teeth should be removed prior to surgery to prevent:**
   A their breakdown
   B biting on the endotracheal tube
   C airway obstruction
   D delay in anaesthetizing the patient.

6. **Approved theatre footwear must be:**
   A fully insulated
   B padded with paper
   C fully conducting for electricity
   D designed to conduct electrostatic charges.

7. **If the surgeon wishes to open the posterior aspect of the skull, the patient may be positioned:**
   A prone
   B supine
   C neck extended
   D in lithotomy.

8. **For haemorrhoidectomy, the patient is placed in the following position:**
   A prone
   B lithotomy
   C supine
   D left lateral.

9. **In which of the following positions is a patient's respiratory function embarrassed?**
   A Trendelenburg
   B supine
   C left lateral
   D reverse Trendelenburg.

10 **In an unconscious patient, lifting only one leg into the lithotomy position at a time may lead to:**
   A sciatic nerve palsy
   B pelvic damage
   C damage of the sacroiliac joint
   D arthritis of the hip joint.

11. **'Wrist drop' is caused by damage to the:**
   A radial nerve
   B medial nerve
   C ulnar nerve
   D femoral nerve.

12. **Continuous pressure on the calf muscles can lead to:**
    A bruising of the skin
    B venous thrombosis
    C ulcers
    D varicose veins.

13. **Which of the following is used during an abdominoperineal resection operation:**
    A perineal post
    B lithotomy poles
    C Lloyd-Davis poles
    D sandbag under the loins.

14. **The maximum safe abduction of an arm on a board is:**
    A 45 degrees
    B 90 degrees
    C 135 degrees
    D 180 degrees.

15. **After tonsillectomy the patient should be recovered in which position:**
    A supine
    B supine with a pillow
    C left lateral
    D prone.

16. **The relative humidity in the operating theatre should be:**
    A 20%
    B 50%
    C 40%
    D 80%.

17. **A hygrometer is used to measure the level of:**
    A hydrogen in atmospheric air
    B mercury in a tube
    C humidity in the operating room
    D urine in the bladder.

18. **The earth or indifferent electrode on a diathermy machine:**
    A makes a wide area of contact with the patient
    B prevents electrical interference of ECG monitors
    C is connected to the patient by a point contact
    D is isolated from patient contact.

19. **Radio-frequency current is used in diathermy to:**
    A prevent muscle stimulation
    B avoid burns
    C prevent electrical interference
    D prevent build up of static electricity.

20. **The air ventilation systems in theatres should be:**
    A hot air
    B water cooled
    C positive pressure
    D negative pressure.

6. Anaesthesia

Anaesthesia is divided into three phases: preoperative period, intraoperative period, postoperative period.

PREOPERATIVE PERIOD

Each patient undergoing surgery is seen by the anaesthetist either a day before (inpatient) or on the day of the surgery (day-bed unit patient).

The anaesthetist interviews the patient with regard to their health, allergies, drug usage, alcohol, smoking, past anaesthetic experience, family problems with anaesthetics (e.g. death due to malignant hyperpyrexia during anaesthesia; following suxamethonium prolonged muscle paralysis due to pseudocholinesterase deficiency), any concurrent illness.

While talking to the patient, the anaesthetist assesses the patient's physical status such as prominent teeth, short neck, immobility of the neck which may cause technical difficulties during anaesthesia (e.g. inability to maintain airway following induction of anaesthesia or difficulty with intubation).

The following investigations are carried out routinely in patients before surgery:

1. Haemoglobin estimation
2. Urine analysis.

If patients are on antihypertensive drugs, diuretics or digoxin, or have suffered from diarrhoea or vomiting, their serum urea and electrolytes are measured.

If patients have cardiac or respiratory disease or are over the age of 40 years, chest X-ray is ordered.

Electrocardiogram (ECG) is performed in patients who have cardiorespiratory disease or who are above the age of 40 years. Lung function tests and arterial blood gas analysis is carried out in patients with lung disease.

X-rays of the neck (cervical region) are carried out in patients who have a severe limitation of the movement of the cervical spine or in patients where endotracheal intubation is anticipated as difficult (e.g. large thyroid goitres).

Physical status of the patient

The patient's preoperative physical condition is classified into five groups, based on the criteria laid down by the American Society of Anaesthesiologists (ASA):

ASA classification	Physical status of patient
1	Normal, healthy
2	Mild to moderate systemic disease, e.g. mild diabetes or anaemia
3	Severe systemic disease which limits activity but is not incapacitating, e.g. severe diabetes, patient with healed myocardial infarction
4	Severe systemic disease which is life-threatening, e.g.

139

	severe cardiac, pulmonary or liver failure
5	Moribund patient with little chance of survival, e.g. patient with ruptured aortic aneurysm, pulmonary embolism
Emergency (E)	Any patient in one of the classes mentioned above who undergoes an emergency operation is considered to be in poor physical condition. The letter E is placed beside the number (e.g. 2E).

Premedication

All patients undergoing surgery are anxious about anaesthesia and the outcome of the operation. Hence it is important to prescribe benzodiazepines to decrease anxiety and fear.

The other reasons for prescribing premedication drugs are:

a. To increase the hypnotic effects of general anaesthetics and to reduce postoperative nausea and vomiting.
b. To decrease the volume and raise the pH of the gastric contents in patients in whom the risk of vomiting or regurgitation is high (e.g. patients with hiatus hernia, duodenal ulcer, full stomach).
c. To decrease the vagal effect (acute bradycardia) which can occur due to repeated administration of suxamethonium.

Some of the common premedicant drugs prescribed are listed in Tables 6.1 and Table 6.2

Metoclopramide (Maxolon) and droperidol are prescribed preoperatively to decrease the incidence of nausea and vomiting. Ranitidine (Zantac) 150 mg or cimetidine 200 mg are given orally 90 min before the operation to increase the pH of the gastric contents to above 2.5 and to decrease the gastric volume.

Metoclopramide (Maxolon) hastens gastric emptying. Atropine (0.3–0.6 mg) or glycopyr-

Table 6.1 Commonly prescribed premedicant drugs for healthy adults.

Drug	Route of administration	Dosage	Remarks
Diazepam (Valium)	Oral	10–20 mg	Good anxiolytic
Lorazepam (Ativan)	Oral	2–4 mg	Prolonged action Anterograde amnesia*
Diazepam (Valium)	Oral	10 mg	Metoclopramide acts as an antiemetic and
Metoclopramide (Maxolon)	Oral	10 mg	lowers the tone of lower oesophageal sphincter
Temazepam	Oral	10–20 mg	Temazepam is used
Metoclopramide	Oral	10 mg	because of its short duration of action
Papaveretum (Omnopon)	Intramuscular	20 mg	Causes good sedation
Hyoscine (Scopolamine)	Intramuscular	0.4 mg	Causes good sedation

* Loss of memory for immediate past events.

Table 6.2 Commonly prescribed premedication for children.

Weight of child	Drug	Dosage (/kg body weight)	Route	Timing (before op.)
Less than 10 kg	Chloral hydrate	50 mg	Oral	45 min
Above 10 kg	Triclofos	25 mg	Oral	60 min
10–15 kg	Diazepam Droperidol (Droleptan)	5 mg 2.5 mg	Oral Oral	90 min 90 min
Above 15 kg	Diazepam Droperidol	5 mg 2.5 mg	Oral Oral	90 min 90 min
Any age	Temazepam	0.5–1 mg	Oral	90 min

ronium (Robinul) 0.2–0.4 mg are given intramuscularly or intravenously to prevent the occurrence of bradycardia. After adequate starvation and premedication (see p. 140) the patient is brought into the anaesthetic room.

The type of anaesthesia, either general or regional, is selected based on the type of operation and the anaesthetist's choice.

INTRAOPERATIVE PERIOD

It is always essential that the anaesthetists and the theatre personnel have an adequate knowledge of the anaesthetic machine and other equipment. These should be checked every time before use. Figure 6.1 shows an ideal setting of anaesthetic room with adequate space.

ANAESTHETIC MACHINE (Fig. 6.2)

The anaesthetic machine comprises: a supply of compressed gases; a method of metering and releasing the gases; a method of vaporizing volatile anaesthesia agents; equipment for delivering

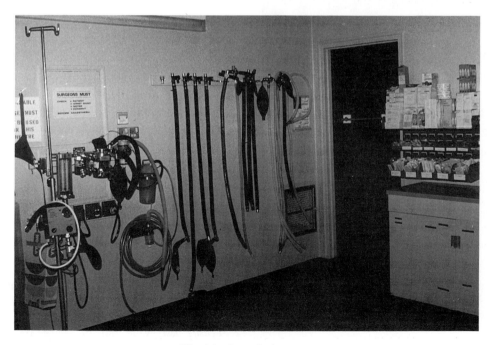

Fig. 6.1 Anaesthetic room.

vapours and gases to the patient (breathing systems); a means for scavenging anaesthetic gases; alarms to indicate the delivery of hypoxic mixtures.

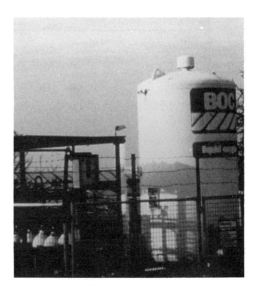

Fig. 6.3 Liquid oxygen tank.

Compressed gases

Oxygen

Oxygen is supplied to the anaesthetic machine as a compressed gas in cylinders of various sizes or from a pipeline source. In large hospitals, pipeline oxygen comes from a liquid oxygen store. Liquid oxygen is stored at a temperature of −165°C at 10.5 bar in a giant thermos flask—a vacuum insulated evaporator (VIE) (Fig. 6.3).

Constant pressure is maintained by transfer of gaseous oxygen into the pipeline system.

In some hospitals, instead of a liquid oxygen store, the hospital pipeline is supplied by a double bank of large cylinders. In addition to oxygen, gases such as compressed air, nitrous oxide and Entonox are piped.

Oxygen is stored as a gas in compressed form at a pressure of 137 bar (1987 lbf/in^2★). It follows the principle of Boyle's law (p. 100) and the pressure gauge gives a reliable indication of the proportion of the original contents still remaining. ★(pound foot per square inch)

The cylinders are made of molybdenum steel. They are checked at intervals by the manufacturer for defects by carrying out the following tests.

Tensile test. One out of every 100 cylinders manufactured is picked up, strips are cut and

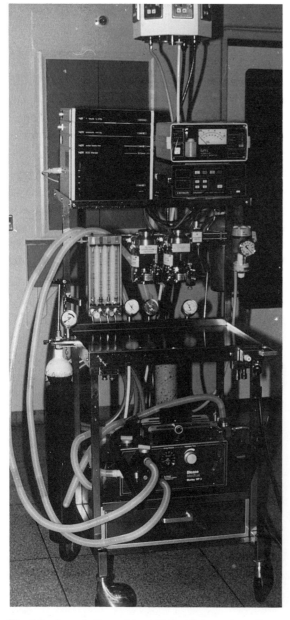

Fig. 6.2 Anaesthetic machine with ventilator and monitors.

stretched—the 'yield point' should not be less than 15 tons in^2.

Hydraulic or pressure test. This is a water-jacket test. The filling ratio of a cylinder is the ratio of weight of gas in the cylinder to the weight of water the cylinder could hold.

Flattening impact and bend tests. These tests are carried out on at least one out of every 100 cylinders made.

Oxygen cylinders supplied are colour-coded as black for the cylinder body, with white shoulders. (See Appendix for details.)

Nitrous oxide

This is supplied in cylinder colour-coded blue. It is liquid at room temperature when compressed, and exerts a pressure of 44 bar (638 lb/in^2) at 15°C. The liquid nitrous oxide evaporates into the gaseous phase when it is released from the cylinder.

When all the liquid nitrous oxide evaporates, the nitrous oxide pressure gauge starts to indicate a decrease, showing imminent emptying of the cylinder. The filling ratio of nitrous oxide cylinders is 0.75.

Entonox

A mixture of nitrous oxide and oxygen (50:50) supplied in cylinders colour-coded blue with white segments on the shoulder, it is stored at a pressure of 137 bar (1987 lb/in^2) at 15°C. The constituent gases in cylinder separate at −7°C. Such a cylinder whose gases have separated delivers initially a mixture rich in oxygen and, as the cylinder empties, a mixture deficient in oxygen.

Before use, cylinders are kept horizontally at a temperature above 10°C for 24 h. If the cylinders are required urgently, they should be stored at a temperature above 10°C for 2 h and then inverted three times.

Carbon dioxide

This is a colourless gas supplied in cylinders painted grey. The filling ratio is 0.75 in temperate and 0.67 in tropical climates. It occupies 90–95% of the cylinder in a liquid form.

Air

Supplied either via a pipeline or in cylinders painted grey with black and white shoulder quadrants, air is stored at 137 bar (1987 lbf/in^2).

Types of cylinder

There are five sizes of nitrous oxide cylinders (sizes C, D, E, F, G) and six sizes of oxygen cylinders (sizes C, D, E, F, G and J).

The larger oxygen cylinders are fitted with a bull-nose valve which can be connected to the pipeline manifold.

The largest nitrous oxide cylinders (F and G) are fitted with a handwheel valve.

Piped gas supplies

For reasons of economy and to avoid frequent changing of gas cylinders in busy theatres, gases are piped from a remote storage area. The central source of oxygen may be a liquid oxygen tank (Fig. 6.3) or a cylinder manifold. This storage area is outside the main hospital buildings, because of the increased fire risk in all areas where oxygen is stored.

Nitrous oxide

This is stored in a bank in the form of a cylinder manifold and piped to the operating theatres (Fig. 6.4). Each cylinder is connected to a pipeline by a coiled tube which passes to a central control box. The high pressure gauges on the left and right sides of the box indicate the contents of the cylinder banks, and below are high pressure valves which reduce the cylinder pressure of 137 bar to approximately 10 bar. There is a changeover valve which switches automatically from the in-use bank, to the reserve bank of cylinders when the pressure falls below a certain value. Attached are two electric warning devices which are activated by the valve and they switch on warning lights or audible alarms at a control box and remote points to indicate the need to change the empty bank of cylinders. At the outlet of the changeover valve is a second stage valve to reduce the pressure from 10 bar to 4.1 bar, the normal pipeline pressure.

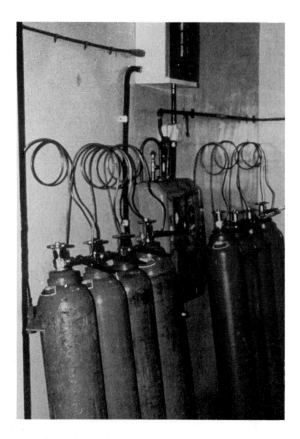

Fig. 6.4   Manifold of nitrous oxide cylinders.

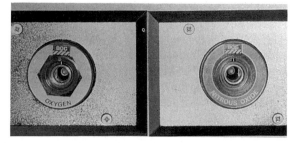

Fig. 6.5   Schraeder outlet.

vacuum inlet and diaphragm. Suction units provide a maximum flow of 40 litres/min at a vacuum of 0.53 bar (53 kPa).

Schraeder Valves

In the UK, all the piped supplies to operating theatres finish in special terminal units with a non-interchangeable coupling called a Schraeder valve. The Schraeder outlet (Fig. 6.5) is labelled and colour-coded and contains an internal non-return valve which seals the gas supply until the probe is plugged in.

Pin-index system (Fig. 6.6)

This is designed to prevent incorrect placing of a cylinder into the wrong yoke. Two pins located in the yoke should fit into corresponding holes drilled into the cylinder neck. The design of these pins and corresponding holes is unique for each gas. The pin index system applies to small gas cylinders mounted on anaesthetic machines.

Pressure regulators (reducing valves) (Fig. 6.7)

In the anaesthetic machine, it is important to provide a controlled and steady low pressure (0.53 bar) from a high pressure source such as a cylinder. This is carried out by a pressure regulator.

Flow restrictors and working pressures

The anaesthetic machines work at pipeline pressures (60 psi, 4 bar). To prevent sudden rises in

Air is supplied to the theatres through pipelines. They can be provided from a manifold of cylinders or a central compressor plant.

A centralized vacuum system is installed along with O_2, N_2O and air. It consists of a pump, large receiver and a filter unit. Air from the theatres is drawn into drainage traps and bacterial filters to dry and clean it. The air then passes through a constant suction which maintains a vacuum of around 0.53 bar (400 mmHg) below the standard atmospheric pressure of 1.01 bar (760 mmHg). The exhaust gases from the pump pass through a silencer before being discharged from air intakes or active scavenging system.

Suction apparatus

This is connected to the vacuum pipeline. The apparatus consists of a collector jar, filter, float, gauge in the patient circuit indicates the airway pressure.

Oxygen pressure failure safety valves

Some anaesthetic machines have a pressure safety system (fail-safe system). The fail-safe system consists of a master pressure regulator which controls slave pressure regulators present in the nitrous oxide line. It is situated between the gas inlet of the anaesthetic machine and the device that controls and measures gas flow. The regulator valve shuts off the nitrous oxide if the pressure in the oxygen line falls below a preset value.

Method of metering and releasing the gases

The gas is directed to the flow delivery unit from the gas supply via the fail-safe system. There are two ways for the delivery and control of gas mixture: a gas mixing and a gas proportioning system.

Most anaesthetic machines use a gas mixing technique in which the flow rate of each gas is independently controlled and measured by a delivery unit. In most machines, the delivery unit is made up of a needle valve and a variable orifice flowmeter. The needle valve acts as a flow controller and a means of turning gas on and off.

In a gas proportioning system, the gases delivered are set in definite ratio.

Flowmeters (Fig. 6.8)

The commonest flowmeter used in the anaesthetic machine is a tapered glass tube containing a bobbin, which indicates the flow rate on a scale engraved on the tapered glass tube. Gas flow is introduced at the bottom of the rotameter tube. As the flow increases, the flow indicator rises.

Flow control valves (needle valves)

The needle valve is placed at the bottom of the corresponding flow tube. It has an on/off function, in addition to regulation of gas flow rate.

High flow oxygen flush (Fig. 6.9)

Sometimes during anaesthesia, it is necessary to fill

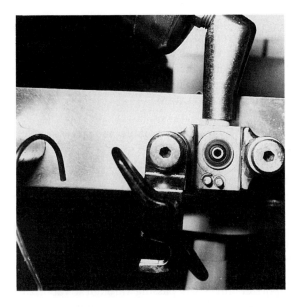

Fig. 6.6   Pin-Index system.

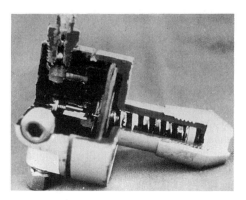

Fig. 6.7   Pressure reducing valve (cross-section).

pressures at the downstream end of the machine, flow restrictors are introduced in the gas line before the needle valve. This valve protects the machine rather than the patient.

Pressure gauges

Pressure gauges are attached to the anaesthetic machines in two places, one at the gas inlet side to indicate the pressure in the gas cylinders or pipelines, and the other in the patient circuit. The

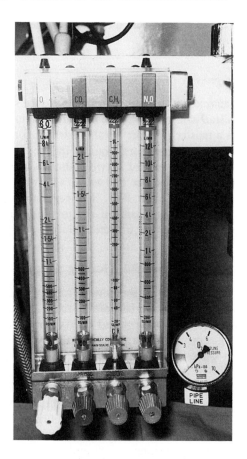

Fig. 6.8 Flowmeters. Conical shaped with flow control valves (needle valves) at the bottom which regulate the flow of gases.

the breathing system with oxygen at a higher rate than the rotameter can deliver. This situation arises when there is a leak between the face mask and the patient's face, or in an emergency. Oxygen is delivered at a high pressure (20–45 psi) at the rate of 30–70 litres/min.

Method of vaporizing volatile anaesthesia agent

Vaporizers

A vaporizer is a device which adds the necessary concentration of anaesthetic vapour to a stream of carrier gas (oxygen and nitrous oxide).

The saturated vapour pressure (SVP) (p. 99) of a volatile anaesthetic such as halothane at room temperature is many times higher than that necessary to produce anaesthesia, hence the vaporizer mixes gas passing through a vaporizing chamber with gas containing no vapour to produce a final mixture with the appropriate concentration. This is carried out by splitting the flow of gas to the vaporizer into two streams—one stream passes through the chamber containing the volatile anaesthesia agent and the other bypasses the chamber. Both these streams reunite and are delivered to the patient.

A gas can be made to pass through a vaporizer by applying positive pressure before the vaporizer, e.g. by gas from the flowmeter, so that gas is pushed through as in the plenum vaporizer.

Plenum vaporizer (Fig. 6.10). (The plenum is a chamber in which the pressure is higher inside than it is outside.)

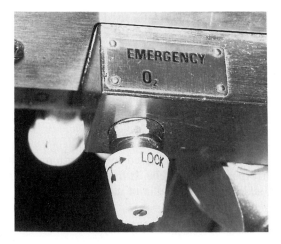

Fig. 6.9 High flow oxygen flush.

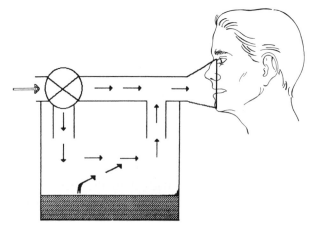

Fig. 6.10 Plenum vaporizer.

A Boyle's bottle is a typical example of the plenum vaporizer. In this vaporizer, the liquid anaesthetic is kept in a glass bottle and a part of the gas flowing through the bypass is controlled by a rotary valve. The problems associated with this type of vaporizer are that the saturation of the gas leaving the chamber depends on the flow rate; and as the anaesthesia agent vaporizes, the temperature falls, which in turn drops the SVP of the agent, thus decreasing the concentration of vapour delivered to the patient.

The development of vaporizers has solved the problem of flow rate dependence and temperature fall.

Flow rate dependence. It is overcome and full saturation achieved effectively by placing fabric

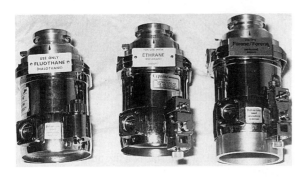

Fig. 6.11 Mark 3 vaporizers. Left to right, halothane, enflurane, isoflurane.

wicks or metal in the vaporizing chamber, one end of which dips into the anaesthetic liquid while the other end projects into the chamber. This method is used in most vaporizers, e.g. Abingdon, Fluotec vaporizers.

Temperature control. Modern vaporizers are made of metal which has good thermal conductivity and which therefore allows heat to be transferred from the surroundings to the vaporizing chamber.

Temperature compensation. This problem is solved by allowing the splitting ratio of the gas to change with temperature, so that more gas flows through the vaporizing chamber if the temperature falls. This adjustment gives a steady concentration. Most vaporizers contain a temperature-controlled valve which adjusts the splitting ratio. This valve consists of two metals with different coefficients of thermal expansion which are joined together. As the temperature changes, the shape of the two metal strips (bimetallic strip) alters so that it bends or straightens.

This mechanism is seen in Enfluratec, Isotec and Fluotec vaporizers (Figs 6.11 and 6.12).

Vaporizer position and controls. On the anaesthetic machine, the vaporizer is placed between the flowmeter block and the emergency oxygen flush control. This prevents the high flow of oxygen being delivered through the vaporizer.

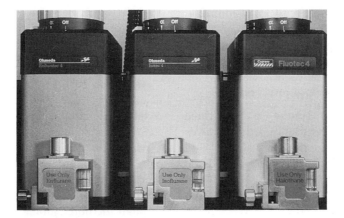

Fig. 6.12 Mark 4 vaporizers. Left to right, enflurane, isoflurane, halothane.

Care of vaporizers. According to the manufacturer's recommendation, the vaporizer needs to be serviced every year. Halothane vaporizers are drained and refilled at regular intervals (weekly) to prevent accumulation of preservatives such as thymol in the vaporizing chamber.

It is essential to fill vaporizers with the correct anaesthetic liquid and to prevent accidental filling of vaporizers with the wrong liquid. A safety system is available. This consists of filter tubes and caps which only fit the appropriate bottles of anaesthetic and vaporizers.

Equipment for delivering vapours and gases

Anaesthetic breathing systems

The words 'breathing system', or 'circuit', mean an assembly of tubes and valves through which the patient breathes.

Components of a breathing system are:

a. Tubing: Made of rubber to which carbon is added to impart conductivity, it has flexible corrugated walls so that it can bend into acute angles without kinking.
b. Rubber reservoir bag: It is a compliant bag which allows accumulation of gas during expiration so that a reservoir for peak volumes is available for the next inspiration. The other use of this bag is a visual monitor in a spontaneously breathing patient, to facilitate ventilating the apnoeic patient manually.
c. Valves: The anaesthetic circuits may contain either non-breathing, unidirectional breathing or adjustable pressure-limiting valves. Non-breathing valves are attached close to the patient. The valve discs and springs are tight, to reduce resistance.

In the circle absorber system (p. 149) three valves exist; two unidirectional breathing valves and the adjustable pressure-limiting valve.

In 1954, W W Mapleson classified anaesthetic breathing systems into five groups: A, B, C, D, E. These are classed as semi-closed systems in which partial rebreathing may occur.

Mapleson A (Fig. 6.13). The most commonly used version is the Magill circuit. It is effective in

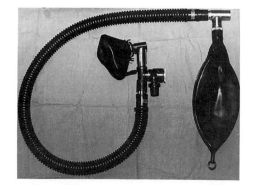

Fig. 6.13   Magill circuit (Mapleson A system).

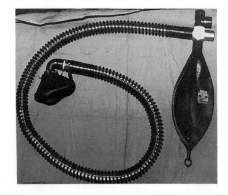

Fig. 6.14   LACK circuit (note the non-breathing valve away from the patient).

patients breathing spontaneously and is not ideal for IPPV.

A modification of Mapleson A circuit is the LACK circuit (Fig. 6.14), which consists of a long tubing which lies inside a corrugated tube making up a co-axial circuit. Through the inner tubing expiration occurs and inspiration takes place through the outer tubing.

A fresh gas flow rate equivalent to the patient's total minute volume is required in these circuits.

Mapleson B and C. These systems are more efficient than the Mapleson A during IPPV. Mapleson C circuit (Fig. 6.15) is usually seen in the recovery room.

Mapleson D. The Bain co-axial system (Fig. 6.16) is the commonest version of Mapleson D. In this system, the fresh gases pass through the inner tubing to the patient and expired gases pass through the outer tubing.

During spontaneous ventilation, the fresh gas flow should be about 2.5 times the minute volume

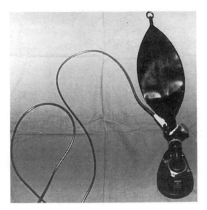

Fig. 6.15 Mapleson C circuit (see in the recovery room).

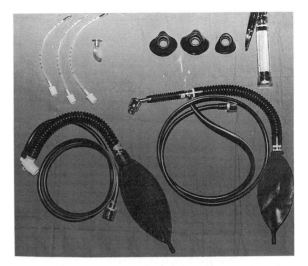

Fig. 6.17 Top row: Paediatric ET tubes, airway, Rendall Baker mask. Bottom row: Jackson Rees modification of Ayres T piece.

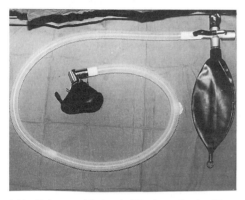

Fig. 6.16 Bain co-axial circuit (Mapleson D circuit).

of the patient. For IPPV, a fresh gas flow of 75–80 ml/kg/min is adequate.

Mapleson E. Also known as Ayres T-piece without a reservoir bag, it is used in babies and children less than 25 kg body weight. The fresh gas flow should be 2.5 to 3 times the minute volume (minimum 4 litres/min). The Ayres T-piece can be used for IPPV, by intermittently occluding the end of the reservoir tube with the thumb.

Mapleson F (Fig. 6.17). This was added by Jackson-Rees as a modification of Ayres T-piece (an open-ended bag being added to the end of the reservoir limb). It provides a method for carrying out IPPV, and as visual evidence that the child is breathing.

Humphrey A, D, E circuit. This circuit can be effectively used in adults and children, as its principles are similar to the Mapleson A, D, and E systems.

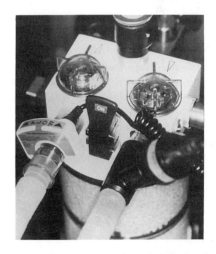

Fig. 6.18 Soda lime absorber (also called Circle absorber).

Circle absorber system (Fig. 6.18). It consists of an inspiratory hose, an expiratory hose, a soda lime cannister, two unidirectional valves, a reservoir bag on the end of a third hose, pressure relief valves and an inflow tube.

In this system, carbon dioxide is removed chemically using soda lime or baralyme.

Soda lime consists of: $Ca(OH)_2$, NaOH, KOH, and silica, with a moisture content of 14–19%.

It is firmly packed in the cannister, avoiding any gaps which can lead to channelling of gases and rebreathing.

Absorption of CO_2 occurs by the following chemical reactions:

$$CO_2 + 2\,NaOH \rightarrow Na_2\,CO_3 + H_2O + Heat$$
$$Na_2CO_3 + Ca(OH)_2 \rightarrow 2NaOH + CaCO_3$$

When the soda lime is becoming exhausted, the indicator, e.g. 'durasorb', changes its colour from pink to white.

Trichloroethylene (Trilene) is not used in soda lime absorber as toxic substances like phosgene, dichloracetylene and carbon monoxide are produced if the vapour comes into contact with hot soda lime granules.

Ventilators

The principle of operation of the ventilator is described by its functional analysis, i.e. how it works during each phase of the respiratory cycle: inspiration, changeover from inspiration to expiration, expiration, changeover from expiration to inspiration.

Inspiration

Ventilators produce inspiration by passing a predetermined pressure (pressure generators) or predetermined flow of gas (flow generators).

Pressure generators. In this type of ventilator, e.g. Manley (Fig. 6.19), the machine delivers gases to the patient at a constant pressure. If there is an increased resistance to the flow due to bronchospasm or kinking of the tube, the gases will not be delivered to the patient.

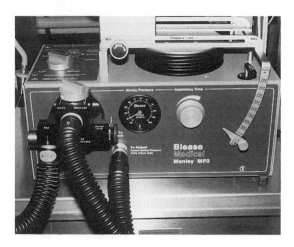

Fig. 6.19 Manley ventilator.

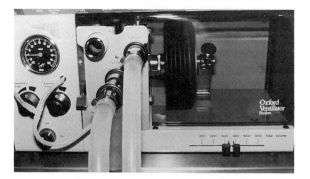

Fig. 6.20 Oxford ventilator.

Flow generators. These types of ventilators deliver gases to the patient at a constant flow irrespective of the changing compliance and resistance of the lungs. An example is the Oxford Penlon ventilator (Fig. 6.20), in which the flow of gases is initiated by a piston compressing the bellows.

Changeover from inspiration to expiration

This can occur either by volume cycling (when the predetermined volume is delivered), time cycling or pressure cycling.

Expiration

The patient is allowed to exhale to atmospheric pressure. Some ventilators can provide positive end expiratory pressure (PEEP), to reduce danger of pulmonary collapse.

Changeover from expiration to inspiration

This can occur either by volume cycling, time cycling or pressure cycling.

Scavenging of anaesthetic gases

The pollution of atmospheric air in the operating theatres is due to gas discharged from the ventilators, the breathing circuits, leaks from equipment, and spillage which occurs when filling the anaesthetic vaporizers.

The pollution can have an adverse effect on the staff working in the operating theatre and recovery room.

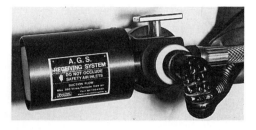

Fig. 6.21 Active scavenging system.

Scavenging of anaesthetic gases can be achieved using:

a. Active systems (Fig. 6.21). This means that active suction is applied near to the expiratory part of the anaesthetic breathing system to remove waste gases. The exhaust is able to accommodate 75 litres/min continuous flow with a peak of 130 litres/min.

b. Passive systems. These allow the venting of patients' expired gas from the anaesthetic system to the outside atmosphere or to a ventilation extract duct. It is important to avoid long tubings.

Alarms

Anaesthetic machines are provided with an oxygen-failing warning device—a battery-powered buzzer activated by a decrease in oxygen pressure.

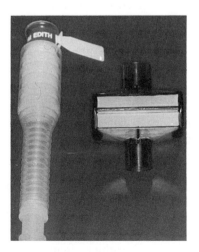

Fig. 6.22 Edith humidifier and condenser.

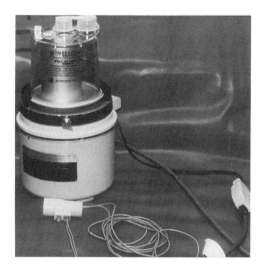

Fig. 6.23 Fischer-Peykel humidifier.

Some devices are activated by the pressure of nitrous oxide to operate a whistle, the valve opens if the oxygen pressure falls.

Humidification of gases

In the operating theatre, inspired gases are humidified using a condensor humidifier, also called an artificial nose (Fig. 6.22). The humidifier conserves the water normally lost on expiration. When the warm, moist expired gases pass through the humidifier they become cooled and the water condenses, only to be evaporated again on the next inspiration. Other systems use a water bath (Fig. 6.23).

Testing anaesthetic machines

Before commencing the anaesthetic, the anaesthetist should test the anaesthetic machine. This ranges from a simple 'tug test' (testing the joints by vigorously pulling on the hoses) to a sophisticated procedure, as follows: (Before starting the tests, the machine is disconnected from all piped medical gas supplies, with oxygen and nitrous oxide cylinders turned off.)

1. Check that full cylinders of O_2 and N_2O are properly attached to the yokes on the anaesthetic machine and that the cylinders are turned off.

2. Open the O_2 and N_2O flowmeter valves; no flows should be seen.
3. Turn on the O_2 cylinder and the O_2 flowmeter registers a flow. If the N_2O flowmeter registers a flow, reject the machine.
4. Turn on the N_2O cylinder and check that the N_2O flowmeter registers a flow. If O_2 flowmeter registers a flow, reject the machine.
5. Set the O_2 failure warning device in operation.
6. Turn off the O_2 cylinder and check that the O_2 failure warning device works.
7. Insert the O_2 probe of the hose into the piped O_2 supply connection at the wall (terminal unit). This must cancel the noise of the O_2 failure alarm. Apply the 'tug test' to this connection.
8. Turn off the N_2O cylinder. See if there is any change in the O_2 flowmeter bobbin setting as the N_2O flowmeter bobbin falls. If the O_2 flowmeter bobbin shows any change, reject the machine.
9. Insert the N_2O probe from the anaesthetic machine into the piped N_2O supply connection at the wall (terminal unit). Apply the 'tug test' to this connection.
10. To complete the check, test for leaks by occluding the outlet from the machine until the pressure relief valve on the backbar is seen or heard to operate. The anaesthetic machine is now ready for use.

Checking the Bain circuit

The end of the little finger or the plunger of a 2 ml syringe is used to occlude momentarily the spout of the inner tube of the Bain circuit while gas is passing through the tube. Sounds indicate if this manoeuvre causes a build-up of pressure and confirms that the inner tube is intact.

PREPARING FOR ANAESTHESIA

Before the patient receives an anaesthetic, it is important to complete this check list:

a. Type of anaesthetic to be given: (i) general,

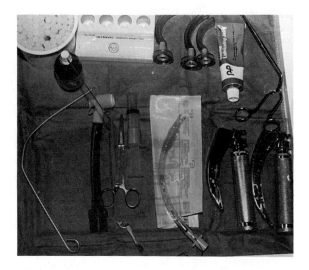

Fig. 6.24 Trolley for endotracheal intubation. Top row: Dental rolls, rack to keep thiopentone, lignocaine spray, Guedel airway. Bottom row: Introducer, catheter mount, artery forceps, syringe for inflation, endotracheal tube, laryngoscopes, short blade, long blade.

(ii) regional
b. Drugs and equipment needed for anaesthesia and monitoring
c. Intravenous fluids and blood for transfusion
d. Postoperative care and recovery facilities.

At the beginning of the operating list, the anaesthetist checks the anaesthetic machine (p. 151) and the equipment which will be used.

An ideal trolley for endotracheal intubation is shown in Figure 6.24. The equipment consists of:

Endotracheal tubes of correct size and a smaller size
Laryngoscopes, small blade and long blade
Endotracheal tube connector
Gum elastic bougies and wire stilette.
Cuff inflating syringe
Magill forceps
Artery forceps
Bandage or tape to secure endotracheal tube
Catheter mount
Local anaesthetic spray (4% lignocaine)
Tube of lubricant
Face masks, breathing circuit
Throat pack.

GENERAL ANAESTHESIA

When administering anaesthesia, it is important to fulfill a triad of anaesthesia, analgesia and muscular relaxation.

INDUCTION OF ANAESTHESIA

A patient can be induced either by intravenous or inhalational technique.

Intravenous (IV) induction

IV induction is suitable for all routine surgical cases and is particularly important during emergency surgery where there is a high risk of regurgitation of gastric contents.

All the drugs necessary for anaesthesia are prepared and the syringes labelled. A butterfly needle or intravenous cannula is inserted in the back of the hand, or a large bore cannula (14G or 16G) is inserted in the forearm vein for transfusion of blood and fluids. Before inserting a large bore cannula, the skin is infiltrated with 1–2 ml of 1% plain lignocaine.

In an emergency, before commencing induction, pre-oxygenation is carried out by administration of 100% oxygen by face mask.

The common induction agents (Fig. 6.25), along with their dosages, are given below:

Thiopentone (Pentothal)	3–5 mg/kg body weight
Methohexitone (Brietal)	1.0–1.5 mg/kg
Etomidate (Hypnomidate)	0.3 mg/kg
Propofol (Diprivan)	1.5–2 mg/kg
Ketamine (Ketalar)	2 mg/kg

The details of induction agents are described on page 58. After attaching the patient to the ECG and blood pressure monitor, induction is commenced. Induction occurs within one arm–brain circulation time (12–30 s) and the anaesthesia is maintained with an inhalational agent (such as halothane, enflurane, isoflurane), oxygen (33%) and nitrous oxide (66%).

The complications which can occur with IV induction are:

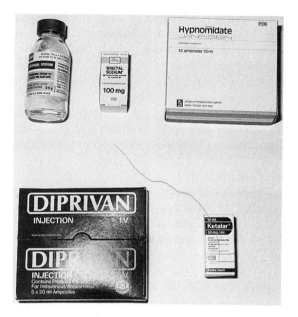

Fig. 6.25 Induction agents. Top row: Thiopentone (Intraval), Methohexitone (Brietal), Etomidate (Hypnomidate). Bottom row: Propofol (Diprivan), Ketamine (Ketalar).

a. Regurgitation and vomiting
b. Injection around vein in the subcutaneous tissue
c. Cardiovascular and respiratory depression
d. Intra-arterial injection of thiopentone
e. Reaction to individual drugs such as hiccup (methohexitone), involuntary movements (methohexitone, etomidate).

Inhalational induction

The indications for inhalational induction are:

a. Uncooperative or very young children
b. Bronchopleural fistula
c. Upper airway obstruction, e.g. epiglottitis
d. Lower airway obstruction with foreign body.

A 'no mask' technique using a cupped hand around the gas delivery tube is used in young children. This hand and later on mask are gradually brought closer to the face until the patient goes to sleep. Initially, high concentrations of halothane (1–4%) or enflurane (1–4%) are used and, once the patient goes to sleep, the concentrations of halothane and enflurane are decreased. Recently, a new device which looks like a telephone has been introduced. The child is asked to speak into the 'phone' as gas is passed through the speaking end of the phone.

Anaesthesia is maintained by firmly placing the mask on the face as consciousness is lost. Once anaesthesia is established, either an oropharyngeal airway (Guedel) or a nasopharyngeal or a laryngeal mask are inserted.

The problems which can occur with inhalational induction are salivation, airway obstruction, laryngeal spasm, hiccups, raised intracranial pressure, and malignant hyperpyrexia (page 190).

MAINTENANCE OF ANAESTHESIA

Anaesthesia can be continued using inhalational agents (O_2, N_2O and volatile agents), total IV infusion anaesthesia (Propofol infusion with air/O_2 mixture) or a combination.

The patient may breathe spontaneously or by ventilation controlled with an endotracheal tube and muscle relaxants.

If a patient is breathing spontaneously, a face mask (with a Guedel or nasopharyngeal airway (Fig. 6.26) or a laryngeal mask are used. In some procedures (dental, ENT) the patient is paralysed with suxamethonium and an endotracheal tube is inserted. Once the patient recovers from suxamethonium, he/she breathes spontaneously.

Endotracheal intubation

The indications for endotracheal intubation are:

a. Operations on the head and neck (e.g. ENT, dental) where a nasotracheal tube may have been inserted.
b. To provide a clear airway.
c. When the patient is going to be in an unusual position, such as prone or sitting, a reinforced, non-kinking tube is used.
d. Protection of the upper respiratory tract from food and vomitus during emergency surgery or from blood during oral and dental surgery.

Before beginning the anaesthesia, the anaesthetist checks appropriate sized endotracheal tubes, and the laryngoscopes.

Endotracheal tubes (Fig. 6.27)

In the majority of hospitals plastic (e.g. Portex, Mallinckrodt) tubes are used and some hospitals continue to use red rubber tubes. In patients who are undergoing surgery in unusual positions (prone, sitting) an armoured tube is used, whereas in plastic surgery preformed RAE tubes are used. In thoracic surgery, a double lumen tube (e.g. Robertshaw) is used (Fig. 6.28). For the sizes and lengths of tubes see Appendix.

An appropriate connector (Fig. 6.29) is required between the endotracheal tube and the anaesthetic circuit, e.g. Magill nasal for nasotracheal tubes,

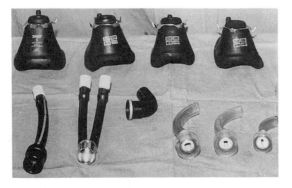

Fig. 6.26 Face masks, catheter mounts, angle piece, Guedel oropharyngeal airway.

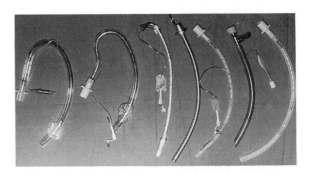

Fig. 6.27 Endotracheal tubes. Left to right: RAE tube, preformed (for plastic), tube with aluminium foil, metal tube, microlaryngoscopy tube, armoured, uncuffed tube.

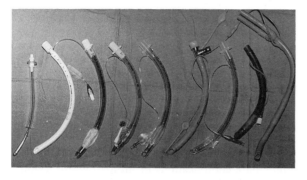

Fig. 6.28 Endotracheal tubes and airways. Left to right: Nasopharyngeal airway, uncuffed ETT, sizes 8 and 9 high volume low-pressure cuff tubes, red rubber tube, Hi-Lo ET tube, armoured tube, Robertshaw tube.

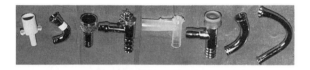

Fig. 6.29 Connectors.

Cobb or Rowbotham connectors for cases where endotracheal suction is necessary. A catheter mount connects the endotracheal connector to either the breathing circuit or the ventilator.

Laryngoscopes (Fig. 6.24)

There are two basic blades, curved and straight. The curved blade (Macintosh) lies anterior to the epiglottis in the vallecula and by lifting exposes the larynx and vocal cords.

The straight blade (Magill) is used in children whose epiglottis is floppy. The blade passes posterior to the epiglottis and lifts it anteriorly exposing the larynx.

Other available laryngoscope blades are the Polia blade, left-handed blade, and blades with a prism. These are used in difficult intubation if a fibreoptic laryngoscope (Fig. 6.30) is not available.

Figure 6.17 shows the Magill laryngoscope for use in children.

Endotracheal intubation is performed: with the patient awake (neonate), under local anaesthesia, after inhalational anaesthesia, blind nasal intubation or with the aid of a fibreoptic laryngoscope or following muscle relaxants.

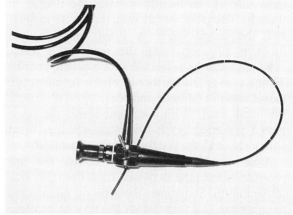

Fig. 6.30 Fibreoptic laryngoscope.

The muscle relaxants used for intubation are suxamethonium (1.5 mg/kg) in emergency surgery or when the patient is allowed to breathe spontaneously. A small dose of non-depolarizing muscle relaxant (gallamine 20 mg) is given before the injection of suxamethonium to avoid postoperative muscle pains in young, fit patients.

Conduct of laryngoscopy

After injecting the induction agent and the muscle relaxant, the patient's head and neck are positioned. The neck is flexed and the head extended with a pillow as a support. This brings the oral, pharyngeal and tracheal axes into one line (Fig. 6.31). The laryngoscope is introduced into the

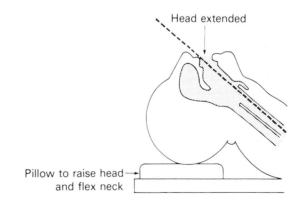

Fig. 6.31 Positioning for laryngoscopy.

right side of the mouth, moving the tongue to the left. The blade passes over the whole tongue, and the laryngoscope is lifted upwards and forwards avoiding using the teeth as a lever. (The teeth can be protected with a plastic guard.) With a curved blade, the tip of the laryngoscope passes into the vallecula and pressure on it exposes the vocal cords. With a straight blade, the tip is passed posterior to the epiglottis, which is lifted anteriorly, and the vocal cords are visualized.

After visualizing the vocal cords, the appropriate sized tube is passed from the right side of the mouth. Sometimes the assistant might have to apply external pressure on the thyroid cartilage to bring the larynx into view. On other occasions, a semirigid stillete (gum elastic bougie) is used to provide the correct degree of curvature of the endotracheal tube to allow intubation. Once in place, the endotracheal tube cuff is inflated to prevent audible gas leak on inflation. The position of the tube is checked by auscultation, to prevent right bronchial intubation.

Some anaesthetists prefer to spray the vocal cords with 4% lignocaine or to have the tubes lubricated with lignocaine jelly.

Nasal intubation

This is carried out for ENT and dental operations. A slightly smaller tube (8.0 mm for man and 7.0 mm for women) is used. This lubricated tube is passed through the right nostril and when it reaches the pharynx, a laryngoscopy is carried out. The tube is passed into the trachea by grasping the tip with Magill intubating forceps or by manipulation of the proximal tube. In dental operations, a moist gauge throat pack is introduced into the pharynx after intubation. A 'tail' of the pack is left protruding from the mouth and the anaesthetist makes a note to remove it at the end of the operation.

Difficult intubation. Difficulty in intubation may be expected or unexpected. As described on p. 139, in the preoperative visit the anaesthetist assesses the patient's airway and, if difficulty is expected, precautions are taken in the form of using a fibreoptic laryngoscope, awake intubation with local analgesia, retrograde intu-

bation using an epidural catheter and a Tuohy needle which is passed through the cricothyroid membrane into the mouth.

If the difficult intubation is unexpected, the anaesthetist uses bougies and manipulates the cricoid pressure; if the patient cannot be intubated in spite of this, he follows a 'failed intubation drill' (p. 182).

Complications of endotracheal intubation. The immediate complications of intubation are trauma to lips, teeth or dental crowns, jaw dislocation, trauma to larynx and vocal cords. If a red rubber tube is used, the cuff exerts a high pressure on tracheal mucosa which can be damaging. Hence, plastic tubes with high volumes and low pressures are used.

ANALGESIA

The patient who is anaesthetized (N_2O, O_2, volatile agent) is given an analgesic intraoperatively in the form of opiates and non-opiates (Fig. 6.32).

The opiates will be alfentanil (Rapifen), fentanyl (Sublimaze), phenoperidine (Operidine), pethidine, nalbuphine (Nubain), morphine or diamorphine. This can be given as a bolus or as an infusion, see page 56 for dosages. The analgesia can be extended into the postoperative period (p. 218).

The non-opiate analgesic used commonly is diclofenac (Voltarol) 1 mg/kg IM.

Analgesics can also be given as regional blocks, epidural and intrathecal opiates (p. 219).

MUSCULAR RELAXATION

Muscle relaxants allow the use of lighter planes of anaesthesia and preservation of autonomic reflexes. Muscle relaxants (with IPPV) are used for major intracranial, thoracic and abdominal operations.

The muscle relaxants are used as follows.

If a difficult intubation is expected or in an emergency, suxamethonium is given after the induction of anaesthesia and endotracheal intubation is completed. Once the effects of suxamethonium wear off, non-depolarizing muscle relaxants are

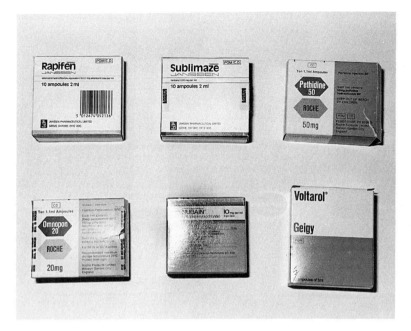

Fig. 6.32   Analgesics. Top row: Alfentanil (Rapifen), fentanyl (Sublimaze), Pethidine. Bottom row: Papaveretum (Omnopon), nalbuphine (Nubain), diclofenac (Voltarol).

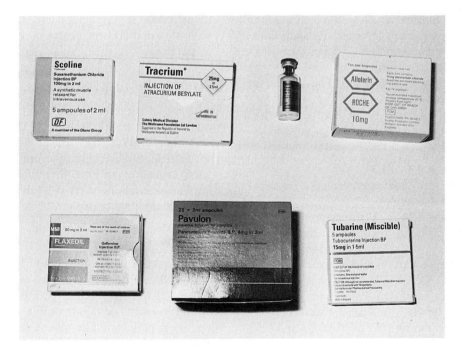

Fig. 6.33   Muscle relaxants. Top row: Suxamethonium (Scoline), atracurium (Tracrium), vecuronium (Norcuron), alcuronium (Alloferin). Bottom row: Gallamine (Flaxedil), pancuronium (Pavulon), Curare (Tubarine).

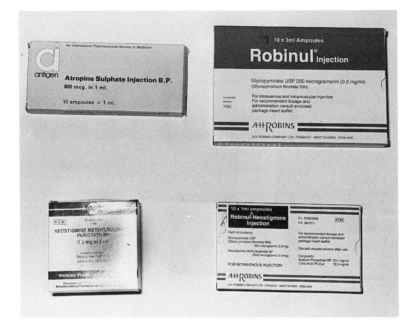

Fig. 6.34 Anticholinergics and anticholinesterases. Top row: Atropine, glycopyrronium (Robinul). Bottom row: Neostigmine, neostigmine plus glycopyrronium.

given. The choice ranges from atracurium (Tracrium), vecuronium (Norcuron), alcuronium (Alloferin) to pancuronium (Pavulon), tubocurarine (Tubarine) (Fig. 6.33). The first two drugs can be given as an infusion. The dosages are mentioned on page 72.

IPPV is maintained by a ventilator which delivers appropriate minute and tidal volume.

During anaesthesia, the following points are checked:

1. Awareness—this can be prevented by using inhalational agents.
2. Adequate anaesthesia. If the patient has received inadequate anaesthesia ('light') he may show signs such as lacrimation, sweating, hypertension and tachycardia.
3. Adequate ventilation. If the patient is inadequately ventilated, he/she may have raised CO_2 levels which cause excessive oozing from the wound, tachycardia and hypertension.
4. Adequate muscle relaxation. If the muscle relaxant is wearing off, the muscle tone increases, the ventilator airway pressure increases. A peripheral nerve stimulator (Fig. 6.45) can detect the degree of muscular paralysis.

END OF SURGERY

At the end of surgery, the residual neuromuscular block is reversed with atropine (0.02 mg/kg) and neostigmine (0.05 mg/kg) (Fig. 6.34). In patients with cardiac disease, glycopyrronium (Robinul) is used instead of atropine to antagonize the side effects of neostigmine such as bradycardia, salivation and abdominal cramps.

Extubation

When spontaneous breathing is resumed, tracheobronchial suction is carried out and extubation carried out in a lateral position (in patients with full stomach) or supine or in a sitting up position (obese patients). The tube is removed during inspiration when the larynx dilates, the cuff is deflated and the tube withdrawn. At this stage, if a throat pack was inserted it is removed before the tube is taken out.

Emergence

Once extubation takes place, the patient receives 100% oxygen by a face mask till he or she is ready to move to the recovery area.

MONITORING DURING ANAESTHESIA

A monitor is 'one who warns', or something that gives warning or reminds. A monitor used during the course of an anaesthetic will measure, display or record the information provided. Some monitors give an alarm if the measured values during anaesthesia fall outside previously defined limits.

It is important to monitor a patient from the time of induction till he/she is discharged from the recovery area. In a fully equipped hospital, monitors are found in the anaesthetic room as well as in the operating theatre. If this is not the case, provision should be made to wheel the monitoring equipment into the anaesthetic room or anaesthetize the patient in the operating theatre.

The anaesthetist is an important monitor, who can care for the patient during anaesthesia, and the instruments used by the anaesthetist:

a. Warn about changes in the state of the patient.
b. Help the anaesthetist in the maintenance of physiological conditions.
c. Warn about the changes in the function of anaesthetic equipment, including the supply of gases and vapours.

Monitoring can be carried out with or without equipment.

Without equipment

The anaesthetist can observe:

a. pupillary size for hypoxia or depth of anaesthesia
b. the breathing pattern, rate, rhythm, and depth
c. the heart rate and peripheral perfusion by feeling the pulse
d. a cold clammy skin, which indicates poor perfusion

e. the rotameters, vaporizer settings and reservoir bag on the anaesthetic machine
f. The anaesthetist can listen to the movements of a ventilator and thus gain warning about disconnection, obstruction or return of spontaneous breathing.

With equipment

All the body systems can be monitored during anaesthesia. The common monitoring, as carried out in everyday working surroundings, is briefly described below.

Cardiovascular system

Electrocardiogram

Two- or three-lead bipolar ECG monitors are used, of which lead II is popular. With the ECG monitors, heart rate and dysrhythmias can be detected. A CM5 lead (lead placed on the fifth intercostal region near the manubrium sterni of the chest) can detect myocardial ischaemia.

Arterial blood pressure

Blood pressure (BP) can be monitored non-invasively or invasively.

Non-invasive monitoring

In routine surgical cases, BP is monitored non-invasively using an oscillotonometer (Fig. 6.35) or an automated oscillotonometer, e.g. Dinamap (Fig. 6.36).

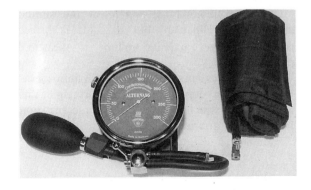

Fig. 6.35 An oscillotonometer.

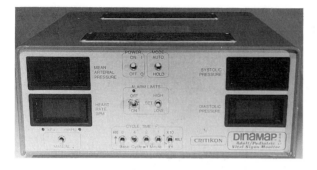

Fig. 6.36 Dinamap.

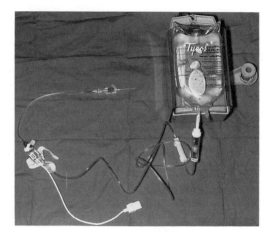

Fig. 6.37 Catheter transducer system.

In an oscillotonometer, the principles of the aneroid pressure gauge are used. It has two cuffs: the upper cuff measures the pressure around the upper arm; the lower cuff measures the pressure differential between the cuffs in order to detect the flow of blood from under the upper cuff. The disadvantage of a non-automated oscillotonometer is that it does not measure the BP when it is low.

An automated oscillotonometer (e.g. Dinamap) consists of a single cuff connected to a display and control box. Inside the box, one length of the tubing is connected to a pump which inflates the cuff and a bleed valve which deflates the cuff. The output from the pressure transducer is connected to either an AC coupled or DC coupled amplifier. This output of the DC amplifier produces a voltage which indicates the pressure in the cuff. The AC coupled amplifier detects oscillations due to blood passing under the cuff. The first oscillations in the cuff are taken as systolic pressure, largest pulsations as mean blood pressure and the least pulsations as diastolic pressure.

The Ohmeda Finapres is a continuous non-invasive BP monitor. It works on the similar principles as Dinamap, but the cuff is placed around a finger and its volume is measured photometrically.

Other instruments available are: Arteriosonde, which uses the doppler ultrasound principle; and Infrasonade, which uses the ultrasonic principle for detecting arterial wall motion.

Invasive monitoring

Direct measurement of BP is the most accurate method. It requires the use of a catheter placed in an artery, associated tubing, pressure transducer and an electronic processor (Fig. 6.37).

All these instruments need to be internally zeroed and transducers are kept at the level of the right atrium during measurement.

The system is affected by the connecting tube between the arterial cannula and the transducer. The terms used are 'underdamping' or 'overdamping'. An 'underdamped trace' shows ringing of waveform with overshooting of systolic and undershooting of diastolic pressures. This occurs due to excessive length of tubing, which can be corrected using a short tubing.

An 'overdamped' trace shows lowered systolic and higher diastolic pressure with an accurate mean arterial pressure. This is due to air bubbles in the tubing, which need to be removed to give accurate results.

The indications for direct intra-arterial monitoring are:

a. Cardiac surgery, aortic surgery, carotid surgery
b. Aneurysmal repair in the brain
c. Thoracic surgery, requiring one-lung ventilation
d. For controlled hypotensive technique (induced hypotension, see p. 183).

The arterial sites used are: radial, ulnar, brachial, axillary, femoral or dorsalis pedis arteries. When the radial artery is cannulated,

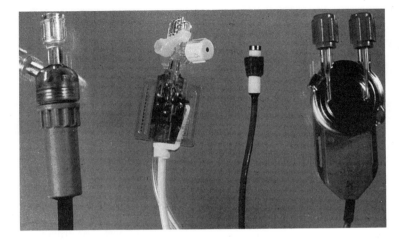

Fig. 6.38 Transducers.

Allen's test is performed before the insertion of cannula to detect the adequacy of collateral blood flow from the ulnar artery.

A number of transducers are available (Fig. 6.38). The catheter transducer system is filled with heparinized saline. 500 IU of heparin are added to 500 ml of normal saline, which is connected to the catheter transducer system after being pressurized by a bag. The pressure in the bag is maintained at 50 mmHg above the systolic pressure. The flush releases 1–3 ml/h saline into the cannula to keep it patent.

Central venous pressure (CVP)

CVP is the pressure in the right atrium and it reflects the volume entering it (preload). The CVP is normally less than 6 mmHg.

A central venous catheter can be inserted either through the internal or the external jugular vein in the neck or subclavian or cephalic veins. Either a single lumen or a triple lumen catheter is inserted. A guide wire is passed into the vein after localization; the catheter is passed over it and the wire is removed (Seldinger technique).

The indications for CVP monitoring are:

a. Assessment of blood volume in septic shock, hypovolaemic shock
b. Difficult venous access
c. In cardiac tamponade, lung disease

d. Neurosurgery (craniotomy in sitting position, see p. 126).

A CVP reading higher than 6 mmHg indicates increased volume, pulmonary hypertension, pneumothorax, left heart disease or tricuspid stenosis.

A CVP less than 6 mmHg indicates hypovolaemia or a normal variation during respiration.

During IPPV, at the end of expiration and in spontaneous ventilation at the end of inspiration, the CVP is low.

The complications associated with central venous cannulation are pneumothorax, air embolism, carotid artery puncture and thoracic duct injury (when CVP is carried out on the left side).

The waves seen in the CVP are: an *a* wave due to atrial contraction, a *c* wave due to bulging of tricuspid valve into the right atrium, and a *v* wave due to right atrial filling.

Pulmonary artery pressure monitoring (PAP)

Pulmonary artery pressure monitoring devices were made popular by Swan and Ganz in the 1970s using multilumen, balloon-tipped, radio-opaque catheters. These are passed via the internal jugular vein or subclavian vein, passing the right atrium and right ventricle into the pulmonary artery (Fig. 6.39).

A pulmonary artery balloon-flotation catheter is shown in Figure 6.40.

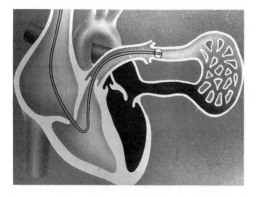

Fig. 6.39 A multilumen balloon-tipped flotation catheter which has been passed through right atrium and right ventricle into pulmonary artery.

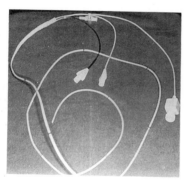

Fig. 6.40 A typical pulmonary artery balloon flotation catheter.

The indications for PAP monitoring are:

a. Cardiac surgery, valve replacement, coronary artery bypass
b. Shock requiring massive blood transfusion, inotrope therapy
c. Severe pulmonary disease, requiring surgery
d. Acute myocardial infarction, cardiomegaly.

The PAP catheter is connected to a pressure–transducer system via the tubing containing heparinized saline. The internal jugular vein or subclavian vein is located and a dilator sheath introduced over a guide wire (Seldinger technique). The PAP catheter is introduced, once the sheath and wire are removed through a protective sheath. As the PAP catheter passes through various cham-

Fig. 6.41 Tracings when the PA catheter passes through various chambers of the heart. RV = right ventricle, PA = pulmonary artery, PCWP = pulmonary capillary wedge pressure.

bers of the heart, the tracing changes (Fig. 6.41). Once the catheter is in the pulmonary artery, the balloon is inflated to get a wedge pressure reading. (Pulmonary capillary wedge pressure = PCWP.) The PCWP reflects the pressure in the left atrium (after load).

The complications associated with insertion of a PAP catheter are similar to CVP monitoring, along with infarction of the pulmonary artery if the balloon is inflated for long periods.

The pressures in various chambers of the heart are listed in Table 6.3.

Table 6.3 Pressures in the heart.

	Systolic pressure (mmHg)	Diastolic pressure (mmHg)	Mean
Right atrium	—	—	−2 to +6
Right ventricle	15–30	0–5	5–15
Pulmonary artery	20–25	10–15	0–12
Left atrium	—	—	0–12
Left ventricle	100–140	60–90	70–105

Cardiac output measurement

Cardiac output is measured by the thermodilution principle using a pulmonary artery catheter (see above). The other methods available are dye dilution, the Fick principle or use of a flowmeter.

Respiratory system

Pulmonary ventilation

This can be effectively monitored as follows:

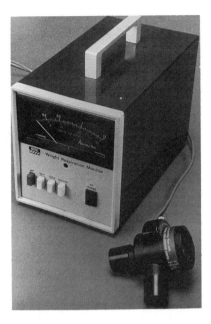

Fig. 6.42 Wright respirometer.

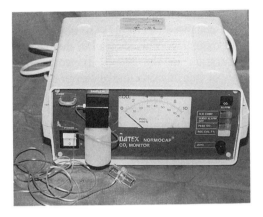

Fig. 6.43 Capnograph (end tidal carbon dioxide monitor).

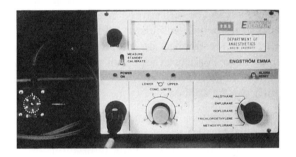

Fig. 6.44 Engström Emma vapour analyser.

Movement of the chest wall. Impedance plethysmography and inductance plethysmographs are used for research purposes.

Movement of air in and out of the lungs. It can be detected using: (i) Fleisch tube respirometer, which has a fixed orifice principle; water vapour condensation gives inaccurate results. (ii) Wright respirometer (Fig. 6.42) which uses the turbine principle. It is a simple instrument. The other example in this category is the Magtrak, which is an electronic form of the Wright respirometer.

Airway pressure. Measurement with either an aneroid gauge or an electric manometer is the most effective way of detecting a disconnection in the patient circuit in a patient receiving IPPV.

Composition of respired gases:

1. Oxygen concentration of the inspired gas. This can be measured using oxygen analysers with either fuel cells, polarographs or paramagnetic analysers.
2. Carbon dioxide concentration in the expired gas (end-tidal). This measures the adequacy of ventilation during anaesthesia. The values of CO_2 seen on a capnograph, a CO_2 monitor (Fig. 6.43), are an indirect measure of the arterial P_{CO_2}.

A sudden fall in end-tidal P_{CO_2} may be due to apnoea, cardiac arrest, pulmonary embolus or air embolism (see p. 180). The capnograph is also useful in detecting the correct placement of an endotracheal tube.

3. Mass spectrometry. This powerful machine, when used, analyses up to eight gases and vapours simultaneously. This is only available in large centres and acts as a research tool.
4. Anaesthetic gases and vapours: All volatile anaesthetic agents have absorption bands in the infrared spectrum. Instruments such as Datex Normocap and Engström Emma (Fig. 6.44) use this principle. The instruments detect all the anaesthetic vapours.
5. Arterial blood gases. In major surgical procedures, such as cardiac or thoracic, arterial blood

gases are estimated at regular intervals when the lungs are collapsed (see p. 178) to allow surgery.

6. Pulse oximetry. This shows the degree of oxygen saturation in the blood. It works on the principle of transmission and absorption of light of various wavelengths across the finger. This device has become highly popular and is seen in anaesthetic rooms, operating theatres and recovery areas.

7. Measurement of transcutaneous Pco_2 and Po_2. By applying CO_2 and O_2 sensitive electrodes to the skin, indirect measurements of arterial gases are made.

Neuromuscular junction

The degree of neuromuscular block using muscle relaxants can be effectively measured using a peripheral nerve stimulator (Fig. 6.45). The electrodes are applied on the skin at the wrist (ulnar nerve) or lateral aspect of the knee (lateral popliteal nerve). There are three types of stimulus which can be applied.

a. Single impulse. This can be used to detect if the patient has recovered from a single dose of suxamethonium following intubation.
b. Tetany. This involves stimulating at 50–100 Hz; post-tetanic facilitation is defined as stimulating the nerve with 50 Hz for 1 s followed by a single twitch. If the patient has residual paralysis due to a non-depolarizing relaxant, the height of the response to a single twitch will be higher than the tetany.
c. Train of four. Four stimuli at 0.5 Hz are given over a period of 2 s. In a patient who

has been given a non-depolarizing muscle relaxant, the twitches will be successively reduced.

Measurement of temperature

Body temperature (core and peripheral) are measured using thermistors or thermocouples (p. 104) in operating theatres. Temperature probes are inserted in the oesophagus (to measure core temperature), nasopharynx (brain temperature); or are attached to the toe (peripheral temperature).

Measurement of blood loss

Blood loss can be measured by observing the degree of bleeding, weighing the swabs (1 ml of blood = 1 g) and measuring the volume of blood collected in the suction bottle. As a rough guide, if a swab is lightly stained, blood loss is 5 ml, 10 ml if moderately stained, 15 ml if heavily stained. Three abdominal packs heavily soaked can contain about 500 ml.

The other methods of measuring blood loss are colorimetric methods, haemoglobin extraction dilution methods.

Measurement of urinary output

Urinary output can be measured using an indwelling catheter in prolonged surgery or where severe blood loss is anticipated. Roughly, the amount of urine excreted per hour is 0.5–1.0 ml/kg body weight.

Cerebral function and monitoring depth of anaesthesia

To detect cerebral hypoxia, an electroencephalogram is valuable, while a cerebral function analysing monitor (CFAM) can be used to assess the depth of anaesthesia.

REGIONAL ANAESTHESIA

History

Cocaine was the first anaesthetic agent introduced into medical practice by Koller in 1884. Uhlmann

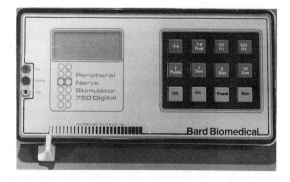

Fig. 6.45 A peripheral nerve stimulator.

and Merscher introduced nupercaine in 1929, and lignocaine was synthezised in 1943 by Lundquist and Lofgren. See page 71 regarding mode of action of local anaesthesia agents.

Although there are a number of regional techniques, only those which are carried out frequently are described here.

General considerations

Before commencing regional techniques, it is essential to check that equipment for resuscitation is ready (anaesthetic machine, drugs such as thiopentone, suxamethonium, midazolam, ephedrine, and endotracheal tubes) and that an indwelling intravenous cannula is inserted in the vein.

BLOCKS OF UPPER EXTREMITY

Brachial plexus block (BPB)

Anatomy. The brachial plexus is formed from the anterior primary divisions of C5, C6, C7, C8 and T1. It forms the motor and sensory nerve supply to the arm (see p. 17 for details).

Indication. The BPB is carried out for blocking the upper extremity and shoulder.

Technique. The brachial plexus can be blocked by one of the following methods:

Interscalene approach. The patient lies supine with head rotated to the opposite side of the block. The cricoid cartilage (C6) is felt and the finger moved laterally till the interscalene groove is felt posterior to the sternomastoid muscle at this level. A 2.5 cm needle is inserted in the groove, and once paraesthesia is elicited approximately 20–30 ml of 0.5% plain bupivacaine is injected after negative aspiration.

Supraclavicular approach. The aim of this approach is to block the brachial plexus at the midclavicular point between the skin and the first rib. The patient lies supine with head rotated to the opposite side of the block and the arm and shoulder depressed. A needle is inserted through a weal 1 cm above the midpoint of the clavicle. The direction of the needle being downwards, in-

wards and backwards. If paraesthesia is felt, the needle is stabilized and 30 ml to 40 ml of 0.5% plain bupivacaine is injected after a negative aspiration. If paraesthesia is felt, anaesthesia is rapid, if not it takes 20 min.

Axillary approach. In the axilla, the nerves of the brachial plexus and the axillary artery are enclosed in a fibrous neuromuscular facial sheath. The aim of the axillary block is to inject the local anaesthetic around the axillary artery into the fibrous neurovascular sheath. The patient lies supine with the arm abducted at a right angle, the skin of the axilla is shaved, cleaned and a weal raised at the highest point of the axilla at which arterial pulsation is felt. Through the weal a 2.5 cm needle (blue needle) is inserted until a click is felt which shows that the needle has entered the neurovascular sheath. After negative aspiration, 30 ml of 0.5% plain bupivacaine or prilocaine is injected. It takes about 30 min for the block to be effective.

Advantages. In the interscalene and axillary approach, the dangers of pneumothorax are avoided. There is a single landmark for the axillary approach, i.e. axillary artery.

Disadvantages. In the interscalene approach there is a risk of injection into the cervical epidural space, the CSF or the vertebral artery.

In the supraclavicular approach there is a high incidence of pneumothorax, puncture of the subclavian artery, and paralysis of the phrenic nerve.

Wrist block

Indication. It is carried out for blocking the digits in tendon repair. Median, ulnar, and radial nerves supply the wrist.

Technique. Circular lines of intradermal and subcutaneous infiltration are carried out just above the wrist joint.

Total intravenous regional analgesia (TIVR) (Bier's block)

TIVR consists of injection of a local anaesthetic into a vein of a limb which has been made ischaemic by a tourniquet. The site of action of the drug is on the peripheral nerve endings.

Indication: It is carried out for operations on arms and also on legs.

Technique: A butterfly needle or a Venflon is inserted into a vein on the dorsum of the hand and firmly secured. The limb is drained of blood by elevation for 5 min or by using an Esmarch's bandage. A double cuff is placed on the upper arm, and the upper cuff inflated to a pressure a little above the systolic blood pressure before removing the tourniquet. Approximately 40 ml of 0.5% prilocaine (Citanest) is injected, and for 5 min the lower cuff is inflated and the upper one released to minimize discomfort.

Cuff deflation should be done slowly, at least 30 min after the injection. Signs of local anaesthesia agent toxicity (see p. 71) can be seen if the cuff is deflated before this period passes. The patient is carefully observed for 10 min after the release of the cuff.

Contraindications. The contraindications are sickle-cell disease, scleroderma, Raynaud's disease.

BLOCKS OF LOWER EXTREMITY

Femoral nerve block

This is carried out for pain relief following a fractured neck of the femur.

Technique. A weal is raised, just below the inguinal ligament, a finger breadth lateral to the femoral artery. A needle is inserted for 3–4 cm and 20 ml of 0.5% plain bupavacine is injected.

Sciatic nerve block

Carried out for reduction of fractures around the ankle and in combination with femoral nerve block for ligation of varicose veins.

Technique. The patient lies on the sound side with the hip slightly flexed. There are a number of approaches to this block and a rough guide to the position of the sciatic nerve is the midpoint of a line joining the posterior superior iliac spine to the ischial tuberosity. After eliciting paraesthesia, 10–20 ml of 0.25% plain bupivacaine is injected.

Ankle block

Carried out for reduction of fractures, toe surgery or postoperative analgesia.

The nerves which supply the ankle are the anterior tibial nerve, musculocutaneous nerve, saphenous nerve, sural nerve and posterior tibial nerve.

These nerves can be blocked by a subcutaneous and intradermal weal raised circumferentially around the ankle between the medial and lateral malleolus behind the malleoli.

The total amount of local anaesthesia agent used is 20–30 ml of 0.5% plain bupivacaine.

SPINAL ANALGESIA

History. The first spinal analgesic was given by Leonard Corning in New York in 1885. First planned spinal analgesia for surgery was undertaken by August Bier in 1898, using cocaine.

Indications

a. Orthopaedic surgery, hip replacements, knee replacements
b. Urological surgery, transurethral resection of prostate
c. Haemorrhoidectomy, vaginal repair
d. Obstetric anaesthesia.

Contraindications

a. Blood clotting disorders
b. Local skin sepsis
c. Deformed backs
d. Abnormality of nervous system, e.g. expanding cerebral lesion, tumour or cyst
e. Patients with enlarged prostate coming for other surgery.

Technique

The patient is told of the procedure which is to be undertaken, and an informed consent is obtained. The anaesthetic room and the equipment necessary for resuscitation is kept ready.

The equipment necessary for conducting spinal analgesia comprises: 22–26 gauge spinal needles with introducer; 2 ml and 5 ml syringes, swabs, swab-holder, antiseptic solution (chlorhexidine) and sterile towels.

The aim of the block consists of entering the lumbar dural sac and injecting the local anaesthetic directly into the cerebrospinal fluid below the termination of the spinal cord. Spinal analgesia can be performed in two positions: (a) lateral and (b) sitting.

Lateral position

The patient is placed with the back at the edge of the table (which can be tilted), parallel to it, knees flexed on to abdomen, head flexed into chest. The hips and shoulders are kept parallel to the table to avoid rotation of the vertebral column.

After preparing the skin, and covering with the towels, the landmarks are identified. The line joining the highest points of the iliac crests which crosses the interspace between L4 and L5 is chosen. (L1 is avoided, because the spinal cord ends here.)

A skin weal is raised at the chosen level and a small incision made to prevent the core of skin being carried out into the intra- or extradural space by the spinal needle.

A Sise introducer, or a 19 gauge needle, is inserted through which the spinal needle is introduced. The needle is then slowly pushed forward at right angles to the back. It passes through the following layers:

> Skin
> Subcutaneous tissue
> Interspinous ligament
> Ligamentum flavum
> Epidural space
> Theca (dura mater).

When the dura mater is pierced, a click is often felt, followed by a free flow of cerebrospinal fluid (CSF) on withdrawal of the stylet. Once the CSF is flowing freely, the local anaesthesia agent is injected.

Sitting position

The patient (especially if obese or pregnant) is placed across the table with feet resting comfortably on a stool. The patient places his/her arms on the assistant's shoulder with spine flexed and chin pressed on the sternum. The procedure as described in the lateral position is carried out during the insertion of the spinal needle.

This position is also helpful if perineal surgery is planned.

Local anaesthesia drug. The local anaesthetic, 0.5% hyperbaric bupivacaine (Marcain) 1–4 ml, is injected. Once the drug is injected in the CSF, the patient is placed in the required position without delay, tilting the table as necessary. For abdominal surgery, the table is levelled as soon as the analgesia reaches the umbilicus (T10) and it should finally reach the subcostal arch (T6–T8).

Other drugs which can be used are: heavy cinchocaine (Nupercain), 1–2 ml; lignocaine 5%, 0.8–1.5 ml.

Factors influencing the height of spinal analgesia:

a. Dose of drug injected: The higher the concentration and dosage, the longer its effect lasts.
b. Position of patient: If the patient is sitting, hypobaric solution tends to rise and hyperbaric solution tends to fall.
c. Volume of fluid injected: The height of analgesia is directly proportional to the amount of local anaesthetic agent.
d. Rate and force of injection: A slow gentle injection is necessary to get good effective block.
e. Barbotage (to mix): By withdrawal and injection of the CSF, the drug is distributed widely.

Physiology of spinal analgesia

1. Nervous system. At the outset of spinal analgesia, the nerve fibres blocked are in this order:

   > Autonomic preganglionic B fibres.
   > Temperature fibres
   > Pinprick fibres
   > Touch fibres
   > Deep pressure fibres
   > Fibres carrying vibratory and proprioceptive impulses.

   During recovery, sympathetic activity returns before sensation.
2. Respiratory system. Phrenic nerve (C3, C4, C5) paralysis can occur, leading to apnoea. The patient is unable to cough effectively and the breathing becomes quiet.
3. Cardiovascular system. Blood pressure fall is seen in the first 20 min after spinal

anaesthesia, which could be due to vasodilatation and depression of vascular smooth muscle.

The heart rate also slows, along with the fall in blood pressure. It is seen if the spinal block reaches T4–T5.

Treatment consists of intravenous fluids, oxygen by face mask, IV ephedrine 5 mg–30 mg, atropine 0.2–0.6 mg or glycopyrronium 0.2 mg if there is bradycardia.

4. Gastrointestinal system. The small gut is contracted owing to vagal influence. Nausea and vomiting can occur due to hypotension, increased peristalsis or traction on the nerve endings in the viscera.

Treatment consists of correcting hypotension, reassurance, antiemetic (metoclopramide 10 mg IM or IV).

5. Genitourinary system. Hypotension can lead to a decreased blood flow. Post-spinal retention of urine, requiring catheterization, may be seen.

6. Body temperature. Vasodilatation causes heat loss, and absence of sweating can lead to hyperpyrexia in hot climates.

Complications during spinal analgesia

Nausea and vomiting
Hiccups
Precordial discomfort
Hypotension
Restlessness
Failed spinal analgesia.

Sequelae

Headache. It is seen in the first 72 hours postoperatively in patients who have endured repeated attempts with spinal needle or the use of a large bore needle. It starts in the occipital region and is made worse by sitting or erect posture.

Treatment consists of (i) oral rehydration, (ii) avoiding strong light, (iii) aspirin. If the headache is severe owing to slow leak of CSF:

— an epidural catheter is inserted through which 1 litre of Hartmann's solution is injected over 24 hours.

— an epidural blood patch with 10–20 ml of autologus blood is administered (patient's own blood injected aseptically in the epidural space).

Retention of urine. This can be treated with either carbachol 0.5–1 mg IM or catheterization.

Paralysis of 6th cranial nerve. Sometimes seen between the fifth and 12th postoperative day in the form of squint, double vision and headache. The patient is treated with bed rest and hydration.

EPIDURAL ANALGESIA (EXTRADURAL BLOCK)

History. It was introduced by Corning in 1885 and made popular in Britain by Massey Dawkins.

Anatomy

The epidural or extradural space lies between the spinal dura mater and the vertebral canal with a diameter of 0.5 cm. Its boundaries are, superiorly, the foramen magnum, inferiorly, the sacrococcygeal membrane, anteriorly the posterior longitudinal ligament and posteriorly the anterior surfaces of the laminae.

The contents of the epidural space include the dural sac, spinal nerve roots, the epidural plexus of veins, spinal arteries, lymphatics and fat.

The epidural space is a potential space with a negative pressure.

Indications

Upper abdominal operations
Lower abdominal operations, such as hernia repair
Operations on the lower limb
Obstetric anaesthesia and analgesia
Postoperative pain relief.

Contraindications

These are the same as for spinal analgesia.

Technique

The patient is told of the procedure and an informed consent is obtained. Equipment necessary

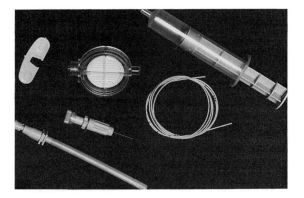

Fig. 6.46 An epidural mini-set showing Tuohy needle, catheter, filter and loss of resistance syringe.

for resuscitation is kept ready and an intravenous cannula is inserted into a vein. The patient is placed in either a lateral or a sitting position (see technique for spinal analgesia).

The back is painted with antiseptic solution and covered by fenestrated towel (towel with a hole to expose the area of needle insertion). The area chosen varies from L1/L2 interspace to L3/L4.

A 16 or 18 gauge Tuohy needle is inserted through the interspace chosen. The needle passes through: skin, subcutaneous tissue, supraspinous and interspinous ligament, ligamentum flavum, epidural space.

The following signs indicate that the needle is in the epidural space:

a. Sudden ease of injection of air or normal saline from a freely running syringe attached to the needle.
b. Sudden loss of resistance to the syringe (Portex loss of resistance syringe).
c. Deflation of Macintosh's epidural space indicator balloon.

Equipment (Fig. 6.46). Sterile pack consisting of towels, Tuohy needle, syringes (10 ml, 20 ml, Portex loss of resistance syringe, catheter and filter).

Local anaesthesia drug

Once the Tuohy needle is in the epidural space, a catheter is inserted through the needle and taped to the skin after removing the needle.

A test dose of 3–5 ml of either 1% lignocaine or 0.25% plain bupivacaine (Marcain) is injected and, if there is no evidence of accidental spinal analgesia, the remaining solution is injected as follows: bupivacaine 0.25% plain 10 ml for obstetric analgesia; and 20–30 ml for abdominal operations, depending on the extent of block required.

Site of action of local anaesthetic. When the local anaesthesia is injected in the epidural space, analgesia is brought about by direct action either on the nerve roots in the epidural space or on the nerve roots in the subarachnoid space.

The nerve fibres which are blocked are anterior and posterior nerve roots, mixed spinal nerves, white and grey rami communicantes.

Factors influencing the spread of epidural analgesia

1. Age of the patient (the elderly require less than the young)
2. Volume of solution
3. Speed of injection.

Management of patient during epidural anaesthesia

The problems and management during epidural analgesia and anaesthesia are similar to those of spinal analgesia.

Complications:

a. Hypotension, which is corrected with IV fluids, ephedrine
b. Inadequate block, which needs to be corrected or supplemented with general anaesthesia
c. Total spinal analgesia, which is treated with IPPV.

Sequelae

— Paraplegia
— Anterior spinal artery syndrome.

INTRAVENOUS FLUIDS

Most patients coming for elective operations are denied food and water for 8–12 h preoperatively. This can result in a considerable loss of water and electrolytes. Water is lost via the kidneys, lungs and skin and a small amount through the gastrointestinal tract. That portion of water lost from the skin and lungs is called 'insensible loss' (which ranges from 800–1000 ml/day in a normal adult). Water is excreted as urine at the hourly rate of 1 ml/kg body weight (about 1700 ml in a 70 kg adult).

Routine IV therapy in elective operations

It is essential to give one third to one half of the estimated fluid requirement during the course of a major operation in the adult, the solutions used being dextrose saline or Hartmann's solution. The maintenance fluid is given at the hourly rate of 2 ml/kg during surgery.

Fluid therapy in dehydrated patient. The patient's degree of dehydration is assessed (see p. 192) and fluids given accordingly.

BLOOD: CONSTITUENTS, TRANSFUSION AND BLOOD SUBSTITUTES

The amount of blood in the human body is approximately 8% of the total body weight. Normal human adult blood volume is 4.5–5.0 litres.
  The functions of blood are:

a. Transport functions: (i) nutrients from the gastrointestinal tract to the cells; (ii) oxygen from the lungs to the cells; (iii) waste products from the cells to the organs of excretion; (iv) heat formed in the more active tissues to all parts of the body thus helping in the regulation of body temperature; (v) hormones transported to all parts of the body.
b. Acid–base balance
c. Immunological reactions.

Constituents of blood

From these functions it can be seen that the blood is a complex fluid containing the nutrients absorbed from the alimentary canal, the oxygen taken up in the lungs, the waste products produced by cellular activity, the hormones, the antibodies, and other substances. It is also clear

that the composition of the blood varies with place and time.
  The composition of blood is as follows:

— plasma (a light yellow liquid), about 55% of the blood volume
— water, 90%
— dissolved solids.

a. Three proteins forming from 6–8% of the plasma are serum albumin (4.5%), serum globulin (2.0%) and fibrinogen (0.3%). They contribute to the viscosity and, to a lesser extent, to the osmotic pressure of the blood. Fibrinogen plays a major role in coagulation. Of the three forms of globulin (alpha, beta and gamma), gammaglobulin is concerned with the immunization of the body against foreign cells and substances.
b. Supplies for cells: glucose (0.1%), fat, amino acids and salts.
c. Cellular products: enzymes, antibodies, and hormones.
d. Cellular waste products (nitrogenous) such as urea and uric acid.

  Gases: oxygen, carbon dioxide, nitrogen.
  Formed elements: these constitute about 45% of the blood volume. They are: red blood cells (RBC, or erythrocytes), carriers of oxygen and carbon dioxide; white blood cells (WBC or leucocytes), scavengers and immunizing agents; platelets, essential for blood coagulation.

Indications for blood transfusion

a. When a person loses considerable amounts of blood owing to haemorrhage, a transfusion is necessary to save his life. The guidelines are loss of 10% or more of blood volume in a child, and loss of 15% or more of blood volume in an adult.
b. To treat anaemias or some blood deficiency such as haemophilia and thrombocytopenia.

Unfortunately, the bloods of different people are not all exactly alike, and failure to transfuse the appropriate type of blood is likely to cause death of a recipient. Hence, it is necessary to know the physiology of blood grouping and matching before giving transfusions.

One of the reasons one person's blood may not be suitable for another person is that the recipient may be allergic to some of the proteins in the blood cells of the donor.

Antibodies in the recipient's plasma can cause agglutination (clumping) and haemolysis (rupture) of the injected cells.

Blood groups

The transfusion of blood became possible after Landsteiner described the main groups of the ABO system in 1900.

The A and B antigens—the agglutinogens:

Two different but related antigens—type A and type B—occur in the cells of different persons. Because of the way these antigens are inherited, a person may have neither of them in the cells, or may have one or both simultaneously.

Some bloods also contain strong antibodies called agglutinins that react specifically with either the type A or type B antigens in the cells, causing agglutination and haemolysis. Because the type A and type B antigens in the cells make the cells susceptible to agglutination these antigens are called *Agglutinogens*.

Table 6.4 Blood groups and their constituent agglutinogens and agglutinins

Blood group	Agglutinogens	Agglutinins
0	–	Anti-A and Anti-B
A	A	Anti-B
B	B	Anti-A
AB	A and B	–

In transfusing blood from one person to another, the bloods of donors and recipients are normally classified into four major groups O, A, B, AB, as illustrated in Table 6.4, depending on the presence or absence of the two agglutinogens.

When neither A nor B agglutinogen is present the blood is group O, when only type A agglutinogen is present the blood is group A. When only type B agglutinogen is present the blood is group B, and when both A and B agglutinogens are present the blood is group AB.

Blood typing

Prior to transfusion, it is necessary to determine the blood group of the recipient and the group of the donor blood so that the bloods will be appropriately matched.

Table 6.5 Blood, plasma and their products available for transfusion.

Presentation	Indication	Useful points
1. Whole blood: Blood 420 ml + acid citrate dextrose 120 ml	a Acute or chronic haemorrhage b. Blood dyscrasias such as aplastic anaemia	For routine preservation, acid citrate dextrose (ACD) is the anticoagulant of choice. Blood life expires in 21 days
2. Concentrated red cells	a. Anaemias in which increased haemoglobin rather than blood volume is needed b. Transfusion in patients with heart failure	Blood life expires in 21 days
3. Freshly drawn whole blood	a. Helpful in exchange transfusion in neonates b. In patients with bleeding owing to thrombocytopenia	Blood life expires in 21 days. It gives viable RBCs and platelets

4. 'Washed' red cells (leucocyte poor)	a. In patients selected for, and post organ transplantation b. Patients with immune deficiency diseases or receiving massive irradiation c. Paroxysmal nocturnal haemoglobinuria	When manual techniques are used, this form is viable for 6 h
5. Fresh frozen plasma (FFP)	a. Haemophilia b. After massive transfusions c. To correct overdose of oral anticoagulants	Chances of serum hepatitis B are increased. The thawed FFP should be used immediately
6. Plasma protein fraction (PPF) concentrate	a. In burns b. To increase the fluid volume	Hepatitis virus is inactivated and the shelf life is 2 years.
7. Albumin (Human albumin)	Hypoalbuminaemia	There is no risk of hepatitis and it should be used within 3 months of preparation
8. Cryoprecipitate	Factor VIII deficiency	There is an increased risk of hepatitis B. Preparation lasts for 3 months
9. Fibrinogen	Low fibrinogen levels following massive bleeding, defective clotting (disseminated intravascular coagulation)	Risk of hepatitis B high
10. Platelet concentration	a. Low platelets (below 40 000/mm^3) before major surgery b. Following massive transfusion c. Bleeding associated with low platelet count	Platelets retain their activity for 2–3 days at 4°C
11. Leucocyte transfusions ('Buffy coat')	a. Leucopenia (low WBCs) in patients on cytotoxics b. Severe infection c. Primary granulocytopenia	Cell separator used on donor blood

Storage and handling of blood (Table 6.5)

Blood for transfusion should be stored at the correct temperature of 4°–6°C. The refrigerator is fitted with an automatic temperature recording device and a battery-operated alarm system. The temperature limits must be rigidly observed, to preserve the red cells and minimize the multiplication of chance bacterial contaminants. Food and pathological specimens must never be stored in the blood refrigerator. Blood for transfusion should not be out of the refrigerator for more than 30 min before transfusion, otherwise it should be discarded.

Bags of blood which have been partly used should always be discarded. Packed red cells, unless concentrated in a sterile plastic transfer pack, must be used within 12 hours, similarly reconstituted plasma, fibrinogen or albumin should be used within 3 hours.

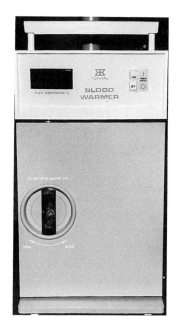

Fig. 6.47 Blood warmer.

Hazards of transfusion

1. Bacterial contamination
Even under aseptic conditions, 2% of stored blood is contaminated by Gram-negative bacteria. Hence blood should be stored at 4–6°C and should be discarded once out of the refrigerator for more than 30 min.

2. Febrile reactions
These are due to pyrogens—polysaccharide products of bacterial metabolism which used to be present in the blood bottles—and have decreased considerably since the use of disposable bags and transfusion sets.

3. Allergic reactions
They occur in 1–2% of all transfusions, and can be controlled with antihistamines such as chlorpheniramine (Piriton).

4. Transmission of disease
In the past, malaria, syphilis, brucellosis and, serum hepatitis were fairly common, but with a careful history and serum tests brucellosis, malaria and syphilis can be excluded. Serum hepatitis and recently, acquired immune deficiency syndrome (AIDS) seem to be the cause of concern in haemophiliac patients who receive multiple factor IX concentrates and cryoprecipitates. HTLV-3 screening has recently been carried out to exclude this virus. Screening of donors for Australian antigen may eventually exclude the hazard of serum hepatitis B, which occurs in 2–5% of blood transfusions in the UK.

5. Incompatibility
Is a term used in transfusion in which the survival of transfused cells is reduced. Normally, the half-life of transfused cells is 32 days, but in 30% of the transfusions the red cells survive only 14–16 days.

6. Acidity of stored blood
Acid citrate dextrose (ACD) blood has a pH of 7.1 and becomes much more acidic (pH 6.6) when stored. Massive transfusion with this type of blood can cause severe metabolic acidosis.

7. Citrate toxicity
Stored blood contains 120 ml ACD solution. Rapid transfusions of large volumes may cause metabolic acidosis, leading to cardiac arrhythmias in patients with severe shock, liver failure or in newborn babies.

8. Problems with cold blood
Administration of cold blood to anaesthetized patients or children can cause hypothermia and cardiac arrhythmias. Hence blood should be warmed, using a blood warmer, during transfusion (Fig. 6.47).

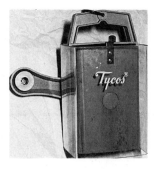

Fig. 6.48 Pressure infusor.

9. Haemolytic reactions

These reactions are due to incompatibility of blood groups and occur in 0.2–0.3% of transfusions.

10. Potassium toxicity

Freshly drawn and stored blood contains approximately 4–5 mEq/litre of plasma potassium, which increases up to 30 mEq/litre by the expiry date.

Blood filters are routinely used during blood transfusion, to prevent microaggregates from the stored blood entering the patient's circulation. For massive blood transfusion in a short time, a pressure infusor is used (Fig. 6.48).

Method of detection of a blood transfusion reaction

If a minor allergic or febrile reaction occurs during a blood transfusion, an antihistamine such as chlorpheniramine (Piriton) is given, and the transfusion continued cautiously.

If a severe febrile or haemolytic reaction is detected or suspected, the transfusion is stopped, and the remainder of the transfused blood and the giving set returned to the blood bank, accompanied by a fresh specimen of blood from the patient.

The basic scheme followed is:

Reports of grouping,
cross-matching, and the blood bag
label are checked

↓

Blood grouping and
cross-matching of the post-
transfusion blood from
patient is repeated

↓

Transfusion set is cultured
for organisms

↓

Transfusion bag is
cultured for anaerobic
or aerobic organisms.
Expiry date of blood bag
is checked

↓

Urine from the patient
is examined for
haemoglobin and
breakdown products.

Table 6.6 Plasma substitutes (volume expanders).

Presentation		Indication	Useful points
1.	Dextran 110 Dextran 70 Dextran 40	a Effective blood or plasma substitute	Maintain blood volume for up to 3 days
		b Dextran 40 (low molecular weight) prevents sludging of RBCs in deep vein thrombosis	Interfere with cross-matching, hence blood should be taken for cross-match before giving dextran
2.	Cross-linked Gelatin (Haemaccel)	Shock due to haemorrhage burns, etc.	It has similar viscosity and osmotic pressure as plasma, and does not interfere with cross-matching.
3.	Hetastarch (Hespan)	Volume expander	Remains in the body for 24–36 h. Is contraindicated in bleeding disorders
4.	Gelofusine	Volume expander	

SPECIALTIES OF ANAESTHESIA

ENT anaesthesia

Most of the patients undergoing ENT surgery are children and young adults, and a number of operations are performed as day cases. The airway (mouth, pharynx) is shared by both the surgeon and the anaesthetist. The important procedures carried out are:

Adenoidectomy and tonsillectomy

Premedication consists of trimeprazine (Vallergan) or diazepam (see p. 141 for details). An oral endotracheal tube is passed after inhalational or IV induction. In adults, nasotracheal intubation is preferred for tonsillectomy.

Postoperative analgesia is given and tracheal extubation carried out with patient slightly head down in a lateral position.

For the management of the postoperative bleeding tonsil see p. 198.

Nasal operations

Submucous resection, rhinoplasty, submucous diathermy and excision of nasal polyps are the common nasal operations.

A standard general anaesthetic employing an oral endotracheal tube and spontaneous or controlled ventilation is employed. A throat pack is inserted during surgery and the patient is positioned 10 degrees head up.

Preoperatively, the nose is prepared by the surgeon using cocaine, lignocaine and adrenaline to decrease the vascularity of the nose.

Microlaryngoscopy

Anaesthesia is induced and a small size (5.5 or 6.0 mm) cuffed ET tube is passed; this allows the surgeon to examine the larynx (Fig. 6.28). Either intermittent suxamethonium or atracurium is used for relaxation of the vocal cords.

Laryngectomy

If respiratory obstruction is expected, then inhalational induction is used and intubation with a small size tube carried out. When the larynx is

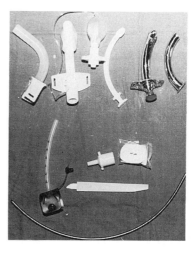

Fig. 6.49 Tracheostomy tubes. Top row: Plastic tracheostomy tubes with introducer and metal tracheostomy tube. Bottom row: Mini tracheostomy set.

dissected out, a sterile tracheostomy tube and connections are kept ready before the trachea is divided (Fig. 6.49). The patient's lungs are ventilated with 100% oxygen for 2 min, the tracheal tube is withdrawn into the larynx, the tracheostomy tube is inserted by the surgeon in the divided trachea and secured firmly. Anaesthesia is carried out through the tracheostomy tube till the end of the surgery.

Laser surgery

A laser is used to remove tumours or polyps from the vocal cords. Because the laser beam ignites polyvinyl chloride (PVC), the microlaryngoscopy tubes are either wrapped with protective silver foil or metal tubes are used (Fig. 6.26).

All personnel in theatre are advised to wear protective spectacles to prevent retinal damage.

Myringotomy

Children and some adults with secretory otitis media undergo examination of the ears, together with myringotomy and insertion of grommets under general anaesthesia. As these patients are treated as day-stay cases, spontaneous ventilation with a face mask is used.

Middle ear surgery

For middle ear surgery, hypotensive anaesthesia (p. 183) is employed. A standard general anaesthesia is administered and a non-kinking oral endotracheal tube passed. The operative site should be bloodless, hence blood pressure is reduced using IPPV, halothane or isoflurance with a 10 degrees head-up tilt. Sometimes drugs such as trimetaphan (Arfonad) or labetalol (Trandate) are employed to cause a fall in blood pressure.

Dental anaesthesia

Dental extractions are carried out on an outpatient basis in a majority of cases; a few are admitted as inpatients.

The majority of patients requiring outpatients' anaesthesia are children who are either too young to be cooperative with local analgesia or who are mentally handicapped.

Induction of anaesthesia is inhalational in the majority of children. Halothane is introduced early during induction with oxygen (30%) and nitrous oxide (70%).

A mouth prop and a throat pack are inserted by the dentist once the jaw relaxes. The anaesthetist observes the reservoir bag and makes sure that the airway is not blocked by the pack and that mouth breathing is avoided. At the end of the procedure, the pack is removed and the patient is transferred to the recovery room. After complete recovery, the patient is discharged.

The problems associated with dental anaesthesia are:

a. Sharing the airway. The anaesthetist overcomes this by holding the jaw forward with the middle and ring fingers of both hands and holding the mask with both thumbs.
b. Horizontal/sitting position. A sitting-up position in the dental chair can cause hypoxia due to fainting, and in a horizontal position blood and debris can pass down the throat cavity.
c. Arrhythmias. In approximately 25–30% of patients transient arrhythmias such as ventricular extrasystoles are seen.

Intravenous induction using methohexitone is employed and a nasotracheal intubation may be re-

quired in adults presenting for dental extractions who either have oral infection, which prevents the use of a local anaesthetic, or who are mentally handicapped.

Inpatient anaesthesia for extraction of wisdom teeth or maxillofacial surgery requires general anaesthesia with a nasotracheal tube and throat pack.

Patients anaesthetized for maxillofacial surgery receive antiemetics as a routine measure.

Paediatric anaesthesia

There are a number of anatomical and physiological differences between adults and children. A few major features are listed here:

Anatomy and physiology. The larynx is higher in children (C3–C4) than in adults. The epiglottis is floppy, and a straight laryngoscope blade elevates the epiglottis to visualise the vocal cords (C5–6). Respiration is rapid (about 30/min in the newborn to 16–20/min in a 2-year-old child) and tidal volume is 7 ml/kg. Mean heart rate ranges from 140 beats/min in the neonate to 100 beats/min in a 6-year-old. Babies do not tolerate bradycardia, as cardiac output depends on heart rate. Blood pressure is around 90/60 mmHg, reaching 120/70 mmHg at around 16 years of age. Blood volume at birth is 90 ml/kg, reaching 80 ml/kg in the infant and 75 ml/kg in a 6-year-old child. Blood transfusion is recommended if the blood loss exceeds 10% of blood volume.

The daily fluid requirements are 100 ml/kg in infants below 10 kg body weight, between 10 and 20 kg 1000 ml and 50 × (wt in kg −10) ml/kg in a child below the age of 1 year. One quarter strength saline is used and then half-strength saline, or Ringer lactate. Buretrols are used for IV infusion.

Neonates lose body heat rapidly from the exposed head, hence the operating theatre temperature is raised to reduce this heat loss. A fall in body temperature can to lead to respiratory depression, a fall in cardiac output and prolonged action of drugs.

Anaesthetic management

The child is premedicated according to body weight (see p. 142). Anaesthesia is induced with an inhalational, IV or IM technique. Inhalational induction is carried out directly by mask or by placing the T-piece in the anaesthetist's hands.

IV induction is made pain-free by the application of EMLA cream on the back of hands 30–45 min preoperatively. An Ayres T-piece is used for short periods of spontaneous ventilation with a fresh gas flow 2.5 times the minute volume of the child, i.e. tidal volume times respiratory rate (TV × RR).

Jackson Rees' modification of the T-piece consists of an open-ended reservoir bag which can be used for IPPV. The fresh gas flow on the anaesthetic machine is adjusted as follows: 1000 ml + 100 ml/kg body weight per minute. A minimum gas flow of 3 l/min is required for this system.

The endotracheal tube (ETT) used for intubation should be small enough to allow a slight leak of gases during IPPV, and the size of ETT is calculated as age in years ÷ 4 + 4.5 (see p. 252 for tube sizes). The narrowest part of the child's airway is at the cricoid ring, as compared to adults (vocal cords). A cuff on the ETT is not necessary in children below 9 years of age. Figure 6.16 shows the equipment necessary for paediatric anaesthesia.

Monitoring. In addition to observation of the patient, a precordial or oesophageal stethoscope is an essential monitor. The intensity of heart sound picked up by the stethoscope varies with the stroke volume, which in itself acts as an indicator of cardiac output.

Other monitoring devices such as temperature probe, ECG and blood pressure monitors are used.

Drugs

The routine drugs used for adult anaesthesia are also used in children. Postoperative analgesia is prescribed either as paracetamol elixir for mild to moderate pain; to nerve blocks such as caudal epidural or penile block for circumcision; to ilioinguinal block for herniotomies and orchidopexy. Opiates such as papaveretum (Omnopon) or pethidine are given for severe pain.

Neonatal anaesthesia

Neonates coming for surgery are at a great disadvantage because their temperature maintenance mechanisms are immature. The incubator and operating theatre temperatures are increased during the surgical procedure, and the baby's temperature is monitored.

Awake intubation is carried out in a premature baby, and IPPV is commenced with a small concentration of inhalational agents. Drugs are prepared in 1 or 2 ml syringes and a 22 g or 24 g cannula is inserted intravenously. A three-way tap is attached for injection of drugs, plasma and blood.

One of the commonest operations carried out in the neonate in a district general hospital is repair of pyloric stenosis. The babies are 3–8 weeks old and dehydrated and metabolically alkalotic (see p. 234) due to vomiting. An IV infusion is commenced, dehydration and acid base imbalance are corrected and a nasogastric tube is passed. An IV induction and ET intubation are carried out and, as it is a short surgical procedure, intermittent suxamethonium or atracurium are given.

Other specific operations in the neonate are for tracheo-oesophageal fistula, diaphragmatic hernia, exomphalos, hydrocephalus and myelomeningocele.

Ophthalmic anaesthesia

Patients presenting for eye surgery are at the extremes of age. Children present with squint and for examination under anaesthetic for congenital glaucoma. Young adults present with perforating eye injuries and diabetic complications of the eye, and the elderly present with cataract and glaucoma.

The problems associated with ophthalmic anaesthesia are: oculocardiac reflex and maintaining intraocular pressure.

a. Oculocardiac reflex. Bradycardia or cardiac arrest can occur following traction on the internal rectus muscle or pressure on the eyeball. Adequate cardiac monitoring is essential. Prevention of bradyarrhythmias consists of IV injection of atropine 0.3 mg or glycopyrrolonium 0.2 mg.
b. Maintaining intraocular pressure. Ideally, the eye should be soft before the anterior chamber is opened. If the pressure is high, it is lowered by deliberate hypotension or hyperventilation using volatile anaesthetics such as isoflurane and mannitol.

A general anesthetic with IPPV is preferred for the majority of cases. Antiemetics, such as prochlorperazine, are given intramuscularly. Some unfit patients or those who prefer it, are given a local analgesic.

Day-stay anaesthesia

Day-stay surgery has become popular because of the short waiting time for surgery and the recovery of patients in their own home. A common day-stay unit consists of a separate ward using the hospital's main operating theatre complex.

Patients in the fitness grade ASA 1 or 2 undergoing operations which do not cause undue haemorrhage and severe postoperative pain are selected.

A letter is sent to the patient undergoing day-stay surgery, describing what she or he should expect. It also includes the following instructions:

a. Patients should not eat or drink for 6 hours before the operation (for 4 hours in children).
b. Patients should be accompanied home.
c. Patients should not drink, drive or work on machinery for 24 h after the operation.

Premedication is avoided to prevent hangover effects; young children are prescribed diazepam and EMLA cream.

Surgery is performed mostly under general anaesthesia and on some occasions regional blocks such as brachial plexus block, individual nerve blocks, intravenous regional anaesthesia, caudal block or penile block are used. Induction agents with the least hangover effects, such as propofol, methohexitone or etomidate, are used. Anaesthesia is maintained with N_2O, oxygen and halothane, enflurane or isoflurane. If an endotracheal intubation is required, atracurium or vecuronium are used. Some anaesthetists use suxamethonium for intubation and maintenance of the procedure. As suxamethonium can cause 'muscle pains', it is essential that a small dose of a non-depolarizing muscle relaxant (such as gallamine 10–20 mg) is used to prevent it. Nowadays, a number of anaesthetists use 'laryngeal masks' to prevent sore throats. Analgesia is provided by short acting analgesics such as fentanyl, alfentanil or diclofenac (Voltarol). When the patient is fully recovered,

oral analgesics such as paracetamol, co-proxamol or co-dydramol are prescribed. Certain patients may require analgesics such as pathidine or papaveretum for severe pain and may even need to be admitted.

Before they are discharged all the day patients are seen by the anaesthetist and once again warned against driving or drinking in the next 24 hours.

Thoracic anaesthesia

The common conditions requiring thoracic surgery are carcinoma of the bronchus, carcinoma of the oesophagus, metastatic disease requiring resection and certain non-malignant conditions. After preoperative assessment and investigation, the patients are prepared for surgery by carrying out physiotherapy, rehydration and correction of acid–base imbalance.

The diagnostic procedures carried out are as follows.

Bronchoscopy

This is carried out using either a fibreoptic bronchoscope or a rigid bronchoscope.

Fibreoptic bronchoscopy is carried out using local anaesthetic solution, or the scope is passed via the endotracheal tube in an anaesthetized patient. Rigid bronchoscopy is carried out by the thoracic surgeons to locate bronchial tumours and for removal of foreign bodies. The most commonly used rigid bronchoscope is the Negus.

A general anaesthetic technique is recommended. In children, deep inhalational anaesthesia with N_2O/O_2 halothane is used, the bronchoscope being passed while the child breathes spontaneously. In adults, intermittent propofol or methohexitone are used to keep the patient asleep and suxamethonium to maintain paralysis.

IPPV is maintained using Venturi bronchoscope injectors. The jet of gas entrains air and produces inflation of the lungs. Expiration occurs through and round the bronchoscope.

Oesophagoscopy

Rigid oesophagoscopy is used to locate oesophageal tumours, to dilate the structures and remove foreign bodies. A general anaesthestic is given. A crash induction technique is employed because of the potential of regurgitation on induction of anaesthesia. A smaller size endotracheal tube is passed to allow the oesophagoscope to pass through the cricopharyngeal sphincter.

Mediastinoscopy

The mediastinoscope is introduced through a small incision in the suprasternal notch. It allows direct inspection and biopsy of mediastinal lesions. A general anaesthetic technique using endotracheal tube and IPPV is employed.

Principles of one-lung anaesthesia

In an awake spontaneously breathing subject lying on one side, the lung nearer to the table (dependent lung) is better perfused with blood supply and has better ventilation. In an anaesthetized patient lying on one side, the functional residual capacity (FRC) is decreased and the upper lung receives better ventilation. During surgery, the upper lung is allowed to collapse to allow better surgical access. This leads to shunting, as the upper lung still receives blood supply but no ventilation. During lung surgery, the diseased lung is uppermost and the dependent lung receives an increased blood flow. In oesophageal surgery, in patients who may have two healthy lungs, collapsing one lung can lead to high intrapulmonary shunting. The intrapulmonary shunting can lead to a fall in arterial oxygen tension (P_aO_2). A P_aO_2 of 9 kPa is acceptable during one-lung anaesthesia. This is achieved by increasing the inspired oxygen concentration to 40% (FIO$_2$, 0.4), adding a positive end-expiratory pressure (PEEP) of 3–5 cm H$_2$O.

The PEEP improves the arterial oxygenation by increasing the functional residual capacity (FRC) in the dependent lung.

Thoracotomy

Double lumen tubes, such as Robertshaw or Carlen bronchocaths (Fig. 6.28), are used to provide separate channels for ventilation and suction of both lungs. A left-sided tube is used for surgery on the right lung. Anaesthetic technique consists of insertion of a large bore IV cannula and induction with a suitable agent.

If the intubation is going to be difficult, suxamethonium is used, otherwise a large dose of non-depolarizing muscle relaxant is used. After the insertion of a double-lumen tube, anaesthesia is maintained with nitrous oxide, oxygen, opiates, and volatile anaesthetic.

ECG and arterial blood pressure (non-invasive) are monitored in the majority of cases. In a few patients who are poor risk or in whom massive haemorrhage is expected, an arterial line and a CVP line are inserted. A warming blanket, blood warmer and temperature monitors are used. The patient is placed in the lateral position, with the diseased side uppermost. Oesophageal surgery is performed with the patient in the lateral or semilateral position.

Analgesia is maintained with IV opiates or intrathecal morphine or extradural opiates.

At the end of thoracotomy, a drain is placed in the pleural cavity to prevent air or fluid accumulating in the thorax in the postoperative period. The lung is reinflated before the thorax is closed and after the closure, the drains are connected to an underwater seal.

The patients are allowed to breathe spontaneously after extubation and are given humidified oxygen (concentration of 40%).

Surgical procedures carried out on the lung are:

Pneumonectomy. This is carried out when a bronchial carcinoma has affected more than one lobe. The bronchus is divided and sutured. The pleural cavity is not drained and the space is filled with serosanguinous fluid and fibrosis.

Bronchopleural fistula. This is a connection between the pleural cavity and the bronchial tree which may occur due to breakdown of a bronchial stump (e.g. following pneumonectomy), trauma, neoplasm.

The patient is dehydrated and toxic owing to the presence of infected fluid in the pleural cavity. The patient's healthy lung can be soiled by the infected fluid, hence IPPV is not commenced until a double lumen tube is inserted and the infected area isolated. Inhalational induction is preferred.

Lobectomy. This is performed for bronchial neoplasm or bronchiectasis. A double lumen tube is used for anaesthesia. When the lobe has been removed, the bronchus is clamped and divided and the remaining part sutured or stapled.

Other surgical procedures carried out on the thorax are:

Repair of hiatus hernia. A left-sided thoracotomy is performed. Either an ordinary endotracheal tube or a double-lumen tube is used.

Oesophageal myotomy. Heller's operation is carried out in the presence of achalasia. This condition results in gross dilatation of the oesophagus with collection in it of large volumes of undigested food. Anaesthetic technique consists of crash induction following treatment with H_2 antagonists and antacids.

Surgery for carcinoma of the oesophagus. If the tumour is in the lower third, a left thoraco-abdominal incision is used. Since the patients are anaemic, dehydrated and hypoproteinaemic, the anaesthetic technique should suit their physical condition.

Neurosurgical anaesthesia

In intracranial operations, the special problems involved are:

Raised intracranial pressure
Maintenance of the airway
Posture such as head-up, sitting or lateral
Length of the operation.

Normal intracranial pressure is about 130 mm H_2O of CSF and the factors which increase the pressure are:

Pressure from outside such as bony tumour
Space occupying lesion such as abscess, neoplasm or haematoma
Cerebral oedema
Venous obstruction
Arterial dilatation due to hypercarbia.

The factors which decrease the intracranial pressure are:

Following blood loss
Following dehydration.

Cerebral blood flow is regulated by the following agents:

a. Arterial CO_2 tension: a rise in P_{CO_2} (8–11 kPa) increases cerebral blood flow (CBF) by 100%, whereas a fall in CO_2 to 3.5 kPa reduces CBF to 30%.
b. Arterial blood pressure: CBF is not altered if the blood pressure is maintained between 90 and 180 mmHg.
c. Anaesthetic agents such as nitrous oxide, halothane and ketamine increase the cerebral blood flow.

Neurological investigations such as carotid angiography, computerized axial tomography (CAT) are nowadays carried out under local analgesia. Children and uncooperative, anxious or confused adults require a general anaesthetic.

Anaesthesia

The patients are assessed preoperatively and, if there are signs of raised intracranial pressure, sedatives and narcotics are withheld. A smooth induction with thiopentone is carried out along with a short-acting analgesic such as alfentanil to prevent fluctuations in blood pressure. Vocal cords are sprayed with 4% lignocaine and an armoured cuffed endotracheal tube is passed. A throat pack may be inserted. IPPV with muscle relaxants, maintaining a P_{CO_2} around 3.5 kPa is achieved. Monitoring consists of ECG, intra-arterial blood pressure, CVP (using a drum catheter), end-tidal CO_2 and precordial stethoscope.

Most craniotomies are performed in the supine, brow-up position, posterior fossa surgery is carried out in the sitting position. The head is shaved under anaesthesia, with the patient in the surgical position.

Air embolism. It occurs in 2–30% of patients in the sitting position. Many of the veins in the back of the neck and scalp do not collapse after they have been divided. During neurosurgery, if air enters the veins, it goes via the right side of the heart to the pulmonary artery, resulting in a mill wheel murmur. The patient develops sudden cyanosis, hypotension and tachycardia. Treatment consists of preventing further entry of air into the circulation by compressing neck veins, lowering the head end of the table, oxygenation and keeping the patient on his left side so that bubbles are carried away from the pulmonary artery.

ICP is reduced during anaesthesia using 20% mannitol (0.2–0.5 g/kg body weight) or frusemide 1 mg/kg.

Elective ventilation is carried out in patients who are expected to develop cerebral oedema, otherwise residual neuromuscular blockade is reversed.

Some of the specific operations carried out are:

Intracranial aneurysm surgery. Preoperatively hypertension is treated, a smooth induction and intubation are carried out. Deliberate hypotension is carried out to lower the systolic blood pressure to 50–60 mmHg for short periods.

Hypophysectomy. Pituitary gland is removed for tumours of the gland or for the treatment of metastatic hormone-sensitive tumours. Tracheal intubation can be difficult in patients with acromegaly, hence a 'difficult intubation' set should be made available.

Anaesthesia in head injury cases

Anaesthesia may be needed in patients with head injuries, either for elevation of a depressed fracture, suturing of lacerations or compound fractures of major bones, or laparotomy. A crash induction is carried out, and a cuffed endotracheal tube passed. Necessary precautions are taken to prevent fluctuations in the intracranial pressure.

Obstetric analgesia and anaesthesia

In the labour ward, anaesthetists provide analgesia during labour to the pregnant women and, where indicated, provide anaesthesia for procedures such as caesarean section, removal of retained placenta.

Analgesia

Labour is painful for a variety of reasons such as uterine contractions and dilatation of the cervix. If the pain is abolished, both mother and fetus do well.

The methods of analgesia available during labour are:

Systemic analgesia. This is the commonest method of giving analgesia in about 60–70% of mothers. Pethidine is given IM (dosages 100–150 mg) four hourly until the second stage of labour. The pain relief is inadequate, and babies born to mothers given pethidine may have feeding problems.

Other analgesics which have been used are pentazocine (Fortral) and meptazinol (Meptid).

Inhalational analgesia. This is used widely in the UK and when used properly a large proportion of women get adequate pain relief. The analgesics which are used are as follows:

Entonox: this is a premixed cylinder containing 50% nitrous oxide in oxygen. In antenatal classes, mothers are taught to apply the face mask tightly around the face and to begin inhaling the gas as soon as a contraction is felt. The breathing should be slow and deep. When the contraction ceases, the mask can be taken off.

Trichloroethylene (Trilene) and methoxyflurane were used in the past to achieve analgesia, but they have now been withdrawn. Recently, isoflurane 0.5% has been used with effective results.

Epidural analgesia. It is the most effective method of pain relief during labour. Once the epidural is done and catheter inserted (see p. 168 for details) the anaesthetist gives the first dose of 6–10 ml of 0.25% plain bupivacaine (Marcain). Further top-ups are given by the midwives every 2–4 hours.

Analesgia for vaginal delivery can be effectively given using either a spinal block (see p. 166) or caudal block. Manual removal of the placenta can be achieved effectively by using either an epidural or a spinal block.

Anaesthesia for caesarean section

The indication for caesarean section may be elective or emergency but the anaesthetic procedure is the same in both cases.

The problems associated with pregnancy and anaesthesia are:

Full stomach. More than half the pregnant mothers have gastric contents of more than 40 ml with a pH below 2.5 owing to delayed gastric emptying.

In a number of labour wards, either Mist. mag. trisilicate 15–30 ml every 2 hours or 30 ml of 0.3M sodium citrate are given to increase the pH to above 2.5. The gastric volume can be decreased by giving either cimetidine 200 mg IM or ranitidine 50 mg IV or IM.

Maternal hypotension. If the pregnant mother lies on her back, she can develop hypotension. This is due to the gravid uterus pressing on the vena cava. In some patients, this can be exaggerated.

Anaesthesia can be given either as a regional or a general technique.

Regional anaesthesia. A lumbar epidural or spinal block can be given for elective caesarean section. If the block is already present, it can be used for emergencies. For an epidural block, a catheter is inserted (in a sitting position) and 10 ml of 0.5% plain bupivacaine is injected and the patient is kept sitting for 12 min. Next, the patient is placed supine (with a wedge) and another 15 ml of 0.5% plain bupivacaine is injected slowly to achieve a block up to T6. After an adequate block is established, surgery is commenced.

Spinal anaesthesia using a 25 g or 26 g spinal needle is an effective and quicker way of obtaining anaesthesia in an emergency; 2–4 ml of hyperbaric 0.5% bupivacaine is used. The precautions are the same as on page 166.

Failed intubation

During emergency anaesthesia, intubation of the oesophagus instead of the trachea can lead to the death of the mother.

Tracheal intubation may be difficult owing to:

a. Short neck,
b. Large breasts obscuring the airway
c. Inappropriate application of cricoid pressure

d. Anaesthetist starting to intubate before suxamethonium begins to work
e. Anatomical abnormalities.

Factors (b) to (d) can easily be corrected by the anaesthetist and the assistant whereas for anatomical problems, where the larynx cannot be visualized, a 'failed intubation drill' is carried out. The 'failed intubation drill' consists of:

— maintained cricoid pressure
— put the patient head down in the left lateral position
— maintain oxygenation with 100% oxygen, by IPPV if the effect of suxamethonium has not worn off
— wake up the patient and send for help.

When the senior anaesthetist arrives, the other alternatives which can be tried are:

a. Reintubate with longer bladed laryngoscopes, fibreoptic laryngoscope or retrograde catheterization
b. Spinal anaesthesia or epidural anaesthesia (if the catheter is in situ)
c. Inhalational anaesthesia.

In an emergency, when it is essential to proceed with surgery as soon as possible (e.g. fetal distress or placenta praevia), anaesthesia is maintained by following these measures:

a. Continue application of cricoid pressure
b. Place the patient head down
c. Maintain oxygenation using 40% oxygen nitrous oxide and add a volatile agent (halothane or isoflurane).

Anaesthesia for radiology

In the UK the radiology (X-ray) department is usually situated away from the theatre suite and is supplied with outdated equipment. This in association with unfamiliar environment, poor lighting or total darkness may make the anaesthetist's task difficult. The anaesthetic machine is checked for full cylinders of O_2 and N_2O. Anaesthesia is required for certain diagnostic procedures such as translumbar aortography, air encephalography and bronchography and carotid angiogram. The patient is kept totally immobile and monitoring may be difficult due to inadequate lighting, moving patient or restricted access (e.g. whole body CAT scanning) For CAT scanning, young children and uncooperative adults are anaesthetized. Long breathing circuits are required as there may be a long distance between the patient and the anaesthetic machine.

Hypotensive anaesthesia

Induced hypotension is defined as the deliberate reduction of blood pressure to facilitate surgery.

The indications for hypotensive anaesthesia are:

a. Microsurgery
b. Major cancer surgery where a bloodless field allows clearance of tumour
c. To lessen blood loss in patients who object to receiving blood transfusion (e.g. Jehovah's Witnesses).

The methods of inducing hypotension are:

— Hyperventilation
— Head-up position
— Use of halothane or isoflurane
— Use of drugs such as labetalol (Trandate), phentolamine (Rogitine), hydralazine (Apresoline), sodium nitroprusside (Nipride), and glyceryl trinitrate.

When induced hypotension is used, ECG monitoring and intra-arterial blood pressure monitoring are carried out.

At the end of the surgical procedure, the blood pressure may still be low, hence it is essential to keep the patient in the recovery room till the blood pressure rises to the preoperative level.

ANAESTHESIA IN PATIENTS WITH CONCURRENT DISEASE

Haematology

Sickle-cell anaemia and sickle-cell trait. A haemolytic anaemia which is inherited and transmitted by both sexes, this is seen in patients of West Indian or African origin and sometimes in Greeks.

It is due to the replacement of normal haemoglobin A by abnormal haemoglobin S. In sickle-cell anaemia, 90% of the haemoglobin is of S type and the patients are typed as homozygotes (SS). In sickle-cell trait, haemoglobin S is approximately 30–40%.

During anaesthesia, body temperature, hydration (IV fluids) and renal output is maintained. Postoperatively, oxygen therapy (35% by face mask) is carried out.

Haemophilia. This is a sex-linked recessive disorder. Females are carriers and the males suffer. It is due to the deficiency of factor VIII, which can lead to intra- and postoperative bleeding.

Before surgery, factor VIII is corrected using fresh frozen plasma, factor VIII concentrate or cryoprecipitate.

Endocrine system

Diabetes. This is a disease which affects the beta cells of the pancreas (see p. 35), altering the metabolism of fat and sugar. The rise in blood sugar can lead to peripheral vascular disease, nephropathy and neuropathy. Diabetics are treated either by diet, oral hypoglycaemics, or insulin (p. 68).

Preoperatively, if the patient is on chlorpropamide (Diabinese) the drug is stopped the day before surgery. Other hypoglycaemics are stopped on the day of surgery. If the patient is on a mixture of insulin, the treatment is aimed at controlling blood sugar using soluble insulin on a sliding scale.

If the patient is a poorly controlled diabetic, elective surgery is postponed until the blood sugar is controlled.

Steroid therapy. The adrenocortical reserve is diminished in Addison's disease, following bilateral adrenalectomy, during steroid therapy, and when a patient has received steroids in the past.

A short treatment with steroids for one week can produce depression of the adrenal cortex for as long as 1–2 years.

If such a patient is scheduled for surgery,

hydrocortisone (Ef-Cortelan) 100 gm is given IM 1 hour preoperatively and continued for 3 days in major surgery and for 24 hours following minor operations.

Carcinoid tumours. They arise from argentaffin cells of the crypts of Lieberkuhn of the gastrointestinal tract; 50–80% originate in the appendix. These tumours do not secrete hormones nor do they metastasize. Tumours which arise away from the appendix are malignant and produce hormones such as serotonin (5-hydroxytryptamine) and bradykinin.

Problems encountered in these patients whose tumour secretes serotonin during anaesthesia are: (i) delayed awakening from anaesthesia; (ii) episodes of tachycardia and/or hypertension, (iii) a raised blood sugar, (iv) hyperpnoea.

Patients in whom the tumour secretes bradykinin present with (i) flushing of the skin leading to hypotension and shock, (ii) bronchospasm.

Preoperative preparation includes using aprotinin (Trasylol) 200 000 units (started 1 h before surgery) if the tumour is bradykinin-secreting. If the tumour is secreting serotonin, methotrimeprazine 2.5–5.0 mg IV or cyproheptadine is used before the operation.

During surgery, morphine, spinal anaesthesia, and vasopressors are avoided. Aprotinin (Trasylol) and steroids can be used. ECG and BP are monitored.

Cardiovascular disease

Anaesthesia in patients with cardiovascular disease may be hazardous.

Heart failure. These patients are at serious risk. Preoperatively the heart failure is corrected using digitalis and frusemide. Most anaesthesic agents make the cardiac failure worse, whereas opiates are well tolerated by the patient.

If the operation is an emergency, the patient is preoxygenated, induction agents such as etomidate or methohexitone are used. Analgesics such as alfentanil or morphine are well tolerated. The fluid input and output is carefully monitored using central venous pressure (CVP) and urine output.

These patients benefit from elective ventilation postoperatively in the intensive care unit.

Hypertension. If the patient is an undiagnosed hypertensive, the operation is postponed until the blood pressure is controlled. Tracheal intubation or pain can raise the blood pressure, which can be controlled using alfentanil or fentanyl during intubation and any analgesic for pain relief.

Myocardial infarction and coronary artery disease. Patients who suffer from coronary artery disease are given the treatment even on the day of the surgery.

Monitoring is carried out very carefully (ECG, BP) throughout the surgery and in the immediate postoperative period.

Operations within three months of a myocardial infarction carry a 35% risk of reinfarction in the immediate postoperative period. Thoracic and upper abdominal operations carry a high risk. Full oxygenation, prevention of hypotension and hypoxia are important.

Presence of a pacemaker. The pacemaker is checked to see whether it is a fixed or demand type. A 'cutting' type of diathermy current is not used in patients with pacemakers. For all operations, the diathermy plates and electrodes are kept well away from the pacemaker.

Heart block. This can occur due to valvular disease or previous cardiac surgery. The patients have a fixed cardiac output, so the heart cannot increase the output in response to stress.

Second degree heart block can proceed to complete block under general anaesthesia. Patients with bifascicular block require a temporary pacemaker before anaesthesia.

Musculoskeletal disease

Myasthenia gravis. This is a chronic disease, possibly an autoimmune reaction. Muscles all over the body are affected which can give rise to ptosis, easy fatiguability of the muscles and dysphagia.

It is due to qualitative reduction in acetylcholine receptors. The treatment of myasthenia gravis consists of administration of anticholinesterase pyridostigmine (Mestinon) and prednisolone. If a patient is scheduled for an operation, on the day of surgery, anticholinesterases are stopped. If general anaesthesia is to be administered, depolarising and certain non-depolarizing muscle relaxants are avoided.

The patient is resistant to the action of suxamethonium and sensitive to all the non-depolarizing muscle relaxants except atracurium (Tracrium). Regional techniques such as epidural or spinal blocks are suitable. The patients are transferred to the ITU for either monitoring or ventilation in the postoperative period.

Rheumatoid arthritis. An autoimmune disorder which occurs at any age. The difficulties arise from:

— Deformity of cervical vertebrae and temporomandibular joint making laryngoscopy difficult
— Involvement of small joints of larynx
— Respiratory depression and pneumonia following surgery
— Involvement of heart, liver
— Steroid therapy.

If a difficult intubation is anticipated, then precautions are taken (p. 156) regarding management.

Ankylosing spondylitis. Stiffness of the cervical spine and the atlanto-occipital joint can cause difficulty during intubation.

Obesity

Obesity is due either to overeating or to endocrine disorder. The problems encountered in obese patients are as follows.

Respiratory system

There is decreased vital capacity, functional residual capacity and an increase in closing volume. Some parts of the lung are underventilated, causing shunting and hypoxia. Postoperative chest complications are common.

Cardiovascular system

Hypertension, coronary artery disease and post-operative thrombosis are common. Total blood volume and cardiac work are increased.

Difficulties

Technically, obese patients are difficult to lift and nurse. A short, thick neck can make intubation difficult. Regional anaesthesia such as epidural and spinal may be patchy and unsatisfactory.

In the postoperative period, some of these patients may not breathe adequately and may need elective ventilation in the intensive therapy unit (ITU).

Respiratory system

In patients with chest disease, defects occur in gas transport, gas mixing and blood distribution.

Bronchitis. Patients who are labelled as 'chronic bronchitics' should have preoperative physiotherapy. The induction of anaesthesia should be smooth to avoid coughing, straining and bronchospasm.

Regional blocks are preferred as the sole technique or as a combination (e.g. general anaesthesia with thoracic epidural). This will allow the patient to breathe adequately without much pain. Some patients may require ventilation in the ITU.

Asthma. Preoperatively, the patients should receive physiotherapy and bronchodilators (salbutamol as an inhaler or nebulizer). Agents which provoke bronchospasm are avoided (e.g. thiopentone, curare, morphine, pethidine). In experienced hands, IV induction with thiopentone is uneventful. If bronchospasm develops after induction, the patient is treated with aminophylline 5 mg/kg (approximately 250–500 mg) given IV slowly or 100–200 mg hydrocortisone IV.

RARE DISEASES WHICH CAN CAUSE PROBLEMS DURING ANAESTHESIA

Condition	*Difficulties*
Achondroplasia	Difficult intubation
Acromegaly	Diabetes, difficult airway and intubation

Condition	Difficulties	Condition	Difficulties
Alcoholism	Resistance to anaesthetics and delirium tremens (withdrawal crisis)	Marfan's syndrome	Cataracts, high arched palate (making intubation difficult), aortic and mitral regurgitation, kyphoscoliosis
Amyotonia congenita	Sensitive to thiopentone and muscle relaxants	Neurofibromatosis	Difficulty in intubation due to fibromas in larynx. Sensitive to muscle relaxants
Burns	Hypovolaemia, shock, problems with intubation (sometimes) and hyperkalaemia following the use of suxamethonium	Pharyngeal pouch	Regurgitation of stomach contents not controlled by cricoid pressure
Choanal atresia	Nasal obstruction	Porphyria	Paralytic crises precipitated by barbiturates, anticonvulsants
Conn syndrome	Hypokalaemia, hypertension and oedema		
Cushing's syndrome	Hypertension, diabetes and hypokalaemia	Scleroderma	Difficulty in intubation owing to restricted mouth opening, difficult veins, regurgitation, hypotension, respiratory failure, renal failure
Cystic fibrosis	Lung infection, bleeding tendency. Atropine dries secretions		
Down's syndrome (mongolism)	Difficulty in sedating, small mouth, large tongue, intubation difficult	Thalassaemia	Haemolytic anaemias
		Werdnig-Hoffman disease (infantile muscular atrophy)	Sensitive to thiopentone, opiates and relaxants
Dystrophia myotonica	Hypertonic muscles. Prolonged muscle spasm after suxamethonium and neostigmine	Wolff-Parkinson-White syndrome	ECG shows prolonged QRS and short P–R interval. Tachycardia produces S–T depression, so glycopyrronium is preferred to atropine.
Klippel-Feil syndrome	Difficult intubation due to congenital fusion of cervical vertebrae		

COMPLICATIONS AND ACCIDENTS DURING ANAESTHESIA

Deaths associated with anaesthesia make up about 2% of overall surgical deaths. The causes being: complications of intubation, respiratory depression after neuromuscular blockers, hypovolaemia and inadequate postoperative care.

The complications of anaesthesia can be described as follows:

Cardiovascular system:

a. Shock
b. Cardiac arrest (see p. 227)
c. Cardiac dysrhythmias: The following dysrhythmias are commonly seen:

— Bradycardia—responds to glycopyrronium 0.2 mg or atropine 0.1–0.3 mg
— Sinus tachycardia, which responds to adequate analgesia and anaesthesia and to fluid and blood replacement
— Atrial or ventricular extrasystoles occur in the presence of high CO_2 levels, and increasing the ventilation and decreasing the concentration of inhalation agents corrects it
— Supraventricular or ventricular tachycardia
— Nodal rhythm.

d. Hypertension in the recovery area; it could be due to (i) pain, (ii) raised CO_2 levels, (iii) following aortic aneurysm repairs, (iv) emergence delirium (e.g. ketamine anaesthesia).
e. Air embolism.

Respiratory system

During anaesthesia

Obstruction:

a. Obstruction by the lips—use oropharyngeal airways.
b. Obstruction by the tongue—the jaw is lifted forwards and upwards (see p. 228 on CPR).
c. Obstruction above the glottis—this could be due to a tooth, foreign body, vomitus, blood. The treatment consists of suction and lifting the jaw.

d. Obstruction at the glottis—this could be due to laryngeal spasm or foreign body impaction (e.g. teeth, vomitus).
e. Bronchospasm—could be due to irritant agents (enflurane, thiopentone, atracurium), anaphylactic reaction or triggering an asthmatic patient. The treatment consists of aminophylline 250 mg IV or salbutamol 1 mg IV for bronchospasm and hydrocortisone 100–500 mg IV for anaphylactic reaction.
f. Faulty apparatus—such as kinking of the endotracheal tube or impacted foreign body (vomitus, sputum) in the endotracheal tube.

Coughing. It occurs in patients who are not deeply anaesthestized with inhalational agents and in those who are heavy smokers.

Hiccup. This is due to intermittent spasm of the diaphragm, followed by a sudden closure of the glottis.

It is seen during surgery around the oesophagus and around the stomach when the phrenic nerve (which supplies the diaphragm) is stimulated. The treatment consists of:

a. Deepening anaesthesia
b. Inhalation of amyl nitrate
c. Methylamphetamine 4–8 mg IV
d. Metoclopramide (Maxolon) 5–10 mg IV.

Sweating. Is usually noticed on the face and forehead. It could be that the patient is hot, or is lightly anaesthestized or in shock or under-ventilated.

Treatment consists of deepening anaesthesia, increasing the ventilation or treating the shock.

Complications and accident after anaesthesia:

Pneumothorax. This may occur owing to accidental opening of pleura during rib resection or nephrectomy. The treatment consists of inserting a chest drain with underwater seal drainage.

Hypoxaemia. A fall in arterial oxygen tension (P_aO_2) occurs in patients, based on the site of operation, age, obesity, and the duration of the operation. The fall in P_aO_2 is due to a fall in the functional residual capacity, a mismatch of ventilation–perfusion and a shunt.

Oxygen by a face mask is given to all ill patients who have undergone major abdominal operations.

Sputum retention. Some patients may not be able to cough their sputum up effectively owing to (i) pain, (ii) sedatives, (iii) reduced movements of the diaphragm, or (iv) a tight binder or dressing.

This can lead to sputum retention and atelectasis (collapse) of the lung. The treatment consists of physiotherapy to the chest and inserting a mini-tracheostomy tube (Fig. 6.49).

Aspiration pneumonitis. Stomach contents may be aspirated into the lungs before, during or after the operation. Mendelson was the first to describe the 'acid aspiration syndrome' during pregnancy in 1946. The stomach contents which have a pH less than 2.5 can cause (i) cyanosis not relieved by oxygen therapy, (ii) tachypnoea (increased respiratory rate), (iii) tachycardia, (iv) rhonchi on auscultation of chest. The treatment consists of oxygen therapy, hydrocortisone, antibiotics, physiotherapy and intensive care treatment.

Vomiting and regurgitation

The problem of aspiration of gastric contents into the lungs is always present during induction, maintenance and immediately after anaesthesia.

Prevention

Metoclopramide (Maxolon) 10 mg IM speeds the emptying of the stomach. Cimetidine (Tagamet) 300 mg IV or ranitidine (Zantac) 50 mg IV 1–2 h before induction of anaesthesia increases the pH of gastric juice and decreases the amount. A dose of 400 mg of cimetidine or 150 mg ranitidine orally has the same effect. Magnesium trisilicate 30 ml or sodium citrate 0.3 molar solution 15–30 ml reduces the danger of aspiration.

Management

If an emergency surgical procedure is to be carried out:

a. A large bore nasogastric tube is passed
(effective in stomach with liquid food material).
b. A stomach tube (12 FG) is passed and solid food material aspirated.
c. A slight head-down position prevents the food material from entering the trachea.
d. Preoxygenation and crash induction with cricoid pressure is carried out.
e. A cuffed endotracheal tube is passed.

If vomiting occurs: (i) the patient is turned on one side or tilted head downwards, thus preventing the contamination of the air passages; (ii) suction of the oropharyngeal region is carried out.

If aspiration occurs: (i) suction of the trachea, followed by bronchosopic suction and lavage is carried out; (ii) IPPV, antibiotics and bronchodilators are given in the ITU.

Neurological complications

Convulsions. Can be seen in patients in whom toxic reaction occurs due to ether, lignocaine or bupivacaine. Treatment consists of IV thiopentone and oxygenation.

Tremors and muscle movements. These are seen following injection of induction agents such as methohexitone (Brietal), etomidate (Hypnomidate) and propofol (Diprivan) in the small veins on the back of the hand.

Prevention and treatment. Treatment consists of injecting in the larger veins and mixing them with 1–2 ml of 1% lignocaine.

Shivering. Myoclonus is seen following halothane anaesthesia. If it occurs, the treatment consists of injecting methylphenidate (Ritalin) IV.

Delayed recovery from anaesthesia. This may be due to:

a. Overdose of narcotic analgesics, volatile agents, infusion of propofol
b. Induced hypotension (see p. 183), hyperventilation during anaesthesia, acid–base imbalance (acidosis)
c. Fat embolism, air embolism and shock
d. Diseases of the patient: e.g. hypoglycaemia,

hyperglycaemia with ketosis, cerebrovascular accident (stroke), myocardial infarction
e. Overdose of atropine (central anticholinergic syndrome), this is treated with physostigmine (eserine) 1–2 mg IV.

Peripheral nerve injuries. These injuries occur due to malposition (stretching and compression of nerves), injection of drugs into or around nerves, use of excessive pressure in the tourniquets.

a. Brachial plexus. This nerve can be stretched by (i) abduction of the arms about the head with the patient supine, (ii) suspension of the arm from a bar when the patient is in lateral position, (iii) abduction, external rotation and dorsal extension of the arm.

It can be compressed when (i) arm is abducted with the patient in Trendelenburg's position, (ii) shoulder braces are used in Trendelenburg's position.

Prevention. The stretching of brachial plexus can be avoided by an arm board covered with pads, prevention of hyperextension and external rotation of elbow, padding the shoulder braces.

b. Ulnar nerve. Can be damaged if the elbow falls over the sharp edge of the table and the nerve is compressed against the medial epicondyle of the humerus.

c. Median nerve. Can be damaged if IV injection of drugs occurs around the median nerve in cubital fossa.

d. Radial nerve. Can be damaged if the arm sags over the side of the table or through use of a vertical screen support.

e. Supraorbital nerve. Can be compressed by a metal endotracheal connector or tight head harness.

f. Facial nerve. Can be damaged by firm compression between the fingers and the mandible while holding a face mask.

g. Lateral popliteal nerve. Can be damaged owing to compression between the head of the fibula and the lithotomy pole resulting in foot drop.

h. Femoral nerve. Can be damaged by the use of a self-retaining retractor during lower abdominal surgery.

Other neurological complications

Postoperative headache. Occurs in 40% of patients after general anaesthesia and in 80% of patients who are prone to develop headache.

Patients who had a spinal or epidural anaesthetic and had undergone repeated attempts in performing the block develop headache. This is due to leakage of cerebrospinal fluid from the holes made by either spinal or epidural needles.

Extrapyramidal effect. Drugs such as phenothiazines, droperidol and metoclopramide (Maxolon) in large doses can cause involuntary movements. Treatment consists of procyclidine (Kemdarin) 10 mg IV.

Awareness. Patients can be aware during any time under general anaesthesia. On induction, the patient must receive N_2O, oxygen and volatile agent before intubation. This should be carried out through the surgery. At the end of the operation, N_2O is turned off only when the patient is breathing adequately. This is to prevent a paralysed and awake patient being aware of events in the immediate postoperative period.

Posture of the patient

The problems which various positions of the patient can cause and their prevention are described below.

Supine. Pressure and stretching of the nerves of the arm can be avoided by:

a. Arms well tucked under the buttock, palm down with the wrists held by a plastic T-shaped splint.
b. Wrist straps are firmly attached to a broad strap surrounding the table.
c. Neck, knees and hips are slightly flexed.
d. Legs are placed flat on the table and not crossed one over the other.

Prone. A pillow is placed under each shoulder and another under the pelvis to allow free breathing and to remove pressure from the abdomen. Obese patients do not tolerate this position well.

Trendelenburg. In short, fat patients steep Trendelenburg's position can cause cyanosis and dyspnoea. Prolonged head-down tilt can cause retinal detachment, and cerebral oedema.

Lateral. It makes the patient's breathing difficult, hence IPPV is used.

Lithotomy. If this position is required, both legs are moved together to prevent strain on the pelvic ligaments. The knee should be outside the metal supports.

Effects of posture on various systems

Blood pressure. A head-up tilt can cause a fall in blood pressure (hypotension). This position is helpful for inducing hypotension in middle ear surgery. Other procedures which cause a fall in blood pressure are: handling and traction of the abdominal viscera, when the table 'break' is applied for the exposure of a kidney.

Respiration. Ventilation is decreased to a large extent in the prone, jack-knife and Trendelenburg's positions and a slight decrease occurs in reverse Trendelenburg's or lateral positions.

Head and neck position. A patient with a low cardiac output or atherosclerotic diseases of the carotid artery can have decreased blood supply to the brain with rotation of the head.

Moving a patient. All anaesthetized patients must be moved smoothly and gently. If a canvas stretcher is not available, at least three to four members of staff should lift the patient.

The patient is placed in the lateral or semiprone position until his protective reflexes return. This helps in monitoring a free airway and prevents aspiration of vomited material into the airway.

Urological complications

Failure to pass urine. A number of patients fail to pass adequate amounts of urine (oliguria) in the first 24 hours. The pathological causes of oliguria are:

a. Prerenal — hypotension, haemorrhage, hypovolaemia
b. Renal — damage to kidneys due to bacterial toxins, mismatched blood transfusion
c. Post-renal — ligation of ureter during pelvic operations (e.g. hysterectomy), bladder neck obstruction.

Difficulty in passing urine. This occurs in about 10–15% of cases after general anaesthesia. It occurs:

— In anxious patients, in patients with an enlarged prostate
— After abdominal and pelvic operations, e.g. haemorrhoidectomy
— In deeply sedated patients.

The treatment consists of encouraging the patient to micturate or to sit up, and if this fails, catheterisation is carried out.

Liver failure

This can occur in the postoperative period owing to a number of anaesthetic and non-anaesthetic causes. Some of them are: (i) halothane, (ii) hypoxia, (iii) blood transfusion, (iv) hypotension, (v) viral hepatitis.

The treatment consists of managing these patients in the ITU with IV amino acid, glucose, and charcoal haemoperfusion.

Postoperative jaundice. This may be due to conjugated or unconjugated hyperbilirubinaemia. Conjugated hyperbilirubinaemia is common and is due to shock, septicaemia, or the use of halothane.

Unconjugated hyperbilirubinaemia is due to haemolysis following blood transfusion.

Rare causes are infection and damage to the biliary tract.

Malignant hyperpyrexia (MH)

A specific condition in which the body temperature rises by at least 2°C/h, this is inherited as an autosomal dominant, characterized by (i) cyanosis, (ii) muscle rigidity (after suxamethonium), (iii) hyperventilation, (iv) hypercarbia, (v) dysrhythmias.

Causes. Drugs such as anaesthetic agents (halothane, suxamethonium), lignocaine and tricylic antidepressants and phenothiazines. It occurs in 1 in 100 000 adult anaesthetics and 1 in 14 000 child anaesthetics.

Predisposing conditions. Patients who suffer from osteogenesis imperfecta, congenital ptosis, hernias, kyphoscoliosis and cleft palate are prone to develop MH. The affected patient is commonly a young athletic male.

Biochemical changes. Calcium is released in excess in the muscle sarcoplasm, i.e. reticulum, which in turn produces uncontrolled muscle spasm. The biochemical changes which occur are hypoxia, hypercarbia, hyperkalaemia, respiratory and metabolic acidosis, disseminated intravascular coagulation.

Diagnosis. MH is suspected when the patient's jaw fails to relax and goes into spasm following the IV injection of suxamethonium, or there is a continuous rise in temperature, or rigidity with the use of halothane.

Management. Management consists of: (i) stopping the anaesthetic mixture and surgery and giving 100% oxygen to the patient; (ii) cooling the patient with ice, fan, cold water, intravenously or as gastric or peritoneal lavage; (iii) injection of dantrolene (Dantrium) 1 mg/kg IV; (iv) checking the blood gases, serum electrolytes, temperature; (v) correction of acidosis with 8.4% $NaHCO_3$, based on the requirements; (vi) 50% glucose, 1 litre and 100 IU soluble insulin IV to correct hyperkalaemia; (vii) dexamethasone 10–20 mg IV.

Management for future operations

Preoperatively, oral dantrolene is given as 4 mg/kg in four doses per 24 hours. A vaporizer-free anaesthetic machine with new hoses is used. Anaesthetic agents such as thiopentone, opiates, atracurium, nitrous oxide are used. Bupivacaine is safer to use as a local anaesthetic agent instead of lignocaine.

Other complications

a. Corneal abrasions when the eyes are not taped during operations and the cornea is exposed
b. Acute glaucoma if atropine is used in the susceptible patients; hence glycopyrronium (Robinul) is used
c. If the operating theatre temperature falls below 21°C, the patient develops postoperative shivering and increased oxygen consumption
d. Postoperative shivering after halothane anaesthetic
e. Minor complications such as trauma to lips, backache owing to lithotomy position.

ANAESTHESIA FOR EMERGENCIES

Patients presenting for emergency anaesthesia may have uncontrolled medical illness, uncertain diagnosis, and metabolic and cardiovascular imbalance. It is essential that they should be adequately assessed, prepared and presented for surgery.

The anaesthetic management consists of: preoperative assessment and preparation; intra-operative management; postoperative management.

Preoperative assessment and preparation

Assessment

As discussed earlier (see p. 139) a relevant past medical and drug history is taken. An enquiry is made about the patient's cardiopulmonary reserve, e.g. breathlessness on exertion, orthopnoea, angina, and productive cough. A quick physical examination is carried out including the assessment of the airway. Laboratory investigations are reviewed and, if necessary, corrections made (e.g. hypokalaemia corrected with potassium supplements).

The major problems in emergency anesthesia are: volaemic status, full stomach.

Volaemic status

It is essential to assess the degree of dehydration and hypovolaemia (e.g. trauma, patients with bowel obstruction and perforated duodenal ulcer) before induction of anaesthesia.

Hypovolaemia. Blood loss (intravascular volume deficit) can be estimated from history,

Table 6.7 Signs of blood loss.

Severity	Mild	Moderate	Severe
Percentage blood volume lost	20%	30%	40%
Approximate blood lost	1000 ml	1500 ml	Above 200 ml
Arterial blood pressure (mmHg)	Orthostatic hypotension	Systolic below 100 mmHg	Systolic below 75 mmHg
Heart rate (beats/min)	100–110	120–140	Above 140
Urinary output (ml)	20–30 ml	10–20 ml	Nil
Peripheral circulation	Cold and pale	Cold and pale	Cold and clammy. Peripheral cyanosis
Central venous pressure (cm H_2O)	−3	−5	−10

Table 6.8 Signs and symptoms of fluid loss.

Signs and symptoms of fluid loss.	Amount of fluid lost (ml/70 kg body weight)	Percentage body weight lost as water
Thirst, dry tongue decreased sweating and reduced skin elasticity	Above 2000 ml	Mild (above 4%)
Thirst, dry tongue, decreased sweating, decreased urine output, low CVP, high packed cell volume (haemoconcentration), hypotension, thready pulse, cold peripheries	Above 5000 ml	Moderate (above 7–8%)
All the above, plus coma, shock	Above 7000 ml	Severe (10–15%)

measured losses, heart rate, pulse pressure, peripheral circulation, central venous pressure and urine output. Signs of severe hypovolaemia become clear (low BP, tachycardia) when blood volume is decreased by 15–20%.

Dehydration. Fluid loss (extracellular volume deficit) is difficult to assess. A rough estimation can be made, based on the time of inadequate water intake, vomiting, duration of intestinal obstruction. For convenience sake, the fluid loss can be estimated, as shown in Table 6.8.

The signs and symptoms in Table 6.8 act as guidelines, and based on these the patient is resuscitated using blood or blood substitutes for

haemorrhage and normal saline (0.9%) or Hartmann's solution for dehydration.

Full stomach

Vomiting or regurgitation of gastric contents followed by aspiration into the tracheobronchial tree when protective laryngeal reflexes are absent is a major disaster which can occur during emergency anaesthesia.

Vomiting occurs during light planes of anesthesia (during induction or recovery from anaesthesia). Regurgitation is a passive process which can occur at any time and is not seen by the anaesthestist.

Aspiration of gastric contents is followed by either minor chest infection or severe aspiration pneumonia.

During an elective surgical list, the patients are adequately starved (at least over 6 hours) but in an emergency it might be essential to induce anaesthesia urgently (e.g. ectopic pregnancy, ruptured aortic aneurysm, caesarean section) before the stomach contents empty. Moreover, the patient's surgical condition (e.g. pain following fractures, intestinal obstruction) can lead to delayed gastric emptying.

The factors which determine whether gastric regurgitation is going to take place are the rate of gastric emptying and the state of the lower oesophageal sphincter.

Gastric emptying. About 1–4% of the total gastric contents empty into the duodenum each minute owing to peristaltic waves. The factors which can effect gastric emptying are:

a. Delayed gastric emptying:
  — Late pregnancy
  — Fear, pain, shock, anxiety
  — Sedation with opiates.
b. Abnormal or absent peristalsis:
  — Peritonitis
  — Hypokalaemia or uraemia.
c. Obstructed peristalsis
  — Pyloric stenosis
  — Gastric cancer
  — Large or small bowel obstruction.

State of lower oesophageal sphincter (LOS)

The LOS lies in the region of the cardia in the stomach; it opens during oesophageal peristalsis to allow food into the stomach. The LOS is the main barrier which prevents stomach contents entering the oesophagus. 'Barrier pressure' is the difference between gastric pressure and LOS pressure. Drugs such as prochlorperazine (Stemetil, anticholinesterases, neostigmine) and suxamethonium increase the barrier pressure.

Drugs such as opiates, thiopentone, alcohol and atropine decrease the barrier pressure, thus increasing the tendency for gastro-oesophageal reflux.

Preparation. The preparation of a patient for emergency anaesthesia consists of resuscitation with fluids, blood and blood products (as mentioned above) and gastric emptying.

Gastric emptying

This is carried out by:

a. Insertion of a nasogastric tube and aspiration of gastric contents which are liquid in nature (e.g. intestinal obstruction).
b. Insertion of a large bore stomach tube for solid food recently eaten.
c. Neutralization of the pH of gastric contents using either Mist. mag. trisilicate (30 ml) or 0.3 m sodium citrate (30 ml). This will raise the pH of gastric contents above 2.5 and if gastric acid aspiration into the lungs occurs accidentally, the damage can be minimal.
d. Decreasing the volume of gastric contents by using cimetidine (Tagamet) or ranitidine (Zantac).
   Cimetidine can be given orally or IM (200–400 mg) and ranitidine orally (150 mg) or IM or IV (50 mg) 1–2 h before operation.
e. Gastric emptying can be carried out using metoclopramide (Maxolon) 10 mg IM or IV.

Intraoperative management

This can be discussed under the headings induction, maintenance, recovery and postoperative care. The anaesthetic machine is checked before starting anaesthesia, all drugs are drawn up into labelled syringes and the ventilator is adjusted to proper settings. Required equipment should be checked.

Induction

As discussed earlier (p. 139) the patient's airway is assessed for likely difficulties whilst performing endotracheal intubation. If the anaesthetist expects a difficult intubation, a senior anaesthetist is called for help by a junior. Techniques such as awake intubation or intubation using a flexible fibreoptic laryngoscope can be carried out.

Crash induction

This is the most regularly employed technique for the patient with a full stomach. The patient is placed on a table or tipping trolley. The patient's head is placed in an ideal 'sniffing position' with the neck flexed on the shoulders and the head extended on the neck.

The anaesthetist is assisted by at least one skilled member of the operating theatre staff (ODA or anaesthetic nurse) to perform cricoid pressure, give endotracheal tube, laryngoscope etc. Before induction of anaesthesia, heart rate and blood pressure are recorded, ECG elecrodes are attached and monitoring commenced. The patient is given 100% oxygen by a face mask for 3–5 min before induction and an IV infusion, using a large bore cannula (14 gauge), is commenced.

The skilled assistant stands on the patient's right side to apply cricoid pressure (also called Sellick's manoeuvre). The assistant identifies the cricoid cartilage which lies below the thyroid cartilage. The thumb and the index finger of the right hand press the cricoid cartilage firmly backwards (posteriorly) thus compressing the oesophagus between the cricoid cartilage and the vertebral column. The cricoid cartilage forms a complete ring as compared to the other cartilage of the trachea (Fig. 6.50).

The patient is informed of the procedure of cricoid pressure. Some anaesthetists prefer to apply it before the IV injection of induction agent, while others apply it as soon as the patient loses consciousness.

With the assistant ready, the anaesthetist injects a sleep dose of induction agent (e.g. thiopentone 3–5 mg/kg body weight or etomidate 0.2–0.3 mg/kg or metohexitone 1–1.5 mg/kg) followed by a paralysing dose of suxamethonium (1.5 mg/kg). As soon as the jaw relaxes, laryngoscopy and tracheal intubation are performed. Cricoid pressure is maintained by the assistant until the anaesthetist inflates the cuff and is certain that the tube is in the trachea, by auscultation of the lungs (Fig. 6.51). Once he is sure, the cricoid pressure can be removed.

The endotracheal tube is then connected to the ventilator and IPPV commenced. The settings on the ventilator are 8–10 ml/kg body weight for tidal volume and 100 ml/kg for minute volume.

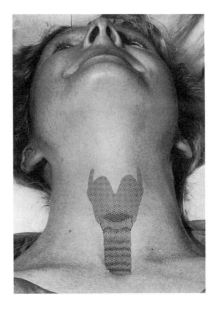

Fig. 6.50 Neck region showing thyroid and cricoid cartilages. Thyroid cartilage is above and cricoid just below it.

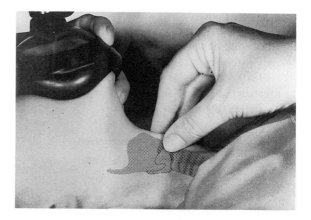

Fig. 6.51 Application of cricoid pressure.

Awake intubation. Carried out in patients with anticipated difficulty in intubation (e.g. ankylosing spondylitis, dental abscess), the intubation can be either oral or nasal, blocking the nasal mucosa, trachea and vocal cords (using local anaesthesia agents (see p. 156)).

Fibreoptic intubation. This is carried out by an anaesthetist experienced in fibreoptic intubation, in patients with anticipated difficulty in intubation. It should not be carried out by an inexperienced anaesthetist for the first time in an emergency. Inhalational induction is performed in patients with faciomaxillary injury or in a child with epiglottitis. Oxygen and halothane via a face mask are used for inhalational induction and when the patient is deeply anaesthetized, endotracheal intubation is attempted.

Regional anaesthesia

Total IV regional anaesthesia (Bier's block) or brachial plexus block (interscalene, axillary approach) are used for orthopaedic procedures on the upper extremity (fracture reductions, repair of tendons).

For surgery on the lower extremity, spinal or epidural anaesthetics are employed. These techniques should not be carried out in patients who are shocked or who seem to have lost a lot of fluids.

Maintenance of anaesthesia

The patient is given a balanced anaesthesia which consists of: anaesthesia, loss of consciousness; muscle relaxation; analgesia.

Anaesthesia. The patient is kept asleep with nitrous oxide 50–66% in oxygen and either 0.5% halothane or isoflurane or 0.5–1% enflurane.

Muscle relaxation. Once the patient recovers from suxamethonium, a non-depolarizing muscle relaxant such as atracurium (Tracrium) 0.45–0.6 mg/kg or vecuronium (Norcuron) 0.1 mg/kg or alcuronium 0.2–0.3 mg/kg is given. The longer acting drugs such as pancuronium (Pavulon) or tubocurarine (Tubarine) are avoided in emergency surgery.

Analgesics. Are administered in small increments (e.g. fentanyl 25–200 mg, papaveretum 2–10 mg) until fluid and blood loss are corrected.

Monitoring

As described in an earlier section (p. 159) all routine monitoring should be carried out.

Fluid and blood therapy

Fluid loss is corrected using Hartmann's solution 2–7 ml/kg and blood loss in excess of 15% blood volume in adults and 10% blood volume in children is corrected by blood transfusions.

Reversal

About 10 min before the surgery is completed, the volatile agent (halothane or enflurane or isoflurane) is turned off. After skin closure and bandaging are carried out, atropine 20 μg/kg and neostigmine 50 μg/kg or glycopyrronium 10 μg/kg and neostigmine 50 μg/kg are given IV to reverse the residual muscular paralysis. Pharyngoscopy is carried out to remove secretions and debris from the pharynx, and if a nasogastric tube was inserted it is aspirated and left unspigoted.

Once the respiratory activity returns and the patient is awake, he/she is turned on one side (if possible) and, at the peak of inspiration, the cuff is deflated and the endotracheal tube removed. Until the patient maintains an adequate airway and has an adequate cough reflex, 100% oxygen is given.

In the recovery room, the patient is given 35–40% oxygen by face mask.

Postoperative period

Postoperatively, all patients who have undergone emergency operations are given oxygen therapy (see p. 220), analgesics (see p. 217) and fluid therapy is written up (see p. 221). Certain patients who have undergone emergency surgery are transferred to the ITU for elective ventilation.

This includes patients with:

a. Extreme obesity
b. Prolonged period of shock
c. Septicaemia
d. Acid aspiration in the lungs
d. Severe lung or heart disease prior to surgery.

Although the technique for emergency anaesthesia is standard as mentioned above, certain surgical emergencies and their management are now described.

General surgery

Perforated peptic ulcer. The patient may be shocked, with his stomach likely to contain vomitable material. Before the patient arrives in the theatre, a nasogastric tube is inserted and gastric contents emptied. IV fluids are given in the form of Hartmann's solution or 0.9% normal saline.

Acute intestinal obstruction. The patient has fluid and electrolyte imbalance, a full stomach and distended abdomen. IV fluids are given based on the degree of fluid loss (see p. 192), a nasogastric tube passed, the stomach emptied, and crash induction employed.

Leaking/ruptured aortic aneurysm. The patient may be in shock, suffering from haematemesis (due to leakage of the aneurysm into the duodenum). Large volumes of blood are needed for transfusion which is given warmed and filtered. The patient is anaesthetized in the operating theatre (rather than the anesthetic room), with the surgeon ready to operate and clamp the aorta. A crash induction technique is used. Monitoring of arterial pressure (direct), central venous pressure and urine output is essential.

Postoperatively these patients are transferred to the ITU for elective ventilation and further resuscitation.

Ear, nose and throat surgery

Post-tonsillectomy bleeding. This is an acute emergency. The patient may be in shock and is likely to have a stomach full of blood clot. The blood loss is assessed by pallor, heart rate and blood pressure. An intravenous infusion is commenced. Blood is grouped and cross-matched and given when necessary.

Anaesthesia is induced with the patient on one side, head down, and the assistant applying cricoid pressure; but some anaesthetists prefer to have the patient lying supine. Once bleeding has been controlled, a gastric tube is passed to empty the stomach contents.

Gynaecology

Ectopic pregnancy. The patient may or may not be shocked. Surgery comprises of ligation of the fallopian tube which is bleeding. Blood may or may not be available. Anaesthesia is induced with a crash induction sequence, and fluids such as Haemaccel and Gelofusine are given to replace blood loss, until the blood derivatives are available.

Ophathalmic surgery

Perforating eye injury. Smooth anaesthesia is essential because of the danger of vitreous loss and possible loss of sight if intraocular pressure rises owing to coughing or straining. For intubation, suxamethonium is rarely used by the anaesthetist nowadays as it causes a transient rise in intraocular pressure. Vecuronium or atracurium are the muscle relaxants of choice.

MULTIPLE CHOICE QUESTIONS

The answers to these questions can be found on page 254.

1. **Which of the following is not a laryngoscope blade?**
   A. Negus
   B. Magill
   C. Shadwell
   D. Macintosh

2. **The size in millimetres (mm) marked on an endotracheal tube is to:**
   A. Maintain a patient's airway during an operation
   B. Maintain an airtight seal with the trachea
   C. Prevent regurgitation of stomach contents
   D. Prevent accidental misplacement of the tube.

3. **The Macintosh laryngoscope:**
   A. Has a straight blade
   B. Is suitable only in neonates

C. Is designed so that its tip lies in the front of the epiglottis when used
D. Is especially designed for a left-handed operator.

4. **Which of the following drugs is an anticholinesterase?**
   A. Hyoscine
   B. Sodium nitroprusside
   C. Neostigmine
   D. Glycopyrronium

5. **Muscle fasciculations indicate that one of the following drugs has been used:**
   A. Atracurium
   B. Suxamethonium
   C. Neostigmine
   D. Thiopentone.

6. **To make a 2.5% solution of thiopentone, the following are mixed together:**
   A. 250 mg thiopentone in 25 ml water
   B. 500 mg thiopentone in 20 ml water
   C. 1 g thiopentone in 25 ml water
   D. 250 mg thiopentone in 40 ml water.

7. **Which of the following is not a muscle relaxant?**
   A. Atracurium
   B. Vecuronium
   C. Physostigmine
   D. Suxamethonium.

8. **The main reasons for humidifying inspired gases is to:**
   A. Keep bronchial secretions moist
   B. Prevent explosions
   C. Maintain the patient's fluid balance
   D. Prevent cross infection.

9. **Which of the following ventilators is a pressure generator?**
   A. Bennett
   B. Servo
   C. Manley
   D. Nuffield.

10. **One of the following drugs causes respiratory depression?**
    A. Doxapram
    B. Morphine
    C. Atropine
    D. Neostigmine.

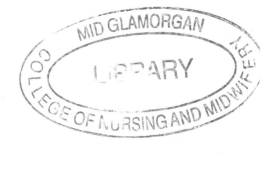

7. Surgery

In this chapter, various incisions and suturing techniques used during surgery are listed, followed by brief descriptions of some important operations.

The patient is made optimally fit for the operation, particular attention being given to weight, nutrition and acid-base balance, anaemia, diabetes, pulmonary and cardiac disabilities.

One to one and half hours prior to surgery the patient is given a premedication (see p. 140); he is then anaesthetized (p. 153), positioned and draped (p. 132) and surgery is commenced.

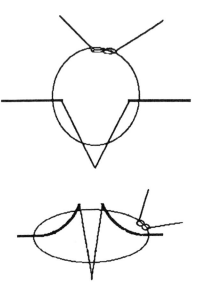

Fig. 7.1 Sutures: through-and-through and vertical mattress. Through-and-through sutures are for simple approximation. Vertical mattress sutures are for accurate edge-to-edge apposition.

Principles of suturing technique

The main types of suture (Fig. 7.1) are as follows:

Simple sutures (through-and-through). These are suitable for almost all wound closures. When applying them it is important to invert one or both skin edges.

Continuous sutures. These are essentially similar to simple interrupted sutures, but care is taken to adjust the tension as it is very easy to make a continuous suture too tight. A continuous subcuticular suture of monofilament material gives a very neat scar.

Vertical mattress sutures. These types of suture are useful in parts of the body where the skin edges tend to invert. In this suture the needle is passed through both skin edges twice.

Abdominal incisions

The principal abdominal incisions (Fig. 7.2) are as follows:

Midline. This is used for operations on the stomach, liver, gallbladder, spleen, lower bowel, uterus and rectum. The incision extends from below the xiphisternum to the umbilicus for high midline incisions and from the umbilicus to the pubis for low midline incisions.

Paramedian. This is used to gain access to one side of the abdomen.

Transverse. This is not often used as there is a danger of damage to the nerves supplying the rectus muscle.

Inguinal. This incision is made for the repair of inguinal hernia.

Pfannenstiel. This incision is used in gynaecological operations.

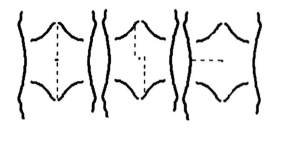

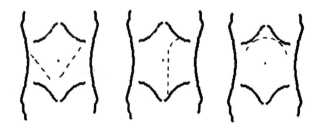

Fig. 7.2 Abdominal incisions. *Top row*:midline, paramedian, transverse. *Middle row*: lumbar, hockey stick, inverted V. *Bottom row*: inguinal, Pfannenstiel, subcostal (Kocher), abdominothoracic.

Subcostal. On the right side, this incision is made to operate on the biliary tract and on the left side, the stomach and spleen.

One other incision used is the Lanz incision for appendicectomy.

Instruments

The general set. The following instruments form the basis of a general set and they need to be arranged according to the kind of operation and preference of the surgeon.

Scalpel handles Nos 3, 4 with Nos 20 and 10 blades × 2

Dissecting forceps, toothed large (Bonney) × 2

Dissecting forceps, toothed small (Lane) × 2

Scissors, straight (Mayo) × 2

Scissors, small and large, curved on flat (Mayo)

Scissors, straight stitch

Artery forceps, straight (Moynihan) × 10

Artery forceps, curved on flat (Kelly, Dunhill) × 10

Photoclips for anchoring soiled dressing bag, diathermy leads or suction tubing etc;

Artery forceps, straight 8 in (Spencer Wells) × 5

Probe, malleable silver
Curetting spoons, medium and large
  (Volkman) × 2
Sponge-holding forceps (Rampley) × 5
Sinus forceps
Needle holder, small (Kilner) × 2
Needle holder, large (Mayo) × 2
Towel clips× 5
Tissue forceps (Allis) × 5
Tissue forceps (Lane) × 5
Retractors, single hook, sharp and blunt ×
  2
Retractors, medium (Langenback) × 2
Retractors, large (Morris) × 2

GENERAL OPERATIONS

Head and neck surgery

Thyroidectomy or removal of thyroid adenoma: removal of the thyroid gland partially or completely. The patient is placed supine with a sandbag under the shoulder blades and the neck extended.

Excision of thyroglossal duct or cyst: removal of a congenital duct between the thyroid gland and the pharynx. The patient is placed as for thyroidectomy.

Excision of parotid tumour: removal of a tumour in the parotid gland. The position is as for thyroid surgery.

Ear, nose and throat surgery

Ear

Myringotomy. Acute otitis media is a common condition occurring in childhood, when the tympanic membrane may be perforated, releasing pus. This discharge is known as otorrhea. Severe cases are treated by myringotomy in which an incision is made in the tympanic membrane.

Mastoidectomy: removal of diseased mastoid air cells. The mastoid air cells communicate with and are found posterior to the middle ear and are protected by the mastoid process of the temporal bone.

Tympanoplasty: repair of the ear drum by myringoplasty (a graft of temporal fascia).

Nose

Reduction of nasal fracture: realignment of the fractured nasal bones.

Nasal polypectomy: removal of the nasal polypi.

Submucous resection of nasal septum: removal of the deflected cartilaginous and bony parts of the nasal septum which block the airway.

Radical antrostomy (Caldwell-Luc operation): making an opening in the antrum via the mouth, leaving a large antrostomy into the nose.

Mouth and throat

Tonsillectomy and adenoidectomy: removal of the tonsils by either dissection or guillotine, and curetting the adenoids. The patient is placed supine with head and neck extended, and a Boyle Davis gag is used.

Direct laryngoscopy: direct examination of the larynx with a laryngoscope.

Tracheostomy: making an opening into the trachea and inserting a tube for the purpose of maintaining an airway. The patient is placed supine with a sandbag under the shoulder blades, the neck extended and the head pushed backwards. The procedure may be performed as planned or as an emergency. Permanent tracheostomies are performed during laryngectomies.

Dental surgery

Dental extraction: removal of a tooth or root. The patient lies supine or sits with the head and neck extended.

Immobilization of fractured mandible: reduction of a fractured mandible, followed by immobilization in which the upper and lower teeth are wired together.

Ophthalmic surgery

Cataract extraction: removal of an opaque crystalline lens.

Trabeculectomy: removal of a short length of the canal of Schlemm allowing the two cut ends of the canal to open directly into aqueous humour. This procedure is carried out to relieve the outflow obstruction of aqueous humour in glaucoma.

Repair of retinal detachment: sealing the retinal breaks using either cryotherapy, scleral encircling or photocoagulation.

Corneal transplants: transplanting a corneal graft from an enucleated eye or a cadaveric eye in the treatment of corneal opacities due to keratoconus.

Enucleation: removal of the entire eyeball because of disease or injury.

Vitrectomy: removal of a diseased vitreous body and adhesions and replacing them with a balanced salt solution. On some occasions, sulphur hexafluoride (SF_6) or silicone oil is injected.

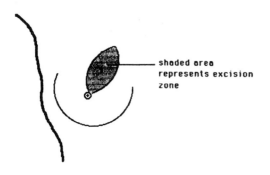

shaded area represents excision zone

Fig. 7.3 Simple mastectomy. An incision is made parallel to the border of the areola and the breast tissue excised as shown by the shaded area.

Breast surgery

Simple mastectomy (Fig. 7.3): removal of a simple adenoma.

Excision of breast lumps. Breast lumps may be cystic or benign tumours (fibroadenoma). If a lump is detected in the breast, initial treatment consists of aspiration with a needle and syringe. A *trucut* biopsy is made to attempt identification of the lesion. In most cases, excision and biopsy of the lump and surrounding tissue are carried out. The biopsy may be sent for frozen section histology. After the pathological diagnosis, several options are available:

— Wedge excision of the affected portion of the breast
— Simple mastectomy as described above
— Radical mastectomy which consists of removing the entire breast and the pectoral muscles and lymph nodes.

Thoracic surgery

Bronchoscopy: examination of the trachea and main bronchus by means of an endoscope.

Thoracotomy: opening the chest cavity to operate on the thoracic organs. The patient is placed in the lateral position.

Lobectomy or pneumonectomy: excision of a lobe of the lung or complete removal of the lung following thoracotomy.

Oesophagoscopy: visualizing the oesophagus for tumours or achalasia.

Oesophagectomy: removal of the portion of the oesophagus affected by carcinoma. The operation is carried out following thoracotomy.

Oesophagogastrectomy (thoracoabdominal approach): removal of part of the oesophagus and stomach for a tumour or a high gastric ulcer, oesophageal varices or oesophageal tumour. The operation is carried out through a combined thoracic and abdominal incision.

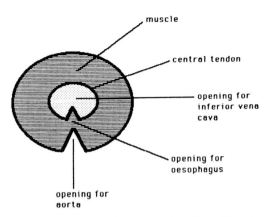

Fig. 7.4 Hiatus hernia. Surgery consists of repairing the defect in the diaphragm to prevent the stomach from entering the chest.

Repair of diaphragmatic hernia (Fig. 7.4): repairing an abnormal opening in the diaphragm which allows a sliding hernia of the stomach to move into the chest. The repair is carried out via the lateral approach following a thoracotomy.

Cardiac surgery

This is a complex specialty requiring a team of surgeons, anaesthetists, nurses, ODAs and perfusion technicians. A number of lesions are operated on and a brief classification of the operations is given below:

Congenital lesions
a. Patent ductus arteriosus which requires ligation and division
b. Coarctation of aorta which requires resection and end-to-end anastomosis or resection and graft
c. Tetralogy of Fallot which requires repair
d. Atrial septal defect and ventricular septal defect which require repair.

Acquired lesions
a. Mitral stenosis which may require either open or closed valvulotomy or valve replacement.
b. Mitral incompetence which requires valvuloplasty or valve replacement.
c. Coronary artery disease which requires either thromboendarterectomy, graft replacement or bypass.

d. Thoracic aortic aneurysm which requires repair and grafting.
e. Chronic heart disease which requires transplantation.

During the corrective procedure on the heart, the patient's circulation is maintained by temporarily bypassing the heart through a heart-lung machine.

The heart-lung machine consists of an oxygenator, arterial and venous pumps, a heat exchanger, a filter and arterial and venous cardiotomy blood reservoirs. The blood is heparinized during bypass and cooled, and at the end of the correction the circulation is established in the body and the heart-lung machine removed. The residual heparin is neutralized with protamine sulphate.

Abdominal surgery

Gastroenterostomy (Fig. 7.5): making an opening between the stomach and the jejunum. A left paramedian or midline incision is used.

Partial gastrectomy (Figs 7.6, 7.7): resection of a part of the stomach with anastomosis between the remaining portion of the stomach and the duodenum or jejunum. It is indicated in carcinoma of the pylorus; the distal three-quarters of the stomach is removed along with the proximal

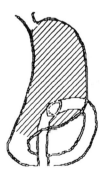

Fig. 7.5 Gastrojejunostomy. A loop of the jejunum is brought nearer to the lower part of the stomach and an anastomosis made between the two.

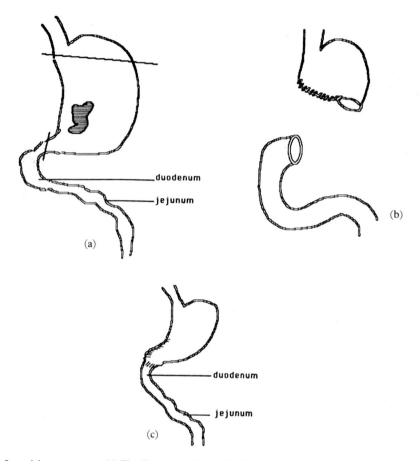

Fig. 7.6 Billroth I partial gastrectomy. (a) The lines show the level of resection. (b) The gastric stump is incompletely closed. (c) The remaining opening of the gastric stump is sutured to the open end of the duodenum (gastroduodenostomy).

2–3 cm of the duodenum. The duodenal stump is closed and a gastrojejunal anastomosis performed. In Billroth I gastrectomy the stomach is attached to the duodenum whilst in Billroth II the stomach is attached to the jejunum.

Total gastrectomy (Fig. 7.8) is performed for malignancy of the body of the stomach, the procedure resembles partial gastrectomy. It is more extensive including 2–3 cm of the lower oesophagus. A Roux-en-Y or Roux loop of 45 cm is formed when the loop of proximal jejunum is anastomosed to the oesophagus.

Vagotomy: division of the vagus nerves in as-

sociation with gastrojejunostomy in the treatment of peptic ulcer.

There are three types of vagotomy:

Truncal in which the two main trunks of the vagus are divided as they travel alongside the oesophagus

Selective in which those fibres supplying the stomach are divided.

Highly selective in which the nerve fibres supplying the antrum and pylorus of the stomach are preserved and the rest divided.

Due to lack of vagal stimulation, after truncal vagotomy or selective vagotomy, the drainage from the pylorus of the stomach is delayed. This is treated with pyloroplasty or gastrojejunostomy.

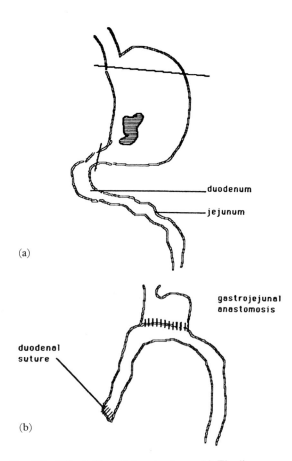

(a)

duodenum

jejunum

gastrojejunal
anastomosis

duodenal
suture

(b)

Fig. 7.7 Billroth II partial gastrectomy. (a) The lines show the level of resection. (b) The duodenal stump is closed and a gastrojejunal anastomosis carried out.

Right hemicolectomy (Fig. 7.9): resection of the right half of the colon.

Appendicectomy (Fig. 7.10) is the commonest emergency operation in younger patients. Through a 'gridiron' or Lanz incision, the appendix is mobilized. Following ligation of the appendicular artery and the mesoappendix, the appendix is ligated and removed.

Volvulus. In this condition in the small bowel, a loop of bowel revolves around its mesentery. The loop becomes distended and may cause complete obstruction. Laparotomy consists of reducing the volvulus; resection and temporary colostomy may be necessary.

Abdominoperineal resection of the rectum (Fig. 7.11): mobilizing the diseased part of the colon which is pushed into the hollow of the pelvis for removal via the perineal route. The patient is left with a permanent colostomy.

Hartmann's procedure (Fig. 7.12): resection of a tumour which lies low in the sigmoid colon or rectum. The resection is carried out with the proximal colon exteriorized as a descending or sigmoid colostomy. The distal stump is oversewn and is left in the pelvis.

Panproctocolectomy (Fig. 7.13): removal of the whole of the colon and rectum and the formation of an ileostomy. It is carried out in the inflamed portion of the colon in patients with ulcerative colitis. If the rectum is not involved and the colitis is not extensive, a total colectomy with ileorectal anastomosis is performed.

Surgery for haemorrhoids is carried out for prolapsed piles (varicosities in the anus). The treatment consists of: injecting phenol (sclerosing agent) through a proctoscope; or applying a rubber band to the neck of the pile through a proctoscope; or freezing with a cryoprobe.

Haemorrhoidectomy consists of ligating and dissecting the pile. 'Lord's procedure' (manual anal dilatation) is carried out under general anaesthetic. Four fingers are inserted to stretch the anus.

Fissurectomy: excision of a sinus or sinuses between the anal canal and the skin in the region of the anus. The patient is placed in the lithotomy or jack-knife position.

Anterior resection of the rectum: sphincter-saving resection of the rectum and part of the colon with re-establishment of continuity by anastomosis.

Colostomy: establishing a temporary or permanent opening in the colon.

Cholecystectomy: removal of the gallbladder.

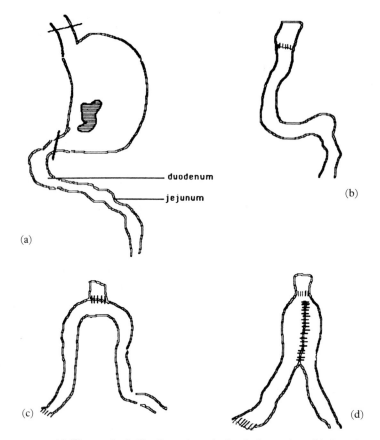

duodenum

jejunum

(a)

(b)

(c)

(d)

Fig. 7.8 Total gastrectomy. (a) First method. The lines show the level of resection. (b) Oesophagoduodenostomy is completed. (c) Second method. The duodenal stump is closed and end-to-side oesophagojejunostomy carried out. (d) Side-to-side jejunostomy is completed.

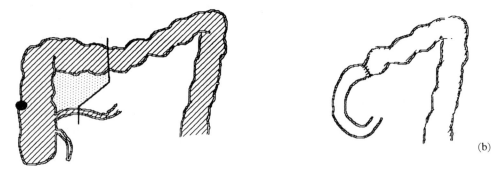

(a)

(b)

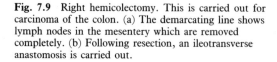

Fig. 7.9 Right hemicolectomy. This is carried out for carcinoma of the colon. (a) The demarcating line shows lymph nodes in the mesentery which are removed completely. (b) Following resection, an ileotransverse anastomosis is carried out.

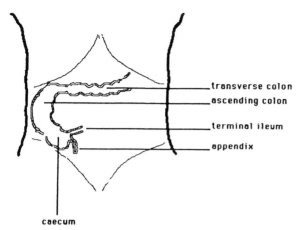

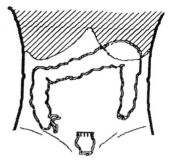

Fig. 7.10 Appendicectomy. The blood supply is ligated and divided. The base of the appendix is invaginated using a purse-string suture.

Fig. 7.12 Hartmann's operation is a modification of an anterior resection. The proximal end is converted into a left iliac colostomy and the lower end in the pelvic cavity is oversewn.

The patient lies supine with the liver bridge elevated occasionally.

Cholecystectomy is indicated in infection of the gallbladder (cholecystitis) along with the presence of gallstones. If a number of stones are detected, there may be a possibility of gallstones in the common bile duct. Hence an on-table cholangiogram (OTC) is carried out in which a radio-opaque dye is injected through a small cannula in the cystic duct. This outlines the biliary tree and the track of the ducts into the duodenum.

Cholecystojejunostomy (Fig. 7.14): anastomosis between the gallbladder and the jejunum, often with jejunojejunostomy.

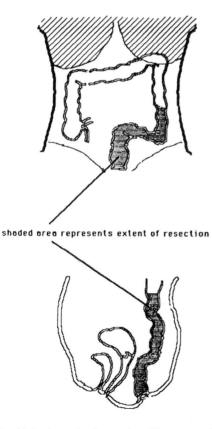

Inguinal herniorrhaphy (Fig. 7.15): closing the sac containing viscus which has protruded from the abdomen either as a direct hernia or an indirect hernia through the internal ring of the inguinal canal.

Femoral herniorrhaphy is similar to inguinal hernia, but the sac protrudes through the femoral ring into the femoral canal.

Fig. 7.11 Abdominoperineal resection. The extent of resection is shown by the shaded area. This operation is carried out in low anal and rectal cancer and consists of both an abdominal and a perineal resection.

Vascular surgery

Excision and grafting for aneurysm of abdominal aorta: excision of a dilated portion of the

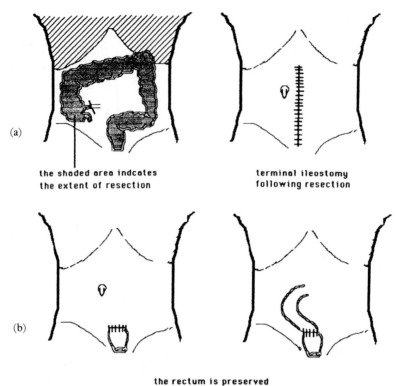

Fig. 7.13 Proctocolectomy. (a) The shaded area represents the extent of gut resection. It is carried out if the rectum needs to be excised. (b) The patient is left with a terminal ileostomy after resection.

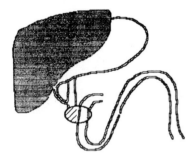

Fig. 7.14 Cholecystojejunostomy: a biliary bypass operation to relieve jaundice. The shaded area represents the liver and the oval structure below it the gall bladder.

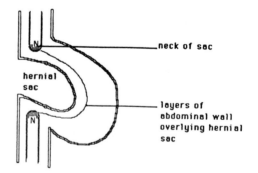

Fig. 7.15 Layers of hernia encountered during inguinal herniorrhaphy.

abdominal aorta and insertion of a synthetic fabric prosthesis e.g. Teflon or Dacron. A midline or left paramedian incision (Fig. 17.2) is made from the xiphisternum to the pubic symphysis.

The aorta is mobilized and the aneurysm is clamped, following which an anastomosis with the prosthesis is made between the portion above the aneurysm and the common iliac arteries.

Embolectomy is a procedure which is carried out to remove a blood clot which has become impacted in an artery or vein and which is interfering with the circulation below that point. The most common site of arterial embolism is the aortic bifurcation into iliac arteries. Venous embolism occurs at the junction of the inferior vena cava with the common iliac veins.

Femoropopliteal bypass graft: creating a passage for arterial blood to bypass an occluded part of the femoral artery. The patient's own saphenous vein or a Dacron graft are used.

Thromboendarterectomy: removal of a central atheromatous obstructive piece of artery, leaving an outer layer which is free of the disease. It is performed on major arteries and subclavian, vertebral and carotid arteries.

Amputations. When vascular reconstructive surgery on the lower limbs fails, amputation is carried out.
Syme's. This type of amputation involves part of the foot being excised, leaving the heel as part of the stump.
Below knee. This type of amputation enables a prosthesis to be fitted.
Gritt-Stokes. The femur is cut above the condyles and the patella is preserved.
Above knee is another form of amputation.
Amputation of legs is also carried out in patients who have developed diabetic complications of the feet or following trauma or in bone tumours.

Gynaecological surgery

Dilatation of cervix and curettage of the uterus: dilatation of the cervix and scraping the uterine mucosa. The patient lies in a lithotomy position and the procedure is carried out for diagnostic purposes.

Excision of the Bartholin cyst: removal of the Bartholin cyst which has formed due to blockage of the duct of the Bartholin gland which lies in the labium majora on either side.

Laparoscopy: inspection of the peritoneal cavity by using a laparoscope introduced through the abdominal wall. Carbon dioxide (3 litres) is passed to lift the abdominal organs. It is carried out to diagnose ectopic pregnancy, infection or infertility.

Abdominal hysterectomy: removal of the uterus, either partially or completely, through an abdominal incision. It is carried out for cancer of the uterus, persistent bleeding or uterine fibroids.

Wertheim's hysterectomy: total hysterectomy and bilateral salpingo-oophorectomy, with removal of the upper part of the vagina and lymphatic glands. It is an extensive procedure carried out for carcinoma of the cervix.

Vaginal hysterectomy: removal of the uterus through the vagina. After hysterectomy the pelvic floor is repaired by closing the peritoneum.

Lower segment caesarean section (LSCS): removal of the fetus through an incision in the abdominal wall and the uterus. LSCS is carried out for fetal distress, placenta praevia or cephalopelvic disproportion.

Orthopaedics and trauma

Fractures

Fractures occur in the following forms:

(i) A complete break due to trauma
(ii) Greenstick fractures in children
(iii) Pathological fractures due in part to pre-existing cancer.

Fractures may be classified as:

(i) Transverse: which occurs due to trauma
(ii) Spiral: which occurs due to a twisting force on the bone
(iii) Comminuted: which occurs when bone is fragmented into three or more pieces.

If a fracture is exposed and the skin broken, it is called an open fracture. If a fracture does not communicate with the surface, it is called a closed fracture.

The treatment of fractures consists of:

a. *Reduction*: fractures may be reduced either by closed or open methods. In the closed method, a force is applied in the opposite direction to the causative force, thus positioning the bone for healing. In the open method, the site of the fracture is operated on and the fracture reduced.
b. *Holding the fracture*: this can be done either by gravity, skin traction or skeletal traction.
c. *Plaster*: plastering is carried out for the majority of fractures.

Internal fixation of a fracture is indicated when:

(i) a bone is prone to non-union e.g. neck of femur
(ii) a bone is prone to malunion e.g. ankle
(iii) a bone is prone to pull apart e.g. olecranon.

Fixation can be achieved using a screw, Kirschner wire, K-nail, plate and screw or dynamic hip screw (DHS).

Fracture of the neck of the femur occurs mainly in elderly women after a fall. There are three types of fractures: subcapital, intertrochanteric and subtrochanteric. Subcapital fractures are classified according to the 'Garden' grading system.

Type I and II subcapital fractures are treated by inserting either Garden screws or a DHS. Type III and IV subcapital fractures are treated by removing the head of the femur. Hemiarthroplasty is carried out using either an Austin-Moore or Thompson prosthesis.

Intertrochanteric fracture. The treatment consists of reducing the fracture under X-ray control and fixation with a dynamic hip screw or McLaughlin pin and plate, or a fixed-angle screw.

Subtrochanteric fracture. These fractures are reduced on the orthopaedic table. A pin and plate (DHS) or a nail such as the Smith-Petersen nail can be used.

Arthroscopy: viewing the interior of a synovial joint with a telescope, usually in the knee joint. The most common injuries which occur are damage to the meniscus. Arthroscopy is per-formed to assess the damage and see whether repairs can be carried out through the scope or whether an open menisectomy should be performed.

Decompression of the carpal tunnel. Carpal tunnel syndrome consists of compression of the median nerve between the forearm and the palm. During surgery, a tourniquet is applied and an incision made from the wrist to the palm. The flexor retinaculum is exposed and divided, thus releasing pressure on the median nerve.

Neurosurgery

Angiography: a serial X-ray examination of the cerebral vascular tree following the injection of a radio-opaque medium into the main artery in the neck.

Craniotomy: an incision through the scalp and underlying muscle to gain access to the brain. The patient is placed supine for frontal, temporal or parietal craniotomies, and prone or in a sitting position for occipital and posterior fossa exposures.

With craniotomy, depressed fractures of the skull vault may be elevated or extradural haematomas can be evacuated.

Insertion of a ventriculo-atrial or ventriculo-peritoneal shunt establishes artificial cerebrospinal fluid drainage to the heart or peritoneal cavity in cases of primary or secondary hydrocephalus.

Plastic surgery

Repair of cleft lip and palate: closing a hare-lip and bringing about the continuity of muscle which is necessary for modelling the underlying bone and producing a cosmetically acceptable lip. Cleft palate closure pushes the soft palate back so that it can come nearer to the posterior pharyngeal wall.

Split thickness Thiersch-type skin graft is a graft which does not include all layers of the skin but only the epidermis and the tips of the papillae of the dermis.

Full thickness Wolfe-type skin graft is a free graft which includes all the skin's layers.

Fasciectomy for Dupuytren's contracture: excision of hypertrophied palmar fascia which has caused contracture of the fingers.

Urological surgery

Circumcision: partial excision of the penile foreskin.

Excision of a hydrocele: removal of a hydrocele sac.

Orchidectomy: removal of the testicle.

Vasectomy (Fig. 7.16): excision of part of the vas deferens.

Cystourethroscopy: examination of the interior of the urethra or urinary bladder with an endoscope.

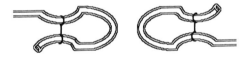

Fig. 7.16 Vasectomy. The two cut ends of the vas deferens are doubly ligated with silk.

Prostatectomy (Fig. 7.17). There are various routes from which the prostate can be removed.

Transurethral prostatectomy: transurethral removal of the prostate gland.

Millin's retropubic prostatectomy: removal of the prostate gland through a suprapubic incision but without opening the bladder.

Total cystectomy: removal of the urinary bladder and implantation of ureters into the sigmoid colon.

Nephrectomy (Fig. 7.18) removal of the kidney. The patient is placed laterally with the kidney bridge elevated.

Nephrolithotomy, pyelolithotomy: removal of a stone from the kidney or pelvis of the ureter.

Ureterolithotomy: removal of a stone from the ureter.

Renal transplantation: transplantation of a kidney from a suitable cadaver or a living related donor.

Paediatric surgery

Repair of hypospadias: plastic repair of the

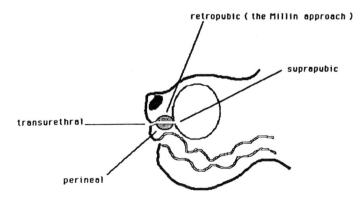

Fig. 7.17 Types of prostatectomy: retropubic (Millin), transurethral, suprapubic and perineal.

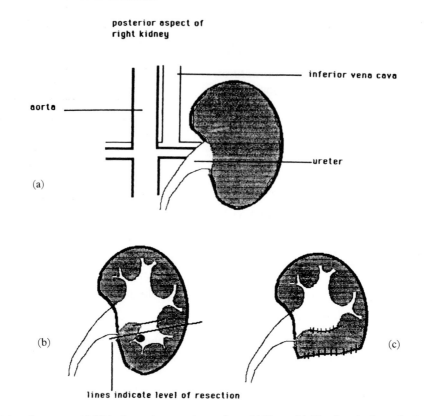

**posterior aspect of
right kidney**

inferior vena cava

aorta

ureter

(a)

(b)

(c)

lines indicate level of resection

Fig. 7.18 Partial nephrectomy. (a) This shows the posterior surface of kidney. (b) The lines indicate the level of transection of the renal calyx and renal substance. (c) Completed partial nephrectomy.

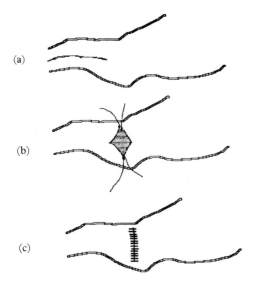

(a)

(b)

(c)

Fig. 7.19 Pyloroplasty. (a) A longitudinal incision is made on the centre of the pylorus. (b) The edges of the incision are stretched. (c) Pyloroplasty is completed by transverse suturing.

urethral opening which is found on the inferior surface of the penis using skin from the shaft of the penis. (Dennis Browne's operation).

Orchidopexy: mobilizing the testis and placing it in the scrotum.

Herniotomy. In children, this consists of excising the hernial sac (herniotomy as compared to repair in adults).

Ramstedt's operation (Fig. 7.19). Also called pyloromyotomy, this is carried out in neonates within the first few weeks of life. After rehydrating and correcting the acid-base balance, the surgery consists of cutting the hypertrophied muscles in the pyloric region of the stomach down to the submucosa. This relieves the stenosis.

MULTIPLE CHOICE QUESTIONS

The answers to these questions can be found on page 254.

1. **Dennis Browne's operation is for:**
   A urethral obstruction
   B epispadias
   C hypospadias
   D ectopia vesicae.

2. **Orchidopexy is an operation for:**
   A acute infection of the testis
   B acute pain in the testicle
   C an undescended testis
   D removing a malignant tumour from the testis.

3. **A Pfannenstiel incision:**
   A involves dividing the external oblique muscle
   B is mainly used for gynaecological operations
   C is a vertical midline incision
   D is a good incision to approach the liver.

4. **A Kocher's incision is used for:**
   A cholecystectomy
   B drainage of an appendicular abscess
   C vagotomy and pyloroplasty
   D gynaecological operations.

5. **Which of the following is undertaken to demonstrate stones in the gallbladder:**
   A cystogram
   B cholecystectomy
   C cholangiogram
   D cystometrogram.

6. **A collection of blood in a tissue is:**
   A epistaxis
   B haematoma
   C haemothorax
   D haematemesis.

7. **In the operations of vagotomy and pyloroplasty, the reason for doing a vagotomy is to:**
   A reduce acid secretion in the stomach
   B prevent pain sensation reaching the brain
   C improve the digestion of fats
   D improve emptying of the stomach.

8. **An abdominoperineal resection:**
   A is indicated in Crohn's disease
   B requires a permanent colostomy
   C requires a temporary colostomy
   D requires a permanent ileostomy.

9. **During a cholecystectomy the on-table-cholangiogram (OTC) is taken to demonstrate:**
   A Hartmann's pouch
   B common bile duct
   C gallbladder
   D cystic duct.

10. **Haemorrhoids are:**
    A benign tumours of the rectum
    B painful ulcers around the anus
    C varicose veins around the anal canal
    D a form of skin warts.

11. **Achalasia of the cardia is a condition of the:**
    A bile ducts
    B rectum
    C heart
    D oesophagus.

12. **A Caldwell-Luc operation is performed to:**
    A drain a pelvic abscess
    B open the maxillary sinus
    C remove a foreign body from the nose
    D repair the pelvic floor.

13. **Ramstedt's operation is performed for:**
    A small bowel volvulus
    B pyloric stenosis
    C duodenal atresia
    D intussusception.

14. In pyelolithotomy, a stone is removed from the:
  A renal pelvis
  B ureter
  C kidney substance
  D gallbladder.

15. A simple mastectomy involves the removal of the:
  A whole breast and lymph nodes
  B breast lump only
  C whole breast but no lymph nodes
  D whole breast, lymph nodes and underlying muscle.

8. Recovery and intensive care

RECOVERY AREA

Patients recovering from a general anaesthestic need to be monitored and nursed until they are fully awake and stable and ready to return to the ward. If these patients are not managed properly, mishaps including death can occur in the immediate recovery period.

Set up of a recovery area

Recovery areas are situated in the theatre suite, supervised by members of the department of anaesthesia. They are usually managed by either a recovery sister or a charge nurse and other nursing staff. The recovery areas are open either for a 24-hour period so that the patient can remain there until the morning after the operation, or until the patient is stable enough to be discharged back to the ward, a high dependency unit (HDU) or intensive therapy unit (ITU) at the end of the operating session.

Equipment required in the recovery area

The patient is nursed on a trolley or bed (if stay of 24 hours is anticipated); both of these can be tilted to a head-down position quickly if a patient vomits.

Within reach of the trolley the following items should be available:

a. Suction apparatus, catheters
b. Oxygen supply, face masks supplying various percentages of oxygen (see p. 220)
c. Electrocardiogram monitors
d. Oscillotonometers/automatic blood pressure monitoring devices, e.g. Dinamap.

For the whole recovery area there should be the following items:

a. Resuscitation equipment, including Ambu bag or a rebreathing bag, face masks, laryngoscopes, endotracheal tubes
b. Defibrillator
c. Equipment for emergency tracheostomy including tracheostomy tubes.

Drugs in the recovery area

Each recovery area should have a cupboard for emergency drugs with facilities to keep controlled drugs.

A list of the drugs which should be available in the recovery area is given below.

General (box/boxes of):

Adrenaline—1 in 1000 1 ml ampoules
Aminophylline—250 mg in 10 ml
Atropine—600 microgram in 1 ml
Calcium chloride—5% in 5 ml
Diazepam (Diazemuls)—10 mg in 2 ml
Dopamine (Intropin)—200 mg in 5 ml
Doxapram (Dopram)—50 mg in 5 ml
Ephedrine—30 mg in 1 ml
Hydrocortisone—100 mg in 1 ml
Isoprenaline
Labetalol (Trandate)
Lignocaine (Xylocaine)—1%, 10 ml ampoules
Metoclopramide (Maxolon)—10 mg in 2 ml
Naloxone (Narcan)—0.4 mg in 1 ml
Neostigmine (Prostigmin)—2.5 mg in 1 ml
Practolol (Eraldin)
Prochlorperazine (Stemetil)—12.5 mg in 1 ml

Propranolol (Inderal)
Sodium bicarbonate—8.4%

Controlled drugs

Diamorphine (Heroin)
Morphine
Pethidine—50 mg in 1 ml
Papaveretum (Omnopon)—20 mg in 1 ml

MANAGEMENT OF THE PATIENT IN THE RECOVERY AREA

At the end of the surgical procedure, the patient is wheeled into the recovery area by the anaesthetist and the recovery nurse. On arrival in the recovery area the patient is attached to an ECG monitor and vital signs such as pulse rate, rhythm, blood pressure, respiratory rate and colour are observed and recorded. In certain recovery areas where ECG facilities are not available, the vital signs mentioned above are monitored.

The following points are observed and procedures carried out carefully from the time the patient arrives in the recovery area until his/her discharge to the ward.

1. Airway maintenance
2. Level of consciousness
3. Postoperative analgesia
4. Oxygen therapy
5. Intravenous fluid therapy
6. Cardiovascular problems
7. Shivering
8. Restlessness and excitement
9. Monitoring urinary output, drains and central venous pressure.

1. Airway maintenance

In the immediate postoperative period patients are semiconscious; and they are prone to have their airway obstructed by the tongue falling backwards and thus occluding the pharynx. The airway is maintained in these patients by either (a) holding the lower jaw upwards and outwards or (b) inserting a Guedel airway into the mouth.

Positioning the patient

Patients are placed in one of four positions depending on the type of surgery and level of consiousness.

— *semiprone*—the patient lies face down with the lower arm placed behind the body, the head turned to one side and the legs flexed in the same direction as the patient's head.
— *Post-tonsillectomy*—this is a similar position to semiprone; in addition a pillow is placed under the chest to prevent the patient rolling forwards.
— *Lateral position*—the patient lies on one side with a pillow placed behind his back. (Fig. 8.1)

The above positions are used in patients who are semiconscious.

— *Supine*. The patient is laid flat on his back when he is fully awake (Fig. 8.2).
— *Sitting-up*. Certain obese patients do not breathe adequately if either lying on their back or on their side because their diaphragm pushes the lungs upwards, thus hindering respiratory attempts. Sitting up pushes the diaphragm downwards and allows the patient to breathe adequately.

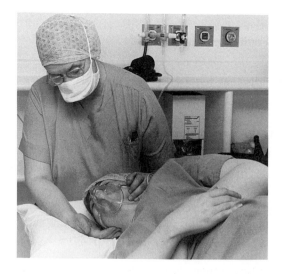

Fig. 8.1 The lateral position.

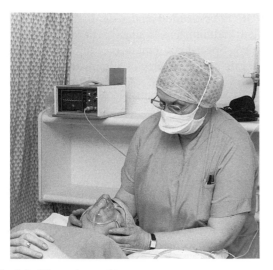

Fig. 8.2 The supine position.

Restrictive or obstructive dressings. Sometimes patients do not breathe adequately due to tight surgical dressings e.g. after a radical mastectomy or after the application of tight dressings or plaster jackets around the head and neck.

In the immediate postoperative period certain patients tend to vomit, so a head-down tilt of the trolley aids in drainage of the vomitus. A suction unit enables the suction of vomitus from the oropharynx using either a wide-hose suction catheter or a Yankaeur sucker.

2. Level of consiousness

A number of patients return to the recovery area in semiconscious state and it is the duty of the recovery nurse to maintain the patient's airway until he is able to do so on his own.

The majority of anaesthestists prescribe oxygen therapy for all patients until consciousness has returned, and in some patients it is continued for 4 to 6 hours in the ward.

3. Postoperative analgesia

Pain is a purely sensory experience. Postoperative pain resulting from tissue injury is acute in nature; it decreases with the healing process. It is of short duration, lasting only hours to days. Acute pain in a patient is accompanied by an increase in heart rate, systolic blood pressure and muscle tension, and a decrease in salivation and gut motility. Some patients become agitated in the presence of acute pain.

The amount of pain experienced by a patient depends to some extent upon the degree of surgery undertaken, but it is also influenced by a previous experience of pain (previous operation), and the social and cultural background of the patient.

Factors which influence the analgesic requirement are:

a. Operative site—patients who have undergone thoracotomy and upper abdominal surgery require pain relief for up to 96 hours whereas those who have undergone lower abdominal, perineal and hip surgery require analgesia for up to 48 hours.
b. Elderly patients require less analgesia.
c. Neurotic patients require a higher dosage; similarly patients operated on for cancer surgery require higher dosages at regular intervals.

The aim of treating acute pain consists of either removing the source of pain or alleviating the symptoms. The latter is the method used routinely following surgery.

Methods of pain relief

The following methods are in use:

   (i) Systemic analgesics—intramuscular, intravenous, bolus or infusion
  (ii) Oral/sublingual analgesics
 (iii) Local and regional techniques—local infiltration, nerve blocks, extradural, intrathecal
 (iv) Transcutaneous nerve stimulation, acupuncture
  (v) Cryoanalgesia
 (vi) Inhalational agents.

Systemic analgesics

These are the most commonly prescribed drugs for postoperative pain relief. The most frequently used opiates are as follows:

a. Opium derivatives, morphine
b. Morphine derivatives—dihydrocodeine, diamorphine (Heroin), codeine
c. Synthetic opiates—alfentanil (Rapifen), fentanyl (Sublimaze), pethidine, phenoperidine (Operidine)
d. Benzomorphinon derivatives—pentazocine (Fortral)
e. Methadone derivatives—dextromoramide (Palfium), dextropropoxyphene (Distalgesic).

Systemic analgesics are prescribed either by the intramuscular or intravenous route.

Intramuscular. Analgesics such as morphine, pethidine, papaveretum (Omnopon) are prescribed on an as required basis (PRN) most commonly in a large number of district general hospitals. This method does not provide adequate pain relief because of poor absorption. There may be a considerable delay between the time the patient asks for analgesia, the drug is checked and injected into the patient, and the onset of effective pain relief. (See p. 56 for drug dosage.)

Intravenous infusion. This is an effective method of pain relief. A loading dose of analgesic is injected followed by its continuous infusion. For example, in a 70 kg man a bolus dose of 7–10 mg of papaveretum (Omnopon) is given followed by an infusion set at a rate of 1 mg to 5 mg per hour (40 mg of papaveretum diluted in 38 ml normal saline).

Patient controlled analgesia. In this method the patient administers analgesic IV to himself as needed. Special equipment is required to limit the dose rate and frequency of administration in order to prevent overdose. Some examples of this method are a Cardiff palliator, an On-Demand Analgesia Computer (ODAC), and a Micropalliator.

Oral sublingual analgesics

Oral opiates such as slow-release morphine (MST) tablets provide pain relief for 6–8 hours. The dose ranges from 10 to 20 mg. Burprenorphine (Temgesic) 0.4 mg when given to an alert cooperative patient gives pain relief lasting up to 8 hours or more.

Side-effects of opiates. All opiates tend to cause nausea and vomiting. Some patients tend to hallucinate following the use of pentazocine (Fortral). If given in large doses respiratory depression can occur and a fall in blood pressure is seen frequently with the use of morphine and pethidine. Meptazinol (Meptid), a non-controlled drug, does not cause hypotension or respiratory depression but has similar analgesic effects to pethidine.

As all opiates tend to cause nausea and vomiting, it is obligatory to prescribe antiemetics. They can be prescribed with the premedication or given intraoperatively or postoperatively with the analgesics. Table 8.1 lists some common antiemetics.

Table 8.1 Common antiemetics prescribed with opiates.

Drug	Dose	Route	Frequency
Premedication:			
Metoclopramide (Maxolon)	10 mg	Oral/IM/IV	6 hourly for IM/IV
Intraoperative:			
Droperidol (Droleptan)	2.5 to 5 mg	Oral/IV	Once
Prochlorperazine (Stemetil)	12.5 mg	IM	6 hourly
Perphenazine (Fentazin)	5 mg	IM	6 hourly
Cyclizine	50 mg	IM	6 hourly

Local and regional techniques

a. Local infiltration of the wound by the surgeon using 0.125–0.25% plain bupivacaine (Marcain) is highly effective in relieving pain. It also decreases the IM/IV analgesics requirement.

b. Nerve blocks. Any nerves/nerve trunks lying near the operative site can be effectively blocked using local anaesthetic agents. Examples of nerve blocks are:

— Upper limb: brachial plexus block, median, ulnar nerve blocks
— Lower limb: sciatic nerve block, paravertebral somatic nerve blocks
— Abdomen: inguinal blocks and penile blocks.

c. Extradural (epidural). A catheter can be introduced into the (epidural) extradural space and a local anaesthetic agent (0.25% plain bupivacaine) injected at regular intervals. Pain relief lasts for up to 4 hours after a single dose. Similarly infusions of local anaesthetic agents (0.25% plain bupivacaine) at the rate of 1–4 ml/hour can be set up to provide continuous analgesia.

Sites where a catheter can be inserted are the thoracic region for upper abdominal surgery and the lumbar region for lower abdominal surgery. Caudal block is performed to provide pain relief in patients undergoing circumcision and haemorrhoidectomy. A dose of 0.3–0.4 ml/kg of 0.25% plain bupivacaine (Marcain) is used in adults whereas 0.5–0.7 ml/kg is used in children.

d. Intrathecal route. Intraoperatively, a subarachnoid block is performed using 25 g or 26 g spinal needles, and preservative-free opiates (e.g. morphine, pethidine or fentanyl) are injected, the dose for morphine being 20 micrograms per kg body weight.

The injection of opiates via this route causes generalized analgesia lasting for 18–24 hours. These patients are nursed either in the high dependency unit (HDU) or in intensive therapy because they have a tendency to develop delayed respiratory depression (after 12–18 hours). Naloxone is given both IV and IM to reverse the respiratory depression. An important feature of giving naloxone is that it does not reverse analgesia.

Extradural opiates. A catheter is inserted into the extradural space and preservative-free opiates are injected. Opiates which are given via an extradural route are as listed below in Table 8.2.

Transcutaneous electrical nerve stimulation (TENS)

A small electric current is passed between surface electrodes (usually two) at frequencies between 0.2 and 100 hertz (Hz). They seem to liberate endorphins (endogenous opiates) which in turn decrease the IM/IV analgesic requirement.

Acupuncture acts in the same fashion as TENS, thus reducing the total analgesic requirement.

Cryoanalgesia

During certain surgical procedures (e.g. thoracotomy), intercostal nerves under direct vision are subjected to intense sub-zero temperatures generated by a cryoprobe (cryo = cold).

Inhalational analgesia

On some occasions, Entonox is used in the postoperative period to allow change of dressings.

Table 8.2 Opiates via the extradural route.

Drug	Dose	Duration
Morphine	2–5 mg	Up to 24 hours
Diamorphine (Heroin)	2.5 mg	Up to 12 hours
Fentanyl (Sublimaze)	0.1 mg	2–4 hours
Pethidine	25–50 mg	1–3 hours

4. Oxygen therapy

In the postoperative period, a number of patients become hypoxic (lack of oxygen). The causes of hypoxia are:

a. Diffusion hypoxia. At the end of the anaesthetic procedure when nitrous oxide is turned off, 'diffusion hypoxia' occurs. The mechanism behind 'diffusion hypoxia' is as follows.

Nitrogen (N_2) is normally present in the blood; nitrous oxide (N_2O) when introduced into the anaesthetic becomes 40 times more soluble than nitrogen. When N_2O is turned off, it leaves the venous blood at higher volumes into the alveoli and this deficiency is not corrected by the volume of nitrogen taken up from the alveoli. This leads to a fall in the alveolar concentration of oxygen resulting in hypoxia.

'Diffusion hypoxia' lasts for about 5–10 minutes in healthy patients but can last longer in patients with lung disease.

b. Ventilation-perfusion abnormalities. This term is coined when ventilation of the lungs does not match blood supply to the lungs (perfusion). If a patient is hypotensive or has collapsed lung alveoli, oxygen arriving at the alveoli does not reach other parts of the body because of low cardiac output. This in turn causes hypoxia.

c. Increased oxygen utilization. This occurs in patients who have had prolonged surgery i.e. those who shiver with increased muscle activity in the postoperative period (as seen following halothane anaesthesia).

d. Hypoventilation. Patients in the postoperative period hypoventilate (decreased respiration) leading to a fall in oxygen delivery to the tissue and retention of carbon dioxide. Some of the important postoperative conditions in which hypoventilation occurs are listed below:

(i) Upper airway obstruction due to laryngospasm or a foreign body
(ii) Bronchospasm

(iii) Intraoperative hyperventilation (lowering of P_aCO_2 and the respiratory drive)
(iv) Respiratory depression due to opiates
(v) Incomplete reversal of neuromuscular blockade leading to muscle weakness
(vi) Pain
(vii) Obesity
(viii) Upper abdominal surgery
(ix) Pneumothorax.

It is essential to administer oxygen in the postoperative period to treat the hypoxia due to the various causes mentioned above. If there is respiratory depression due to opiates, either naloxone (Narcan) or doxapram (Dopram) is given to reverse the depression.

'Oxygen therapy' devices (Fig. 8.3)

These are classified into:

a. Fixed performance devices. These devices deliver an inspired gas mixture of known composition. These are 'patient independent' which means the oxygen concentration delivered does not change with the changing respiratory rate/rhythm of the patient.

(i) Low flow systems—anaesthetic circuits such as Mapleson A circuit will deliver a metered flow of oxygen and air provided the mask is tightly fitting on the face.
(ii) High air flow oxygen enrichment (HAFOE) systems–an oxygen driven injector entrains (traps) a fixed proportion of room air. A high flow rate (between 20–30 litres/min) of premixed gas (O_2 + air) prevents dilution.

Venturi masks. This principle should be used at the recommendation of the manufacturers. Injectors of different sizes are used at varying oxygen flow rates to deliver set oxygen concentrations to the patient.

b. Variable performance devices. These devices are 'patient dependent' which means the oxygen delivered to the patient depends on the respiration of the patient and the dead space between the face and the mask. These devices, although inaccurate, are sufficient for the postoperative period.

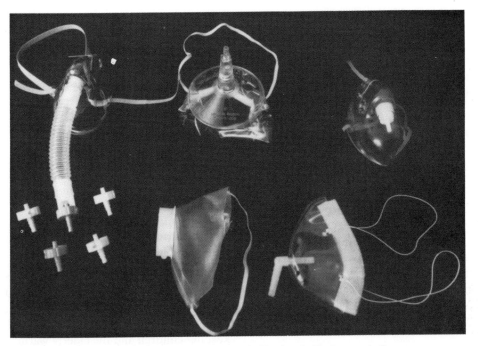

Fig. 8.3 Oxygen masks. Top row: Venturi type mask, Ventimask, Hudson mask. Bottom row: M C mask, Edinburgh mask. (From Smith J, Aitkenhead A R 1989 Textbook of anaesthesia Churchill Livingstone, Edinburgh.)

A list of masks with the approximate oxygen concentration delivered and the flow rates that need to be set are given below.

Masks	Oxygen concentration (%)	Oxygen flow (litre/min)
Mary Caterral (MC)	28–50	2
	41–70	4
	52–74	6
Hudson	24–38	2
	35–45	4
	57–61	6
	61–73	10
Harris	60	6
Edinburgh	25–29	1
	31–25	2
	33–39	3
Nasal catheter	25–29	2
	30–60	4

Choice of masks—a MC mask or Mapleson A circuit are used to increase oxygenation whereas a Ventimask or Edinburgh mask are used to deliver a fixed oxygen concentration (e.g. to a patient with chronic obstructive airway disease).

5. Intravenous fluid therapy

In a large number of cases, intravenous fluid therapy is commenced in theatre. The fluids usually administered are Hartmann's solution, dextrose 4% in normal saline 0.18% or 5% dextrose. The rate of administration intraoperatively is 2 ml/kg/hour of surgery. When the blood loss is more than 10% of blood volume in children and 15% in adults, blood transfusion is started. After checking the unit of blood against the information on the patient's wristband and case notes and the form received from the blood bank, the transfusion is commenced. It is essential to use a blood filter, blood warming coil and blood warmer to prevent the patient receiving debris and cold blood. The transfusion of warm blood prevents the patient from becoming hypothermic.

The anaesthetist completes the fluid therapy chart before handing over the patient to the recovery stage.

6. Cardiovascular problems

a. Hypotension

Most patients on arrival in the recovery area show some degree of hypotension. The usual causes of hypotension are:

(i) Excessive premedication
(ii) Overdose of general anaesthetics (e.g. high concentration of halothane or isoflurane delivered during anaesthesia)
(iii) Vascular absorption of local anaesthetics. (Local anaesthetics depress the myocardium and cause dilatation of peripheral vessels)
(iv) Spinal and epidural anaesthesia
(v) Haemorrhage and blood loss which has not been replaced adequately
(vi) Motion and change of position
(vii) Hypoxia
(viii) Metabolic acidosis
(ix) Pain

Over a period of time, the residual effects of (i), (ii), (iii), (iv) wear off and when blood loss, hypoxaemia and acidosis are corrected, blood pressure returns to within normal limits.

b. Hypertension

When patients become excessively hypertensive in the postoperative period, they may develop a cerebrovascular accident or myocardial infarction as its complication.

The important causes of postoperative hypertension are:

(i) Pain
(ii) Hypoxia, hypercarbia
(iii) Excessive replacement of fluid losses
(iv) Following aortic grafting for abdominal aortic aneurysm.

Adequate analgesia and oxygenation will decrease the blood pressure in conditions (i) and (ii), and the use of vasodilators such as sodium nitroprusside given IV slowly with careful monitoring of blood pressure or chlorpromazine will treat the hypertensive response.

7. Shivering

Patients shiver in the postoperative period due to lowered body temperature which in turn increases heart rate and oxygen consumption.

Heat loss leading to lowered body temperature occurs:

(i) when Magill circuits (open and semi-closed circuit) are used
(ii) when cold IV fluids and blood are used
(iii) when thoracic and abdominal cavities are open for prolonged periods
(iv) in deep planes of anaesthesia
(v) in children and the elderly
(vi) due to air conditioning in theatre and the recovery areas.

Body temperature can be maintained by keeping the room temperature at 21°C or 70°F, using closed circuits, condenser humidifiers and blood warmers, infusing warm fluids and bloods, and keeping children and the elderly warm with heated ripple mattresses.

8. Restlessness and excitement

Patients become agitated in the postoperative period for a number of reasons, some of which are:

(i) Pain
(ii) Anxiety about anaesthetic recovery
(iii) Uncomfortable position and full urinary bladder

Excitement occurs due to:

(i) Hypoxia following thoracic and upper abdominal operations
(ii) Hypotension
(iii) Use of hyoscine, phenothiazines (chlorpromazine), barbiturates and premedicants
(iv) Use of ketamine as an anaesthetic agent leading to postoperative hallucinations.

Management

This consists of relieving pain, changing the uncomfortable position of the patient, emptying the urinary bladder, oxygen therapy for hypoxia, and fluid or blood replacement to correct hypotension.

As the anaesthetic agent is eliminated, the patient becomes quiet gradually. Time and patience are important, and the patient should be comforted throughout this difficult period.

9. Monitoring urinary output, drains and central venous pressure

Urinary output

In recovery areas which are open for 24 hours it is essential to monitor urine output as some patients develop retention of urine postoperatively. In patients who have had urological surgery (prostate resection), bladder irrigation or intermittent washouts are needed to prevent clotting of blood, which in some cases may lead to retention of urine.

Patients who have undergone major surgical procedures (e.g. aneurysmal surgery, cardiac surgery, abdomino-perineal resection) need their bladder catheterized, and hourly monitoring of urine output using a 'urimeter' is carried out.

Wound drainage

In a number of surgical cases a wound is drained and the recovery nurse is made aware of the site of the drain or drains. When patients are positioned on trolleys or beds in the recovery area it is essential that precautions are taken so as not to block or kink the drains.

By observing the drains it is possible to detect early haemorrhage. Following thoracic or cardiac procedures when underwater sealed drains are inserted it is important to check that these are 'swinging' with respiration and that a large volume of blood is not being collected rapidly in the bottle. If either 'swinging' with respiration stops or larger amounts of blood start accumulating, medical help should be sought immediately.

Central venous pressure (CVP)

CVP is measured using a calibrated transducer (for blood pressure) or a manometer line. In the immediate postoperative period, CVP monitoring becomes essential for patients who have undergone major surgical procedures such as repair of an aneurysm, cardiopulmonary bypass or coronary artery bypass and valve replacements.

SPECIAL CONSIDERATIONS IN THE RECOVERY AREA

Most of the problems and management discussed above hold good for a number of surgical procedures, but the following paragraphs are relevant in the recovery of patients from certain surgical procedures.

a. ENT surgery. Children undergoing tonsillectomy should be nursed in the post-tonsillectomy position until they are fully awake.

b. Dental and maxillofacial surgery. Patients who have a fractured jaw indergo surgical fixation followed by wiring of the jaw. The anaesthetist administers an antiemetic intraoperatively (e.g. prochlorperazine (Stemetil). In the recovery area he pulls the nasotracheal tube above the vocal cords allowing it to function as a nasopharyngeal airway. The patient is usually accompanied with wire cutters from the theatre into the recovery area. The nursing staff are informed of which wires to cut in case the patient vomits. The patient is nursed on one side with a slight head-down tilt until he is fully awake. The nasopharyngeal tube is then pulled out.

c. Ophthalmic surgery. Most patients undergoing ophthalmic surgery receive antiemetics during the intraoperative period, as vomiting, coughing and straining can increase the intraocular pressure and damage the eye. They should be nursed on one side until fully awake. Patients who have undergone vitrectomy should be recovered according to the surgeon's recommendation.

d. Bronchoscopy. All patients who have had a local anaesthetic spray on their vocal cords should be observed by the recovery staff at all times as their swallowing and cough reflex are dulled. No oral fluids should be given for at least four hours or longer according to the wishes of the anaesthetist.

Although patients may be fully awake after a

general anaesthetic they may still have difficulties in swallowing and speaking.

If a bronchial biopsy was taken there is a greater danger of haemorrhage. Control of bleeding may be difficult, hence patients are usually nursed on the side from which the biopsy was taken, or in an upright, sitting position.

e. Thoracic surgery. In the recovery room or high dependency unit all vital signs are monitored regularly. Underwater seal drains which are inserted intraoperatively should be seen to be 'swinging' (moving with respiration) and not blocked by surgical debris or a clot. Some anaesthetists clamp the drains when moving a patient to prevent the water from entering the thorax via the tubing.

Clamps should be removed at the earliest opportunity to prevent the development of tension pneumothorax. The drains should always be below the level of the patient's chest. Analgesia in the form of intrathecal morphine, epidural block or infusions are prescribed.

f. Cardiothoracic surgery. A number of patients are transferred directly to the intensive care unit for elective ventilation.

g. Paediatric surgery. Neonates who undergo surgery are quickly replaced in their incubators and returned to the special care baby unit. Larger babies are placed in their preheated cots.

Some babies who are not critically ill can be recovered in the arms of the recovery staff. They are returned to the ward when fully awake. At all times the child's airway is maintained. Although a fair number of anaesthetists do not prescribe analgesia for neonates, it should be prescribed based on the type of surgery the child has undergone. Analgesia in the form of pethidine, papaveretum or regional blocks can be given to older children.

h. Neurosurgery. Patients who undergo major neurosurgical procedures such as posterior fossa exploration or clipping or a cerebral aneurysm are transferred to the intensive care unit.

i. Vascular surgery. Patients who undergo aneurysmal surgery are transferred directly to the intensive care unit. Some patients who have undergone a femoropopliteal bypass graft are sent to the high dependency unit or ward.

Before they are sent to the ward blood loss in the drain should be measured and if necessary a blood transfusion commenced. Once the patient is stabilized he/she can be sent back to the ward.

INTENSIVE THERAPY UNIT

The intensive therapy unit (ITU) is a specialized area in hospital where critically ill patients are given the highest level of continuous care and treatment. As compared to general wards a larger area is allocated for each bed space. Bulky monitoring equipment occupies space; some of this room is also needed for several nurses to attend to the patient at once. Each bed space is provided with piped oxygen, air, suction and a minimum of two electric power sockets. Each bed has sufficient space for storing drugs and carrying out physiotherapy.

Staffing in the ITU

The administrative consultant in charge of the ITU is usually an anaesthetist who, in addition to looking after patients, looks after the day-to-day administration of the unit.

Junior anaesthetists act as 'middle men' in conveying messages from senior staff to nursing staff, who carry out a major part of patient care. The ITU junior anaesthetist liaises with other specialists and acts on the recent test results and changing physiological condition of the patient.

Indications for admission to the ITU

Patients who are admitted to the ITU usually require life support (cardiac, respiratory) either whilst the diagnosis is being made or when it is known.

Other groups of patients who are admitted to the unit are those who have undergone major surgery (neurosurgery, cardiac, transplants of liver, heart) or patients with organ failure (liver failure, renal failure, head injury).

Patients who are admitted to the ITU are monitored continuously using highly sophisticated equipment. This monitoring is summarized below:

Organ	Monitoring
Brain	Electroencephalogram (ECG) Cerebral function analysing monitor (CFAM) Intracranial pressure monitoring (ICP)
Cardiovascular	Electrocardiogram Intra-arterial blood pressure monitoring (invasive/non-invasive) Central venous pressure (CVP) Cardiac output Pulmonary artery pressure monitoring
Respiratory	Tidal volume, minute volume Oxygen delivery (oxygen analyser) Carbon dioxide production (CO_2 monitor) Pulse oximetry Arterial blood gases
Urinary	Urinary catheter
Temperature	Peripheral temperature Core temperature

Charts used in the ITU

As patients are monitored continuously, charts are completed by the nursing staff. They show a record of physiological changes, drugs and fluids given, and laboratory results from which the medical staff can make decisions and institute treatment.

A number of patients are intubated and ventilated to support their cardiovascular and respiratory systems. They tolerate the endotracheal tube and ventilator because sedatives such as midazolam (Hypnovel), analgesics, papaveretum (Omnopon, morphine) are infused continuously.

When the patient gets better he is gradually weaned off the ventilator. Some patients require feeding and this is carried out using total parenteral nutrition (TPN) in patients with gastrointestinal ileus, or enteral nutrition using a nasogastric feeding tube (Clinifeed).

The number of patients who die in the ITU is quite high because of multi-organ failure or severe septicaemia, which may not respond to intensive therapy. Patients who are admitted to the unit after cardiac surgery, neurosurgery or transplantation for postoperative observation are sent back to the ward once they are stabilized.

NB. Multiple choice questions on intensive care can be found on page 235.

MULTIPLE CHOICE QUESTIONS

The answers to these questions can be found on page 254.

1. **All of the following equipment is required in the recovery area except a:**
   A defibrillator
   B suction unit
   C diathermy machine
   D electrocardiograph.

2. **Following tonsillectomy, the patient is nursed in the:**
   A prone position
   B supine position
   C lateral position
   D sitting position.

3. **All of the following are routine postoperative analgesics except:**
   A alfentanil
   B papaveretum
   C pethidine
   D nerve blocks.

4. **All of the following are side-effects of intrathecal morphine except:**
   A pruritus
   B urinary retention
   C delayed respiratory depression
   D hallucinations.

5. **The commonly used local anaesthetic agent is:**
   A bupivacaine
   B lignocaine
   C cinchocaine
   D prilocaine.

6. **All of the following are common causes of postoperative hypoxia except:**
   A hypoventilation
   B hyperventilation
   C bronchospasm
   D diffusion hypoxia.

7. **The common cause of postoperative hypertension is:**
   A pain
   B hypovolaemia
   C residual effect of anaesthetic agent
   D faulty monitoring equipment.

8. **In the recovery area all of the following agents can be used as antiemetics except:**
   A hyoscine
   B metoclopramide
   C prochlorperazine
   D perphenazine.

9. **All of the following are causes of postoperative excitement except:**
   A pain
   B preoperative anxiety
   C preoperative depression
   D full bladder.

10 **All of the following are important causes of postoperative hypotension except:**
   A excessive premedication
   B residual effect of anaesthetic agent
   C following spinal analgesia
   D full urinary bladder.

9. Cardiopulmonary resuscitation

Cardiac arrest is defined as a sudden interruption of cardiac output which may be reversible with appropriate treatment. Hypoventilation (decreased respiration with retention of carbon dioxide), blood loss and airway obstruction are the major causes of death in victims of road traffic accidents and heart attacks.

If the cardiac arrest lasts longer than a few minutes irreversible brain damage can occur, but if resuscitation is commenced immediately this damage can be prevented. Resuscitation can be carried out by individuals ranging from hospital staff to the lay public who have undergone training.

Diagnosis of cardiac arrest

Cardiac arrest can be diagnosed by the following signs:

— Loss of consciousness
— Absent pulses in major arteries (carotid and femoral arteries)
— Pallor or cyanosis.

Cardiopulmonary resuscitation (CPR) is the term used for the management of cardiac arrest. It comprises:

I. Basic life support without equipment i.e. external cardiac compression and expired air resuscitation
II. Advanced cardiac life support with resuscitation equipment.

For simplicity CPR is divided into three phases:

Phase I: Basic life support

This consists of:

A. Airway control
B Breathing support
C. Circulatory support.

Phase I is started if the resuscitator does not get an answer to the question 'are you alright?' As soon as Phase I is begun, assistance in the form of a cardiac arrest team in hospital and an ambulance on the roadside is sent for.

Phase II: Advanced cardiac life support

This involves starting spontaneous circulation and stabilizing the cardiopulmonary system.
It consists of:

D. Drugs and fluids via an intravenous infusion
E. Electrocardiogram (monitoring and diagnosis)
F. Fibrillatory treatment (defibrillation).

Phase I and Phase II should be established as soon as possible because external cardiac compression produces only 6–30% of normal blood flow to the brain.

Phase III: Prolonged life support

This consists of:

G. Gauging
H. Human mentation i.e. cerebral resuscitation
I. Intensive care i.e. multiple organ support.

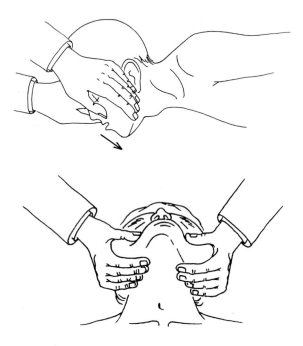

Fig. 9.1 Triple airway manoeuvre. This consists of holding the head backwards, and lifting the chin upwards and forwards.

Phase I Basic life support

A. Airway control

The hypopharynx (the area below the pharynx) is the commonest site of airway obstruction in a victim who has lost consciousness. The tongue falls backwards, thus obstructing the airway; this obstruction is relieved by holding the head tilted backwards with the chin lifted upwards and forwards. This is called the triple airway manoeuvre (Fig. 9.1).

Another cause of obstruction of the airway is the presence of blood or vomitus, and, depending on where it is present, laryngospasm (if the vomitus is near larynx) or bronchospasm (if the vomitus lodges in the bronchial tree) may develop.

The diagnosis and management of acute airway obstruction should be simultaneous. If the victim is unconscious and not breathing, he is placed supine with the head tilted backwards by lifting the neck. If the airway is obstructed, the mouth is forced open and cleared of the foreign material.

In a hospital environment, a foreign body from the oropharynx can be removed by using suction devices with large bore non-kinking tubes (Yankaeur sucker).

B. Breathing

Breathing is supported by either direct mouth-to-mouth or mouth-to-nose ventilation.

For mouth-to-mouth ventilation, the patient's head is tilted backwards and the mouth opened slightly. The rescuer takes a deep breath, seals his mouth around the victim's mouth (mouth and nose in a child), blows forcefully in adults and gently in children and watches the chest expand.

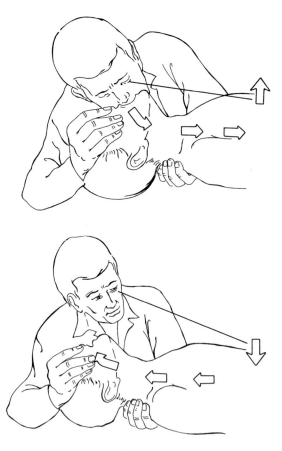

Exhaled air ventilation

Fig. 9.2 Mouth-to-mouth ventilation. This consists of the rescuer sealing his mouth around the victim's mouth and blowing forcefully into the adult patient and watching the chest expand.

When the chest expands, inflation is stopped and the victim is allowed to breathe passively by relaxing the seal on the mouth (Fig. 9.2).

If a victim develops trismus (lock-jaw), a mouth-to-nose ventilation is performed.

In a hospital environment, oxygenation can be carried out using a bag-valve mask. This consists of a self-refilling bag, inlet valve, oxygen reservoir and a breathing valve at the mask end. It facilitates both spontaneous and artificial ventilation.

C. Circulation

Causes of cardiac arrest. The primary causes are ventricular fibrillation (VF) secondary to myocardial ischaemia, and VF and asystole from heart disease, electric shock or drugs. The secondary causes are hypoxia due to pulmonary oedema, shock and acute brain insults.

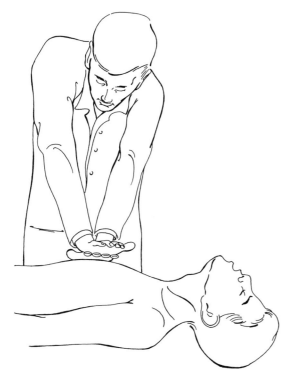

Fig. 9.3 Cardiac massage. This consists of placing the heel of one hand on the lower half of the sternum and the heel of the other hand on top of it. The sternum is compressed downwards towards the spine.

Closed chest CPR. Artificial circulation is readily produced by chest compressions which compress the heart between the sternum and the spine. Blood is forced out of the heart, lungs and aorta when sternal pressure is released. The technique of cardiac compression consists of identifying the xiphoid-sternal junction. The heel of one hand is placed at the lower half of the sternum and the heel of the other hand is placed on top of the first hand (Fig. 9.3).

The sternum is compressed towards the spine 1–2 inches downwards, forcefully enough to produce a good carotid or femoral pulse. The sternum is held down to allow the chest to fill with blood, and the pressure is reapplied every second. The recommended rates vary, based on the number of people resuscitating. If there is one rescuer, the rate is to compress the chest 15 times, alternating with two quick lung inflations a minute. If there are two rescuers, the rate of compression is 60 per minute, with ventilation after fifth compression. The cardiac compression is carried out with the heels of the hands, keeping the fingers raised; this avoids producing rib fractures. In small children, the sternum is compressed with one hand only and in infants, with the tips of two fingers.

Phase II Advanced cardiac life support

After initiating basic life support a spontaneous circulation should be established at the earliest opportunity using IV drugs (step D), ECG diagnosis (step E) and fibrillatory treatment (step F).

D. Drugs and fluids

Drugs and fluids can be given either intravenously, through a central venous line or via a pulmonary route. Drugs such as adrenaline, lignocaine and atropine can also be given transtracheally. Although the intracardiac route is used on a number of occasions, blind injections are not recommended because of the dangers of dysrhythmias when injected into the heart muscle.

If a cardiac arrest is monitored on the ECG in the form of ventricular tachycardia (VT) or ventricular fibrillation (VF), an electric countershock is administered. If it does not restore a spontaneous pulse, CPR is commenced.

Adrenaline, 0.5–1.0 mg, is given IV followed by sodium bicarbonate (NaHCO₃) 1 mmol/kg body weight.

Sodium bicarbonate should not be given if there has been a prompt start of CPR as there is minimal tissue acidosis. If NaHCO₃ is given at the early stage it causes tissue alkalosis which will make VF intractable to treatment.

If a countershock fails to achieve sinus rhythm or if this rhythm reverts rapidly to VF or VT then lignocaine 100–200 mg is given IV slowly followed by an infusion of lignocaine at 1–3 mg per minute. This is followed by a countershock.

If a cardiac arrest is witnessed in asystole then CPR is started followed by IV adrenaline (0.5–1.0 mg). This dose can be repeated every 2–5 minutes. If the cardiac arrest has lasted for more than 2 minutes NaHCO₃ at the rate of 1 mmol/kg is run IV slowly.

Sodium bicarbonate should be given secondary to adrenaline at 1 mmol/kg IV. During CPR the amount of NaHCO₃ required is considerably less but the demand increases after spontaneous circulation is established when the acids formed during hypotension are washed out. Arterial blood gases are estimated and the base deficit (base deficit = excess acid, see also page 233) noted. To correct acidosis NaHCO₃ is given in a large vein. The amount of NaHCO₃ is calculated as follows:

$$\text{Dose of } NaHCO_3 = \text{Base deficit} \times 0.3 \times \text{body weight in kg}$$

Lignocaine is used to treat premature ventricular contractions or VT. The loading dose is 1 mg per kg given IV slowly followed by an infusion at the rate of 1–4 mg per 70 kg body weight per minute via an infusion pump.

Calcium is recommended only for the treatment of electromechanical dissociation. (This means there is electrical activity on ECG, but no output.) Calcium chloride 10% is given in divided doses of 5 ml per 70 kg and repeated if necessary at 10 minute intervals.

Dopamine has an inotropic effect and also increases the renal blood flow. It is set up as infusion to maintain arterial blood pressure at the rate of 2–10 micrograms per kg per minute.

Dobutamine is used to maintain arterial blood pressure in refractory cardiogenic shock at the rate of 2.5–10 micrograms per kg per minute.

Fluids. Intravenous fluids are usually administered to restore normal circulating blood volume after fluid losses, as in dehydration and burns, and to expand the blood volume when cardiac arrest occurs due to hypovolaemia. The choice of IV fluids vary from Hartmann's solution to Haemaccel to blood transfusion.

E. Electrocardiography

As soon as the CPR is started it is essential to attach an ECG monitor to determine the cause i.e. VF, asystole, mechanical asystole with bizarre complexes. Modern defibrillator paddles incorporate ECG pick-up electrodes. Initially the electrodes are placed on the arms and legs and once spontaneous respiration is established the extremity electrodes are replaced with chest electrodes.

F. Fibrillation

Fibrillation is used to treat lethal arrhythmias such as VT and VF. Direct current (DC) shocks are highly effective. The most commonly used energy for external DC shock is 400 J for adults, 100–200 J for children and 50–100 J for infants.

If a cardiac arrest due to VF is witnessed then a countershock is applied within 30–60 seconds of its onset. In an arrest which is not witnessed, CPR is carried out for 2 minutes before an initial attempt is made to defibrillate the patient. If VF persists or recurs after the first two shocks this is repeated several times with CPR in between (Fig. 9.4).

If a countershock fails to correct VF despite CPR, ventilation, adrenaline and NaHCO₃, then it is better to try lignocaine (1 mg per kg body weight). Attempts to defibrillate should not be abandoned

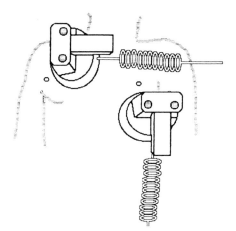

Fig. 9.4 External electrical defibrillation. This consists of applying defibrillator pads on the sternum and at the apex of the heart and applying a direct current shock.

until the acidosis of the patient is adequately corrected.

The suggested initial energy dose for external shock in an adult is 3 joules per kg body weight and 2 joules per kg body weight for children. The highest repeatable dose is 5 joules per kg.

Phase III Prolonged life support

Once the victim is resuscitated, he should be assessed for the damage caused by the cardiac arrest by: gauging, cerebral resuscitation and intensive care support of various organs such as brain, lungs, heart, kidneys.

Cardiac arrest in the operating theatre

If a cardiac arrest occurs in the operating theatre the chances of a successful resuscitation are high because the precipitating causes such as hypoxia, hypovolaemia and electrolyte imbalance are usually reversible. The other factors which help in resuscitation are warning signs in a patient such as cyanosis, bradycardia and hypotension before a cardiac arrest occurs. The presence of trained staff and resuscitation equipment further contributes towards saving a patient.

Ethics of resuscitation

Ideally resuscitation should be attempted only in patients who have a very high chance of successful revival for a comfortable existence. The decision to resuscitate depends on the patient's own wishes, or the opinion of a relative or relatives.

Training in CPR

All health personnel, such as doctors, nurses, theatre personnel and medical students, should be taught the skills of CPR.

To retain knowledge and skills, it is essential to train an individual in advanced cardiac life support for three-hour sessions twice a week.

Training manikins are available to teach both basic and advanced cardiac life support.

NB. Multiple choice questions for this chapter can be found on page 235.

10. Acid–base balance

Acid–base balance is a vast subject and in this chapter an attempt will be made to simplify and correlate a few clinical situations which are seen in operating theatres, recovery rooms and intensive care units.

The biochemistry and physiology of lungs and kidneys are the principal basic sciences involved in acid–base balance. For the maintenance of the normal functioning of body metabolism, the composition of the body surroundings (extracellular) and the contents of cells (intracellular) need to be kept constant or within certain limits. Various processes in the body, such as enzyme activity and the transport of various ions across cell membranes, are pH dependent.

What is pH?

pH denotes the hydrogen ion concentration as its negative logarithm to the base 10. The normal hydrogen ion concentration is between 36 and 44 nanomols (nmol) per litre, whereas the normal range of pH in arterial blood is 7.35–7.44.

The following table shows the corresponding values of hydrogen ion concentration for a set pH.

Hydrogen ions (nmol/litre)	pH (units)
10	8.0
16	7.8
25	7.6
40	7.4
63	7.2
100	7.0

A member of the theatre personnel will be asked to assist the anaesthetist in obtaining an arterial blood sample and then take it to the biochemistry laboratory or the blood gas analyser machine to get the results. The print-out usually shows the following:

	Normal values
pH	36–44
P_{O_2}	11–13.5 kPa
P_{CO_2}	4.6–6.0 kPa
SBC	22–24 mmol/l
ABC	24–26 mmol/l
BE	−2 to +2 mmol/l

pH is the hydrogen ion concentration as described above.

P_{O_2} is the oxygen tension.

P_{CO_2} is the carbon dioxide tension.

SBC is the standard bicarbonate, which is defined as the concentration of bicarbonate in plasma at a P_{CO_2} of 5.3 kPa with haemoglobin fully saturated at 38°C.

ABC is the actual bicarbonate; which is the actual bicarbonate concentration in the plasma at the patient's present body temperature and P_{CO_2} levels.

BE is the base excess which is defined as the amount of acid or base in mmol per litre required to titrate the pH back to 7.40 at a temperature of 38°C with a P_{CO_2} of 5.3 kPa.

After interpreting the above results it can be found out if the patient has a respiratory or metabolic imbalance (alkalosis or acidosis).

The following definitions will further simplify the understanding of the acid–base balance.

— Acidaemia: the hydrogen ion concentration is above the normal range.
— Alkalaemia: the hydrogen ion concentration is below the normal range.

— Acidosis: is a condition which occurs if acidaemia is not corrected.
— Alkalosis: is a condition which occurs if alkalaemia is not corrected.

Alkalosis can be of respiratory (respiratory alkalosis) or metabolic (metabolic alkalosis) origin. Similarly acidosis can be respiratory (respiratory acidosis) or metabolic (metabolic acidosis) in origin. In all these conditions, compensation occurs to varying degrees; it involves a secondary acid–base disturbance which brings the pH changes caused by primary disturbance to within normal limits.

Metabolic alkalosis

This can occur in a patient who has been vomiting with a consequent loss of hydrochloric acid (secreted by the stomach). Metabolic alkalosis is also seen following ingestion of large amounts of sodium bicarbonate. Patients may present with signs of confusion due to a decreased cerebral blood flow and tetany due to a fall in the ionized calcium levels in the plasma. In these patients the body compensates by underventilating and increasing the excretion of bicarbonate in the urine.

A typical arterial blood gas picture in metabolic alkalosis looks as follows:

pH	above 7.45
P_{CO_2}	35–45 mmHg (4.66–5.8 kPa)
Standard bicarbonate	above 26 mmol/litre
Actual bicarbonate	above 26 mmol/litre
Base excess	above + 2 mmol/litre

The P_{O_2} may be high or normal.

When this metabolic alkalosis is compensated by respiratory changes (underventilation), the arterial blood gases look as follows:

pH	7.35–7.45
P_{CO_2}	above 45 mmHg (5.86 kPa)
SBC	above 26 mmol/litre
ABC	above 26 mmol/litre
BE	+ 2 mmol/litre

Respiratory alkalosis

This occurs following hyperventilation with a consequent fall in P_{CO_2} and a rise in pH. The effects of hypocapnia include a decreased cerebral blood flow, clouding of consciousness, and a fall in blood pressure with a lowered ionized calcium and sodium. It prolongs the action of muscle relaxants such as gallamine and shortens the action of curare.

During anaesthesia, a moderate hyperventilation (P_{CO_2} of 3–3.5 kPa) can reduce the requirement of barbiturates, analgesia and potentiate hypotensive anaesthesia (see p. 183).

The side-effects of hypocapnia during anaesthesia include fetal asphyxia (during caesarean section if the mother is hyperventilated), a fall in cardiac output, and cerebral changes in elderly patients due to vasoconstriction of cerebral blood vessels.

A typical arterial blood gas picture in respiratory alkalosis looks like:

pH	7.5
P_{CO_2}	18 mmHg (2.4 kPa)
SBC	20.5 mmol/litre
ABC	14 mmol/litre
BE	−4.5 mmol/litre

Metabolic acidosis

This occurs in diabetic ketoacidosis, starvation, salicylate poisoning and acute renal failure. The clinical signs include: clouding of consciousness, cold blue hands and feet, and gasping respiration.

A typical arterial blood gas picture shows:

pH	7.19
P_{CO_2}	33 (4.4 kPa)
SBC	14 mmol/litre
ABC	13 mmol/litre
BE	−14 mmol/litre

Respiratory acidosis

This occurs during the administration of anaesthesia following underventilation due to respiratory obstruction, narcotic overdose, faulty CO_2 absorption by the soda lime absorber and accidental administration of CO_2. A rise in CO_2 causes an increase in cerebral blood flow and intracranial pressure, and a rise in catecholamines which in turn cause an increase in cardiac output and contraction of the heart. Peripheral resistance is increased.

A typical arterial blood gas picture shows:

pH	7.22
P_{CO_2}	80 mmHg (10.7 kPa)
SBC	26 mmol/litre
ABC	31.5 mmol/litre
BE	+2.5 mmol/litre

MULTIPLE CHOICE QUESTIONS ON CARDIOPULMONARY RESUSCITATION, ACID-BASE BALANCE AND INTENSIVE CARE

The answers to these questions can be found on page 254.

1. **Which one of the following is not a characteristic of cardiac arrest**
   A pin-point pupils
   B death-like appearance
   C absent pulses
   D pallor or cyanosis.

2. **The normal P_{O_2} of arterial blood is:**
   A 95 mmHg
   B 40 mmHg
   C 46 mmHg
   D 110 mmHg.

3. **When two operators are available during cardiopulmonary resuscitation (CPR), the ratio of mouth-to-mouth ventilation to cardiac massage in an adult is:**
   A 2:15
   B 1:5
   C 1:10
   D 1:15.

4. **In the terminology of blood gases SBC stands for:**
   A actual bicarbonate
   B standard bicarbonate
   C base excess
   D base deficit.

5. **Hyperventilation causes:**
   A respiratory acidosis
   B respiratory alkalosis
   C metabolic alkalosis
   D metabolic acidosis.

6. **Metabolic acidosis is seen in all the conditions except:**
   A diabetics
   B salicylate poisoning
   C hyperventilation
   D hypoxia.

7. **In the intensive care unit, junior anaesthetists carry out all duties except:**
   A liaising with senior medical staff and nursing staff
   B liaising with other specialties
   C taking major decisions
   D acting on recent test results.

8. **In cardiopulmonary resuscitation (CPR), adrenaline is given in:**
   A systole
   B ventricular fibrillation
   C ventricular tachycardia
   D electromechanical dissociation.

9. **With regard to defibrillation in cardiac arrest which one of the following is not true?**
   A Commonly used shock is with an AC current
   B Current strength starts at 100 joules
   C The maximum strength which can be used is 5 joules per kg in adult
   D The maximum strength which can be used is 2 joules per kg in a child.

10. **Which one of the following drugs is not used in cardiac arrest?**
    A adrenaline
    B sodium bicarbonate
    C calcium
    D ranitidine.

11. Management of chronic pain

Chronic pain or intractable pain is defined as that pain which is not relieved by conventional treatment such as analgesics or nerve blocks.

Pain relief clinics

There are three types of recognized clinics:

(i) *A single-handed practice* is where an anaesthetist interested in pain relief work sees patients on a limited scale. He/she carries out simple examinations and nerve blocks.

(ii) *A multidisciplinary clinic* is where a number of specialists such as a physician, surgeon, anaesthetist, neurosurgeon, psychiatrist, physiotherapist and social worker are involved. There is an organized outpatient clinic with adequate junior medical and nursing staff. These types of clinics are few in the United Kingdom but are often seen in the USA.

(iii) *The intermediate group,* somewhere between the single-handed practice and multidisciplinary clinic, is most often seen in the UK. This clinic is usually run by one or two consultant anaesthetists, with outpatient facilities, arrangements for investigations, one or two inpatient beds, operating time and radiological facilities to perform nerve blocks.

Who refers the patients?

A number of referrals to pain relief clinics are by general practitioners, orthopaedic surgeons, vascular surgeons and local hospices. To a certain extent ophthalmologists and ENT surgeons also refer patients to the clinic.

What types of patients are referred?

The types of patients referred to the clinic are those suffering from:

A. Vascular conditions:
    (i) Migraine
    (ii) Raynaud's disease
    (iii) Claudication due to thromboangiitis obliterans.
B. Orthopaedic conditions:
    (i) Backache
    (ii) Osteoarthritis.
C. Neurological conditions:
    (i) Trigeminal neuralgia
    (ii) Post-herpetic neuralgia
    (iii) Nerve entrapment syndromes such as scar pain and back pain
    (iv) Pain from neuromas—stump pain
    (v) Central pain e.g. phantom limb pain and thalamic pain.
D. Pain due to carcinoma:
    (i) Arising from primary growth
    (ii) Due to metastasis
    (iii) Following treatment (e.g. radiotherapy)
E. Unknown cause: Atypical facial pain.
F. Psychogenic pain.

These are only a few of the wide range of conditions presented at the clinic.

Assessment of patients with chronic pain

All the patients referred to the pain relief clinic are assessed thoroughly including obtaining a history, clinical examination and investigation, and a definitive diagnosis is made following which treatment is carried out. In some patients, in spite of lengthy investigations no definitive cause can be found and their pain is treated symptomatically.

A number of patients with chronic pain suffer from anxiety and depression. They are assessed by a psychiatrist and treatment is prescribed.

Management of patients with chronic pain

The management of patients with chronic pain depends on their life expectancy. Patients with normal life expectancy suffering from chronic pain are treated differently from patients who have a short life expectancy (e.g. patients with cancer pain).

Patients with normal life expectancy

These patients are usually suffering from backache, post-herpetic neuralgia, Raynaud's disease and postoperative scar pain. The aim of the treatment consists of proper diagnosis and treatment. For example a patient with backache needs to be investigated by either an orthopaedic surgeon or a neurosurgeon, and if there is a cause, surgical correction should be carried out.

If the patient still has pain the following line of treatment is carried out:

1. Drugs. Patients are prescribed non-steroidal anti-inflammatory drugs (NSAIDs). For mild to moderate pains acetylsalicylic acid (Aspirin), codeine or dihydrocodeine, and dextropropoxyphene (Distalgesic) are prescribed, and for severe pain buprenorphine (Temgesic), nalbuphine (Nubain) and meptazinol (Meptid) are prescribed. Potent analgesics such as morphine and diamorphine are not prescribed for fear of addiction.

Other drugs used include carbamazepine (Tegretol), prescribed in the treatment of trigeminal neuralgia, and phenytoin (Dilantin) and sodium valproate (Epilim), prescribed for patients with post-herpetic neuralgia.

2. Nerve blocks. These are carried out with local anaesthetics such as plain 0.25–0.5% bupivacaine (Marcain). The nerve blocks which are performed are local infiltration for scar pain and individual nerve blocks. Epidural blocks are performed for low back pain and sciatica using 0.5% plain Marcain and Depomedrone (methylprednisolone). The epidural blocks are performed at either the cervical, thoracic, lumbar or caudal level.

3. Alternative methods of pain relief. When the pain relief is inadequate in these patients with normal life expectancy, following the use of drugs and nerve blocks, the next line of treatment consists of:

a Transcutaneous nerve stimulation (TNS). A small battery-operated stimulator is used to apply an electrical stimulus to the skin overlying the painful area via flexible electrodes.

b Acupuncture. This treatment is based upon the principle that insertion of needles at certain points of the body can produce analgesia. Acupuncture points are areas of low skin electrical resistance and acupuncture needles are inserted to varying depths at these points.

Hypnosis, biofeedback and operant conditioning are other alternative methods of pain relief.

Patients with short life expectancy

The aim of treatment in this group of patients is to make them pain-free, and the danger of addiction to narcotic drugs and the side-effects of permanent nerve blocks do not take precedence.

The line of management consists of the following:

1. Drug therapy. Potent analgesics (morphine, diamorphine) are given either orally or intramuscularly at regular intervals and not as necessary.

2. Nerve blocks. Before carrying out permanent blocks, temporary nerve blocks using local anaesthetic solutions are carried out. This may confirm whether the block may or may not be effective. An image intensifier is essential to carry out some blocks such as chemical sympathectomy and coeliac plexus blocks.

The following are some of the important nerve blocks:

Trigeminal nerve block. The block of this nerve and its branches is carried out for the relief of facial pain in patients suffering from trigeminal neuralgia.

Intrathecal block. This technique is highly effective if the pain is confined to a few dermatomes. A hyperbaric solution of phenol in glycerine is used. If this block is performed at the sacral region, sphincter control is lost resulting in urinary retention.

Autonomic blocks. Stellate ganglion block is carried out to relieve pain of vascular origin.

Lumbar chemical sympathectomy is carried out to relieve the pain of claudication and improve the blood flow to the lower limbs. It is performed using an image intensifier and 6% aqueous phenol.

Coeliac plexus block is carried out to relieve pain due to malignancy of the abdominal contents. An image intensifier and either 50% alcohol or phenol are used.

3. Cryoanalgesia means destruction of the nerves using cold temperature probes. The probe (called a cryoprobe) consists of an insulated needle and it produces a cooling effect using nitrous oxide as the refrigerant. The probe tip can reach temperatures of up to −80°C, thus producing nerve destruction at the site of application.

4. Radiofrequency lesion. The radiofrequency lesion maker uses a high frequency alternating current which flows from the tip of the electrodes to the tissues. Temperatures above 45°C damage the nerve fibres, thus preventing the conduction of nerve impulses. This radiofrequency generator is used in the treatment of trigeminal neuralgia and percutaneous cervical cordotomy.

5. Cordotomies. Anterolateral cordotomy is a procedure carried out on the anterolateral tracts of the spinal cord where the nerve tracts are sectioned. This relieves the pain on the opposite side.

6. Pituitary ablation. Alcoholic injection in the pituitary gland is carried out in patients with severe cancer pain. This technique involves inserting a needle into the pituitary area via the transphenoidal route. After confirming the position of the needle using a image intensifier, increments of 0.1 ml of absolute alcohol are injected until the desired effect is achieved.

Role of the operating theatre personnel in the pain clinic

Anaesthetic nurses and the ODAs are involved in the organization of trolleys containing needles, syringes and drugs. Similarly, they are involved in the organization of nerve block sessions.

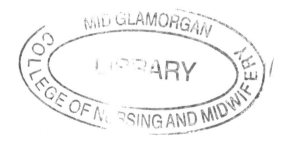

12. National health service

History

In the 17th century, money was raised by the non-elected local authorities through rates to finance the support of blind, lame and disadvantaged people who were without work. Between 1750 and 1800 the number of voluntary or charitable hospitals grew considerably as Britain increased her wealth through foreign trade. However, for the next century, inpatient and outpatient hospital care was used mostly by the poor living in cities. The majority of rich patients were treated at home, and many of the doctors who worked in the voluntary hospitals earned their income from these rich people and gained their clinical experience from the hospitals. In 1808, the Country Asylums Act allowed local authorities to construct and finance institutions for the 'insane'.

In 1867 the Metropolitan Poor Act created a common fund and enabled the non-elected London local authorities to provide separate institutional care for smallpox, tuberculosis and the 'insane'. In 1926 a Royal Commission on National Health Insurance recommended that the health services be financed directly from public funds.

In 1946 Bevan's National Health Service Act was passed and in 1948 the National Health Service (NHS) was formed. In 1974, on the recommendation of Sir Keith Joseph, the first reorganization took place. Local health authorities were created to provide health care whose powers were restricted to environmental services. In 1982 a further reorganization of the NHS eliminated the area health authority tier of the NHS in England. District health authorities became the main operational authorities.

In 1983 the Griffiths management enquiry was established and conducted. The NHS employs more than 1.2 million full-time and part-time staff. It is the nation's largest institution, utilizing about 6% of manpower resources. In the last 40 years the NHS has undergone considerable changes.

Scotland, Northern Ireland and Wales have slightly different NHS arrangements to England, though many of the general points made can be related to the NHS in England (see Fig. 12.1).

The NHS in Scotland (with a population of 5.2 million) involved the creation of 15 area health boards immediately below the Home and Health Department, the ultimate authority lying with the Secretary of State who is advised by the Scottish Health Service Planning Council. At a sub-area level the Scottish boards were allowed to establish as many districts as possible. Thus the Greater Glasgow Health Board, serving 1.1 million people, set up five district boards. In the 1980s restructuring of the health care system occurred in Scotland. All 15 health boards eliminated their districts, and unit level management was introduced and strengthened.

In Northern Ireland, with a population of 1.5 million people, reorganization of the NHS took place in October 1973. Under the Ministry of Health and Social Services, four new health and social services boards were set up. There is an advisory central council and the Northern Ireland Central Services Agency handles the administration of issues of common interest.

Each board has districts with their own district executive teams, working in relationship with

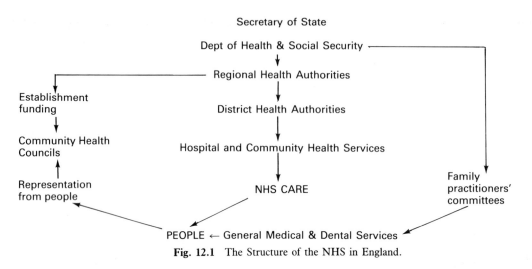

Fig. 12.1   The Structure of the NHS in England.

those above. In the reorganization the four health boards were retained, the districts were eliminated and more powers were delegated to the unit management level.

In Wales, with a population of 2.5 million people, eight area health authorities were created along with a Welsh Health Technical Services Organization. The Secretary of State at the Welsh Office has ultimate authority in the Welsh NHS. During reorganization, the original area health authorities were converted into district health authorities, except in the case of Dyfed which was split into two. Below the District tier, unit organization has been introduced.

After the 1982 reorganization of the NHS, various working parties were set up by the Government on health service information (Korner Working Party), the development of performance indicators and a 'value for money audit'. Gerard Vaughn, the Minister of State for Health in early 1982, emphasized the need for distribution of power in the NHS and the creation of a system directly influenced by consumers' (patients') wishes. He also stressed the importance of cutting administrative costs, with emphasis being placed on the need for better management.

In 1982 Norman Fowler was appointed as Secretary of State for Health and Social Services and government policy shifted towards the NHS being more accountable to Parliament. He commissioned an independent NHS management enquiry led by Roy Griffiths, the managing director of J. Sainsbury PLC. This Griffiths enquiry team decided to focus on matters relating primarily to hospital management and also to recommend reforms which could be achieved within existing legislation. The summary of recommendations of the Griffiths Report is as follows:

> The NHS should be managed more like a business organization. At the DHSS there should be a part-time supervisory board comprising ministers and chief officials, and a full-time management board with a chairman who should perform the functions of a general management at national level with a director of personnel and specialists in other functions. Each regional health authority (RHA) and district health authority (DHA) should appoint a general manager and a similar provision be made for each unit. Emphasis was placed on the importance of the general management function at every level and also the importance of unit budgets and the involvement of doctors in management.

By mid-1985 all regions and nearly all districts had appointed a general manager and the Secretary of State had appointed the chairman of the NHS management board. All the managers are appointed on a short-term contract.

The Griffiths Report was also applied to Wales, Scotland and Northern Ireland.

In January 1989, the government under the Secretary of State for Health published a White Paper, Working for Patients, which set out plans to reform and strengthen the NHS. This proposal is designed with two objectives:

a. To give patients, wherever they live, better health care and a greater choice of the services available
b. To produce greater satisfaction and rewards for NHS staff who successfully respond to local need and preferences.

The White Paper contains seven key measures:

1. More delegation of responsibility to local level to make the service more responsive to patients' needs.
2. Self-governing hospitals. To encourage a better service to patients, hospitals will be able to apply for a new self-governing status within the NHS as NHS hospital trusts.
3. New funding arrangements. To enable hospitals which best meet patients' needs to get the money to do so, the money required to treat patients will be able to cross administrative boundaries (i.e. from one health authority to another).
4. Additional consultants. To reduce waiting times and improve the quality of service, 100 new permanent consultant posts will be created over the next three years.
5. GP practice budgets. To help the family doctor improve his service to patients, large GP practices will be able to apply for their own NHS budgets to obtain a range of services direct from hospitals.
6. Reformed management bodies. To improve the effectiveness of NHS management, regional, district and family practitioner management bodies will be reduced in size and reformed on business lines.
7. Better audit arrangements. To ensure that all who deliver patient services make the best use of resources, quality of service and value for money will be more rigorously audited.

These proposals will be put forward to Parliament for approval. The reforms will take place in three main phases:

Phase I: 1989

1. The Secretary of State for Health will establish a new NHS policy board and reconstitute the management board as a management executive.
2. The health departments and RHAs in England: will identify the first hospitals to become self-governing as NHS hospital trusts and plan for their new status; will devolve further operational responsibility to districts and hospitals; and will begin preparing the grounds for GP practice budgets.
3. The Government will introduce regulations to make it easier for patients to change their GP.
4. The first additional consultant posts will be created; districts will begin agreeing on job descriptions with their consultants; and a new framework for the medical audit will begin to be implemented.
5. The Resource Management Initiative will be extended to more major acute hospitals.
6. Preparations for indicative drug budgets for GPs will begin.
7. The audit commission will begin its work in the NHS.

Phase II: 1990

1. The changes begun in 1989 will gather momentum. Devolving operational responsibility, changing the management of consultants' contracts and extending the medical audit throughout the hospital service will near completion.
2. 'Shadow' boards of the first group of NHS hospital trusts will start to develop their plans for the future.
3. RHAs, DHAs and the FPC will become accountable to RHAs. Regions will begin paying directly for work they do for each other.

Phase III: 1991

1. The first NHS hospital trusts will be established.
2. The first GP practice budget-holders will begin buying services for their patients.

3. The indicative drug budget scheme will be implemented.
4. DHAs will begin paying directly for work they do for each other.

REFERENCE

Working for patients 1989 A summary of the White Paper on the government's proposals following its review of the NHS. HMSO, London

Appendix

(A) SI units (Système International d'Unités)

There are seven base units and they are expressed in SI units as follows:

Base units	SI units	Symbol
Length	metre	m
Mass	kilogram	kg
Time	second	s
Amount of substance	mole	mol
Electric current	ampere	A
Thermodynamic temperature	kelvin	K
Luminous intensity	candela	cd

Other units are derived by multiplying or dividing the base units. For example:

Volume	cubic metre	m^3
Force	newton	N
Pressure (force/area)	pascal	Pa

SI multiples and fractions

Multiples	SI prefix	Symbol
10	deca	da (D)
10^2	hecto	h
10^3	kilo	K
10^6	mega	M
10^9	giga	G
10^{12}	tera	T

Fractions	SI prefix	Symbol
10^{-1}	deci	d
10^{-2}	centi	c
10^{-3}	milli	m
10^{-6}	micro	μ
10^{-9}	nano	n
10^{-12}	pico	p

(B). Haematological values

(These values vary from laboratory to laboratory)

		Normal values	SI units
Red cell count (RBC)	Male	5.5 +/− 1	$\times 10^{12}$/litre
	Female	4.8 +/ − 1	$\times 10^{12}$/litre
Haemoglobin (Hb)	Male	15.5 +/−2.5	g/dl (decilitre)
	Female	14 +/− 2.5	g/dl
Mean corpuscular volume (MCV)		85 +/− 18	
Mean corpuscular haemoglobin (MCH)		29.5 +/−2.5	pg (picogram)

Table continued

	Normal values	SI units
Reticulocytes (0.2–2%)	10–100	$\times\ 10^9$/litre
White cell count (WCC)	7.5 +/− 3.5	$\times\ 10^9$/litre
Differential count		
Lymphocytes (20–45%)	1.5–4.0	$\times\ 10^9$/litre
Neutrophils (40–75%)	2.0–7.5	$\times\ 10^9$/litre
Monocytes (2–10%)	0.2–0.8	$\times\ 10^9$/litre
Eosinophils (1–6%)	0.04–0.4	$\times\ 10^9$/litre
Basophils (less than 1%)	Less than 0.1	$\times\ 10^9$/litre
Platelets	150–400	$\times\ 10^9$/litre
Erythrocyte sedimentation rate (ESR) (Westergren method)	Male up to 5 mm in first hour Female up to 9 mm in first hour	

Coagulation tests

Test	Normal range	What does it test
Bleeding time	1–7 minutes	Behaviour of blood vessels and platelets
Prothrombin time	10–14 seconds	Tests extrinsic system of clotting
Thrombin time	10–12 seconds	Conversion of fibrinogen to fibrin
Total fibrinogen assay	2–4 g/litre	It is decreased in pregnancy and DIC
Fibrin degradation products (FDPs)	Absent or trace <10 mg/litre	Detects fibrinolytic activity; increased in DIC
Partial thromboplastin time	35–45 seconds	

(C) Biochemical values

(These values vary from one laboratory to another)

Plasma	Normal range	Units	Abnormalities
Sodium	135–145	mmol/l	Increased in sodium load and decreased in water excess
Potassium	3.5–5.5	mmol/l	High in acute renal failure, low in patients on diuretics
Chloride	96–106	mmol/l	High in patients with ureters implanted in colon and low in patients with pyloric stenosis

Table continued

Plasma	Normal range	Units	Abnormalities
Bicarbonate	23–29	mmol/l	Low in acute/chronic renal failure and diabetic acidosis
Urea	2.5–7.0	mmol/l	High in renal failure, sodium loss Low in water load
Creatinine	60–120	μmol/l	High in acute and chronic renal failure
Osmolality	280–295	mosmol/kg	High in renal failure and diabetes insipidus.

Serum	Normal range	Units	Abnormalities
Total protein	60–80	g/l	Low in malnutrition,
Albumin	35–50	g/l	and nephrotic syndrome
Globulin	20–40	g/l	Increased in cirrhosis
Total calcium	2.12–2.62	mmol/l	Low in renal failure
Ionized calcium	1.14–1.30	mmol/l	Low in renal failure and during liver transplantation
Phosphate	0.8–1.4	mmol/l	Decreased in malnutrition

(D) Respiratory system

Composition of inspired and expired gases (pressure in kPa)

	Air	Alveolar	Expired
Oxygen	19.9	13–15	15–16
Nitrogen	75.0	78–79	77
Carbon dioxide	–	4–6	2.8–3.7
Water vapour	–	6.3	6.3

Arterial blood gases

	Range
pH	7.35–7.45
H^+	36–44 (nmol/litre)
Oxygen (kPa)	11.9–13.2
Carbon dioxide (kPa)	4.8–6.3
Bicarbonate	
actual	22–30 (mmol/litre)
standard	21–25 (mmol/litre)
Base excess	+/ −2 mmol/litre

Gas exchange

Measurement	Value/range	Unit	Symbol
Respiratory rate	12–20	/minute	f
Minute volume	6–10	l/min	VE
Tidal volume	0.3–0.65	l/min	Vt
Alveolar minute volume	4–7	l/min	VA
Anatomical dead space	2	ml/kg	Vd
Oxygen consumption	11–13	mmol/minute	nO_2
Carbon dioxide production	9–11	mmol/minute	nCO_2
Respiratory quotient	0.8		

Simple lung function tests

Measurement	Range & units		Symbols
	Male	Female	
Forced expiratory volume	3.5 ± 1.5 l/sec	2.5 ± 1.0 l/sec	FEV_1
Forced vital capacity	4.5 ± 1.5 1	3.5 ± 1.0 1	FVC
Peak expiratory flow rate	550 ± 150 l/min	400 ± 100 l/min	PEFR

(The first two measurements are carried out using a spirometer whilst PEFR is carried out using a peak flow meter)

(E) Cardiovascular system

Electrocardiogram

Wave	Duration (sec) Average		Range	What does it mean
P wave	<0.10			Atrial contraction
PR interval	0. 18		0.12–20	Atrial depolarization and conduction throughout AV node
QRS time	0.08	to	0.10	Ventricular depolarization
QT interval	0.40	to	0.43	Ventricular depolarization plus ventricular repolarization
T wave	<0.22			Ventricular repolarization

Normal pressures (mmHg)

	Range	Derived values in haemodynamics
Central venous pressure (CVP)	0–7	
Right atrium (RA)	1–10	5
Right ventricle (RV)		
systolic	14–30	23
diastolic	0–7	9
Pulmonary artery (PA)		
systolic	15–30	25
diastolic	5–12	9
Pulmonary artery wedge press (PAWP)	5–15	10
Left atrium (LA)	8	8

Derived values

		Value (in a 70 kg man)
Stroke volume (SV)	$\dfrac{\text{Cardiac output} \times 1000}{\text{Heart rate}}$	80/ml
Cardiac output (CO)	Stroke volume × heart rate	5 litres/min
Cardiac index (CI)	$\dfrac{\text{Cardiac output}}{\text{Body surface area}}$	3.2 l/min/m^2
Rate pressure product (RPP)	Systolic arterial press. × heart rate	12 000

(F) Fluid composition in body

	Male	Female
Total water content:		
Between 18 and 45 years of age	60%	55%
Above 60 years of age	55%	45%

Volume of extracellular fluid (ECF) is 35% of total water content and the volume of intracellular fluid (ICF) is 65% of total water content.

Blood volumes	
Infant	90 ml/kg body weight
Child	80 ml/kg body weight
Adult female	65 ml/kg body weight
Adult male	75 ml/kg body weight

(G) Composition of commonly used IV fluids in theatre

Fluid	Na	K	Cl	HCO$_3$	others	pH	Glucose
			(all in mmol/litre)				g/litre
Dextrose	0	0	0	0		4.0	50
Dextrose 4% in 0.18% saline	31	0	31	0		4.5	40
Sodium chloride 0.9%	154	0	154	0		5.0	
Lactated Ringer's (Hartmann's)	131	5	112	29	Mg^{++} Ca^{++}		
Sodium bicarbonate 8.4%	1000	0	0	1000		8.0	
Haemaccel	145	5.1	145	0	Ca^{++}		
Dextran 70 in 0.9% NaCl	154	0	154	0		4–7	
Dextran 70 in 5% Dextrose	0	0	0	0		3.5–7	50
HPPF	150	2	120			7.4	40

(H) Conversion from weight per unit volume to mmol/litre

The formula used for this conversion is:

Concentration in mmol/litre =

$$\frac{10 \times \text{concentration in mg/100 ml}}{\text{Molecular weight}}$$

Example: Conversion of glucose 180 mg/100 ml to mmol/litre, the molecular weight of glucose being 180.

$$\frac{10 \times 180 \text{ mg/100 ml}}{180} = 10 \text{ mmol/litre}$$

Other conversions

Height: cm = inches × 2.54
   e.g. 10 in × 2.54 = 25.4 cm
Weight: kg = lb × 0.454
Volume: ml = fl oz × 28.5
Pressure: kPa = mmHg × 0.133
   e.g. 100 mmHg × 0.133 = 13.3 kPa

inches = cm × 0.39
   e.g. 10 cm × 0.39 = 3.9 inches
lb = kg × 2.2
fl oz = ml × 0.035

mmHg = kPa × 7.5
   e.g. 10 kPa × 7.5 = 75 mmHg

Remember:

1 gram (g) = 1000 milligrams (mg)
1 milligram (mg) = 1000 micrograms
1 mega unit = 1 000 000 units (1 million units).

A percentage solution means the number of parts of a drug in a hundred parts of the final solution. The abbreviation %(percent) is used to express it.
   For example, a 5% solution of dextrose means:

5 parts of dextrose in 100 parts of the solution
1 part of dextrose in 20 parts of the solution
5 grams of dextrose in 100 ml of the solution.

On a number of occasions, theatre staff are asked to handle solutions (such as adrenaline, cocaine) which are expressed as dilutions.
   What do these dilutions mean?

1 in 5 solution means 20%
1 in 10 solution means 10%
1 in 40 solution means 2.5%
1 in 100 solution means 1%
1 in 1000 solution means 0.1%

Certain conversions/formulae used to calculate infusion rates

(i) If you want to convert drops/min to ml/hour:

$$\frac{\text{Number of drops per minute} \times 60 \text{ minutes}}{\text{Drops per ml of giving set}}$$

= ml/hour

If a paediatric buretrol (giving set) which gives 60 drops per ml is used and 20 drops per minute are to be given, then ml/hour to be set up is:

$$\frac{20 \times 60}{60} = 20 \text{ ml/hour}$$

(ii) To calculate the number of drops/minute for IV infusion:

$$\frac{\text{Volume (ml) to be infused c drops/ml of giving set}}{\text{Time (minutes) over which volume is to be given}}$$

= drops/minute

(This formula is used daily in recovery rooms and wards postoperatively.)

For example, an infusion of dextrose saline 500 ml is set up via an ordinary giving set which delivers 15 drops/minute and has to be delivered in 6 hours; then drops/minute can be calculated as:

$$\frac{500 \times 15}{360 \text{ minutes}} = 20 \text{ drops/minute}$$

(iii) On a number of occasions staff in the anaesthetic or recovery rooms are asked to assist the anaesthetist in setting up infusions of dopamine, dobutamine or sodium nitroprusside.

Example:

800 mg of dopamine added to 500 ml of 5% dextrose or
250 mg of dobutamine added to 500 ml of 5% dextrose or
50 mg of sodium nitroprusside added to 100 ml of 5% dextrose

The following calculation gives the number of drops/minute to be set up on an infusing device (e.g. IVAC pump) for an infusion of the above-mentioned drugs prescribed in micrograms/kg/minute.

$$\frac{\text{Drops/ml of giving set} \times \text{Dosage prescribed (microgram/kg/min)} \times \text{Volume of diluent}}{\text{Amount of drug (micrograms used in solution)}}$$

$$\frac{60 \times 70 \times 2 \times 500}{800\,000} = 5 \text{ drops per minute}$$

Where 60 is drops/ml of giving set; 70 is body weight in kg; 2 is dosage of dopamine in micrograms/kg/min prescribed; 500 ml is the diluent and 800 000 micrograms of dopamine is used to make up the solution.

Usually wall charts are provided by respective manufacturers to give accurate dosage according to body weights.

Nowadays a number of anaesthetists are using syringe pumps to set up infusions of various drugs such as muscle relaxants (atracurium, vecuronium), propofol (Diprivan) or analgesics such as papaveretum (Omnopon), alfentanil (Rapifen). The dilution of these agents varies with the individual anaesthetists and the types of syringe pumps used.

(I) Physical properties of anaesthetic agents

Name	Formula	BP*(°C)	SVP*	MAC*(%)	Blood gas coefficients
Cyclopropane	C_3H_6	−33	4800	9.2	0.45
Chloroform	$CHCl_3$	61	160	0.5	10
Enflurane	$CHFCl, CF_2CF_2H$	56	175	1.68	1.9
Ether (Diethyl)	$C_2H_5OC_2H_5$	35	425	1.9	12
Halothane	$CF_3CHClBr$	50	243	0.8	2.5

Table continued

Name	Formula	BP*(°C)	SVP*	MAC*(%)	Blood gas coefficients
Isoflurane	$CF_3CHClCF_2H$	49	250	1.15	1.4
Nitrous oxide	N_2O	−88	–	105	0.47
Trichlorethylene	$CHClCCl_2$	87	60	0.17	9.0

*BP = Boiling point (in °C)
*SVP = Saturated vapour pressure at 20°C
*MAC = Minimum alveolar concentration

(J) Endotracheal tube size

(i) Children

The internal diameter of an endotracheal tube for a child may be calculated from the formula:

$$\frac{Age\ (years)}{4} + 4$$

For example an 8-year-old child will require, according to the formula, a size 6.0 endotracheal tube. Ideally it is advisable to use non-cuffed tubes below the age of 10 years and also to use a tube one size smaller than calculated.

However this formula does not hold below the 2 to 3 years age group and also the length of the tube required for each age group varies.

The length of an endotracheal tube for children in the 1 to 3 years' age group is calculated as:

$$\frac{Height\ in\ centimetres}{5} + 12 = cm$$

The formula is not accurate for infants below the age of one year where head circumference (the Liverpool chart) is used.

For simplicity, the chart below may be useful with regard to choosing the length (oral, nasal) and internal diameter of the tubes.

(ii) Adults

An adult female requires a size 8.0 mm or 8.5 mm cuffed endotracheal tube whereas an adult male needs a size 9.0 or 9.5 mm tube.

The length required for size 8.0 or 8.5 mm is 21 cm for oral and 24 cm for nasal tubes. The length for a size 9.0 is 23 cm for oral and 25 cm for nasal tubes.

Endotracheal tube sizes for children

Age	Tube internal diameter (mm)	Length (cm) Oral	Nasal
0–3 months	3.0	10	
3–6 months	3.5	12	15
6–12 months	4.0	12	15
2 years	4.5	13	16
3 years	4.5	13	16
4 years	5.0	14	17
6 years	5.5	15	18
8 years	6.0	16	19
10 years	6.5	17	20
12 years	7.0	18	21

Answers to multiple choice questions

Anatomy and physiology (*page 45*)

1. C	6. B	11. B	16. B
2. A	7. C	12. B	17. C
3. C	8. B	13. B	18. B
4. A	9. A	14. C	19. C
5. C	10. C	15. D	20. B

Pharmacology (*page 76*)

1. D	5. D	9. A	13. D
2. A	6. C	10. B	14. A, C
3. C	7. C	11. B	15. A
4. C	8. D	12. C	

Microbiology (*page 95*)

1. C	6. B	11. B	16. C
2. A	7. C	12. C	17. C
3. B	8. A	13. C	18. B
4. A	9. A	14. A	19. A
5. C	10. B	15. A	20. C

Physics and electronics (*page 120*)

1. A	6. A	11. B	16. B
2. C	7. C	12. B	17. C
3. C	8. C	13. C	18. A
4. A	9. B	14. D	19. B
5. A	10. D	15. B	20. B

Patient care (*page 136*)

1. A	6. D	11. A	16. B
2. A	7. A	12. B	17. C
3. C	8. B	13. C	18. A
4. C	9. A	14. B	19. B
5. C	10. C	15. C	20. C

Anaesthesia (*page 139*)

1. A	4. C	7. C	10. B
2. D	5. B	8. A	
3. C	6. B	9. C	

Surgery (*page 199*)

1. C	5. C	9. B	13. B
2. C	6. B	10. C	14. A
3. B	7. D	11. D	15. B
4. A	8. B	12. B	

Recovery area (*page 225*)

1. C	4. D	7. A	10. D
2. C	5. A	8. A	
3. A	6. B	9. C	

Cardiopulmonary resuscitation and acid base (*page 235*)

1. A	4. B	7. C	10. D
2. A	5. B	8. A	
3. B	6. C	9. A	

Glossary

Abdomen	Largest cavity in the body, lying below the thorax and separated from it by the diaphragm.
Abdominoperineal	Relating to the abdomen and perineum. This term is used in the surgical removal of rectal cancer.
Abduct	To move away from the median line of the body; opposite to adduct.
Ablation	Excision or removal.
Abrasion	Superficial injury to the skin or mucous membrane.
Abscess	A localized collection of pus caused by bacteria.
Acebutolol	A beta-adrenergic blocking drug used in the control of hypertension, angina pectoris and dysrhythmias.
Acetylcholine	A chemical substance (also called neurotransmitter) which is released at the neuromuscular junction resulting in the passage of a nerve impulse.
Actrapid	Neutral insulin.
Adenocarcinoma	A malignant tumour of glandular tissue e.g. breast.
Adenoidectomy	Removal of adenoid tissue from the nasopharynx.
Adenotonsillectomy	Removal of adenoids and tonsils.
Adhesion	Following inflammation, abnormal union of two parts by a fibrous tissue.
Adiposity	Excessive accumulation of fat in the body.
Adrenalectomy	Removal of adrenal gland.
Afebrile	Without fever.
Agglutination	Clumping of red blood cells in the presence of specific immune antibodies called agglutinins.
Allograft	When a part of one person is transplanted into another person.
Amethocaine	A synthetic local anaesthetic.
Anaesthesia	Reversible loss of sensation.
Anaphylaxis	When a body is presented with a foreign protein, it becomes hypersensitive and, following a second exposure, can result in an acute reaction.
Aneurysm	Local dilatation of a blood vessel, usually an artery.
Antacid	An agent which neutralizes acidity e.g. Mist. Mag. Trisilicate or sodium citrate.
Anticholinesterase	An enzyme that destroys acetylcholine at nerve endings. Neostigmine is a drug with this property.
Anticoagulant	An agent which prevents clotting of blood e.g. Heparin
Antiemetic	An agent which prevents nausea and vomiting e.g. metoclopramide (Maxolon) and prochlorperazine (Stemetil).
Antihistamine	An agent that blocks the effect of histamine e.g. chlorpheniramine (Piriton).

Antrostomy	In ENT surgery, an artificial opening is made from the nasal cavity to the antrum of the maxillary sinus to facilitate the drainage of pus.
Arteriogram	A film showing arteries after the injection of an opaque substance in the X-ray department.
Arthroplasty	Creation of an artificial joint.
Arthroscopy	Procedure in which the inside of a joint is visualized.
Ascites	Free fluid in the abdominal cavity.
Autoclave	An apparatus used to sterilize equipment.
Avascular	Bloodless.
Bifurcation	Division into two branches.
Bleeding time	Time required for spontaneous stoppage of bleeding from a skin puncture (normally 1–7 minutes).
Boyle's law	At standard temperature, the volume of a given mass of gas is inversely proportional to the pressure upon it.
Bronchodilator	A drug which dilates the bronchi (plural of bronchus) e.g. aminophylline.
Bronchospasm	Sudden contraction of the bronchial tubes in the presence of irritants.
Buerger's disease	Disease of the peripheral blood vessels.
Bursa	A fibrous sac lined with synovial membrane. Bursae are present between skin and bone, muscle and muscle.
Caecostomy	Surgical procedure in which the caecum is exposed on the abdominal wall.
Caecum	The beginning of the colon; it is attached to the appendix.
Carcinoid syndrome	A benign tumour of the appendix which secretes serotonin. Patient presents with asthma, bronchospasm and diarrhoea.
Cardiomegaly	Enlargement of the heart.
Cardiopulmonary	Related to the heart and lungs. The term 'cardiopulmonary bypass' is used in heart surgery.
Cardioversion	The use of electrical countershock to restore heart rhythm to normal.
Cataract	An opacity of the crystalline lens or its capsule in the eye.
Catgut	Ligature suture of varying thickness prepared from sheep's intestines.
Chemotherapy	Chemical agents used to arrest the progress of disease e.g. leukaemia.
Cholangiogram	A film showing hepatic, cystic and bile ducts.
Cholecystectomy	Surgical removal of the gallbladder.
Cholecystolithiasis	Presence of gallstones in the gallbladder.
Choledocholithotomy	Surgical removal of a stone from the common bile duct.
Cholinergic	Parasympathetic nerves which liberate acetylcholine.
Cholinesterase	An enzyme which breaks down acetylcholine into choline and acetic acid.
Claudication	Limping caused by interference of the blood supply to the limbs. It may present as severe pain when the patient is walking.
Colectomy	Removal of part or the whole of the colon.
Colonoscopy	Use of a fibreoptic instrument (colonoscope) to view the inside of the colon.
Colporrhaphy	Surgical repair of the vaginal wall. Anterior colporrhaphy repairs a cystocele and posterior colporrhaphy repairs a rectocele.
Contracture	Shortening of a muscle.
Coronary	Artery/arteries supplying blood to the heart.

Cryoanalgesia	Pain relief achieved using a cryosurgical probe. This probe is cooled to a very low temperature.
Cryosurgery	Instead of a knife, an intense, controlled cold is used to remove diseased tissue.
Cystectomy	The partial or complete removal of the urinary bladder.
Cystodiathermy	Application of diathermy to the urinary bladder.
Cystometrogram	A record of pressure changes in the urinary bladder.
Cystostomy	Fistulous opening between the urinary bladder and the abdominal wall.
Cystotomy	Incision into the urinary bladder.
Dacryocystorhinostomy	An operation in which the lacrimal sac in the eye is drained into the nose.
Dextrocardia	Transposition of the heart to the right side of the thorax.
Dupuytren's contracture	Contracture of the palmar fascia, which bends one or more fingers.
Dysphagia	Difficulty in swallowing.
ECG	Electrocardiogram.
Eclampsia	A complication of pregnancy, resulting in fits, hypertension and coma.
Ectopic pregnancy	Pregnancy outside the uterus, the fallopian tube being the most common site. The tube ruptures between the 6th and 8th week, leading to a surgical emergency.
Edentulous	Without teeth.
Electrocochleography	Recording of the movement in the fluid in the internal ear.
Embolectomy	Surgical removal of an embolus.
Emetic	Agent which produces vomiting.
Endarterectomy	Surgical removal of an atheromatous plug from an artery.
Endoscope	An instrument used to visualize body cavities.
Epiglottitis	Inflammation of the epiglottis.
Episiotomy	An incision made in the perineum during the birth of a child to allow delivery.
Epispadias	A congenital opening on the upper surface of the penis.
Epistaxis	Bleeding from the nose.
Esmarch's bandage	A rubber bandage which is rolled onto an arm or leg to produce a bloodless operative field.
Ethmoidectomy	Surgical removal of bone (ethmoid) from the lateral wall of the nose.
Evisceration	Removal of internal organs.
Extrapleural	Outside the pleura.
Extraperitoneal	Outside the peritoneum.
Fibroid	A tumour of fibrous and muscular tissue found in the uterus.
Fibrosarcoma	A malignant tumour.
Fissure	A split or cut e.g. anal fissure.
Fistula	An abnormal communication between two body cavities or surfaces e.g. colostomy between the colon and the abdominal wall.
Gallie's operation	Use of fascia from the thigh in the permanent repair of a hernia.

Gastroenterostomy	An anastomosis between the stomach and small intestine.
Gastropexy	Surgical fixation of a displaced stomach.
Haemangioma	An abnormal blood vessel in any part of the body.
Haematuria	Blood in the urine.
Haemodialysis	A technique by which waste products are removed and essential constituents are replaced in the blood.
Hemicolectomy	Removal of half the colon.
Hydronephrosis	Following obstruction, urine fills up the kidney causing distension.
Hyperkalaemia	High levels of potassium in the serum.
Hyperpituitarism	Increased activity of the anterior pituitary causing acromegaly or gigantism.
Hyperthermia	High body temperature.
Hypertrophy	Increase in the size of tissue or muscles.
Iatrogenic	A complication arising following treatment of a primary condition.
Infarction	Death of a section of tissue.
Intra-arterial	Within an artery.
Intrathecal	Into the subarachnoid region.
Intravascular	Within the blood vessels.
Ion	A charged atom.
Jejunostomy	An opening (fistula) made between the jejunum and the anterior abdominal wall for feeding purposes.
Keller's operation	An operation to correct the deformity of the proximal portion of the proximal phalanx.
Keratectomy	Removal of a part of the cornea.
Keratoplasty	Replacing unhealthy corneal tissue with a graft.
Küntscher nail	A nail used for the fixation of fractured long bones e.g. femur.
Labile	Unstable.
Lacrimation	Outflow of tears.
Laminectomy	Removal of part of a degenerated disc between two vertebrae and vertebral laminae to expose the spinal cord.
Laparoscopy	Insertion of an instrument (laparoscope) to visualize the abdominal contents and perform operations such as sterilization.
Laparotomy	Incision of the abdominal wall to expose the contents.
Laryngoscope	An instrument used to visualize the larynx.
Lateral	Away from the midline or on the side.
Ligate	To tie a blood vessel.
Lipoma	A benign tumour containing fatty tissue.
Lithotrite	An instrument used to crush stones in the urinary bladder.

Lugol's solution	An aqueous solution containing potassium iodide and iodine. It is used in the preoperative preparation of patients undergoing thyroid surgery.
Lymphadenopathy	A disease of the lymph nodes.
Lymphosarcoma	A malignant tumour of lymphatic tissue.
Macroglossia	An abnormally large tongue.
Mammography	An X-ray examination of the breast after injection of an opaque agent.
Mastectomy	Surgical removal of the breast.
McBurney's point	A point one third of the way between the anterior superior iliac spine and the umbilicus. This point develops maximum tenderness in acute appendicitis.
Meconium	A greenish-black discharge from the bowel of a newborn baby.
Medial	Near to the middle.
Meibomian glands	Sebaceous glands which lie in the grooves on the inner surface of the eyelids, their ducts opening on the free margins of the lids.
Melaena	Black tar-like stools due to gastrointestinal bleeding.
Multilobular	Possessing many lobes.
Mydriasis	Abnormal dilatation of the pupil of the eye.
Myringoplasty	An operation to close a defect in the tympanic membrane of the ear using a graft (e.g. temporal fascia).
Myringotomy	An incision into the tympanic membrane (ear drum) to drain pus from the middle ear.
Necrosis	Local death of tissue.
Nephrolithotomy	Removal of a kidney stone.
Neuromuscular	Related to nerve and muscle.
Neurotoxic	Poisonous to nervous tissue.
Nuclear magnetic resonance (NMR)	A non-invasive technique which detects and analyses the growth of cancer.
Oedema	Abnormal infiltration of tissues with fluid.
Oesophagectomy	Excision of a part or whole of the oesophagus.
Oncology	Study of neoplasms.
Orthopnoea	Breathlessness necessitating an upright, sitting position for its relief.
Orthostatic	Caused by an upright position.
Osteotome	An instrument used for cutting bone.
Papilloedema	Oedema of the optic disc in the eye, indicating raised intracranial pressure.
Para-aortic	Near the aorta.
Paramedian	Near the middle.
Paraphimosis	The prepuce (foreskin) of the penis is retracted behind the glans; the tightness of this ring interferes with the blood flow in the glans.
Parasympathetic	A part of the autonomic nervous system consisting of cranial and sacral portions of the nerves.
Parathyroidectomy	Excision of one or more parathyroid glands.

Paravertebral	Near the spinal cord.
Parenteral	Not via the gastrointestinal tract.
Patellectomy	Excision of the patella.
Percutaneous	Through the unbroken skin.
Peritoneum	Serous membrane which lines the abdominal and pelvic contents.
Phaeochromocytoma	A tumour of the adrenal medulla or the sympathetic chain. It secretes adrenaline and noradrenaline causing episodes of severe hypertension.
Pharyngectomy	Surgical removal of the pharynx.
Polya operation	Partial gastrectomy.
Polycystic	Consisting of a number of cysts (kidney).
Pott's fracture	A fracture dislocation of the ankle.
Proctocolectomy	Surgical removal of the colon and rectum.
Prolapse	Falling of an organ or structure e.g. prolapse of the uterus or an intervertebral disc.
Prophylaxis	Prevention.
Prosthesis	An artificial replacement for a missing part e.g. a knee prosthesis.
Pyelolithotomy	An operation for the removal of a stone from the renal pelvis.
Quadriplegia	Paralysis of all four limbs.
Quinsy	Acute inflammation of the tonsil with abscess formation.
Radiograph	An X-ray picture which is developed.
Radiology	The study of diagnosis of disease by using X-rays.
Radiologist	One who specializes in X-ray diagnosis.
Radiotherapist	One who specializes in the treatment of disease with X-rays.
Ranula	A cystic swelling below the tongue.
Rectocele	Prolapse of the rectum and its herniation into the posterior vaginal wall.
Referred pain	Pain occurring at a distance from its source e.g. pain from angina pectoris can be felt in the left upper limb.
Renin	An enzyme released into the blood from the kidney in response to sodium loss.
Rennin	A milk-curdling enzyme present in the gastric juice of infants.
Reticulocyte	A young circulating red blood cell with traces of nucleus.
Retrobulbar	Back of the eyeball.
Retrocaecal	Behind the caecum e.g. a retrocaecal appendix.
Retrograde	Going backwards.
Rhinology	A study of disease affecting the nose.
Rhinoplasty	Plastic surgery of the nose.
Rhizotomy	Surgical division of a root, usually the posterior root of a nerve.
Salpingectomy	Surgical removal of a fallopian tube.
Salpingo-oophorectomy	Surgical removal of a fallopian tube and ovary.
Salpingostomy	An operation performed to restore tubal patency.
Sarcoma	A malignant growth of connective tissue, muscle, bone.
Sclerotherapy	Injection of sclerosing agents (e.g. phenol) for the treatment of varicose veins.

Septicaemia	The presence and multiplication of living bacteria in the bloodstream.
Shirodkar's operation	An operation carried out during pregnancy, in which a purse-string suture is placed around an incompetent cervix. This suture is removed when labour starts.
Spirometer	An instrument used to measure the tidal volumes and minute volumes of the lungs.
Stapedectomy	Surgical removal of stapes (a small bone in the middle ear) and replacement with teflon or a vein graft.
Subcostal	Below the rib.
Subdural	Below the dura mater.
Sublingual	Below the tongue.
Suboccipital	Beneath the occiput, in the nape of the neck.
Supraorbital	Above the orbit.
Suprapubic	Above the pubis.
Synovectomy	Excision of the synovial membrane.
Tachypnoea	Abnormal rate of respiration.
Tarsorrhaphy	Suturing of the lids together.
Tetanus	Disease caused by *Clostridium tetani* which develops following accidents. These organisms are present in road dust and manure.
Tetany	A condition in which muscles are hyperexcitable and mild stimuli produce cramps. This is seen in patients with low serum calcium.
Tetralogy of Fallot	A congenital heart defect which consists of narrowing of the pulmonary artery, hypertrophy of the right ventricle, a septal defect between the ventricles and a displacement of the aorta to the right.
Thoracotomy	Surgical exposure of the thoracic cavity.
Thyroglossal	Relating to the thyroid gland and the back of the tongue.
Thyroidectomy	Surgical removal of the thyroid gland.
Trabeculectomy	Operation carried out for glaucoma. A channel is created through the trabecular meshwork from the canal of Schlemm to the angle of the anterior chamber.
Tympanoplasty	A reconstructive operation carried out on the middle ear to improve hearing.
Ultrasonic	Relating to mechanical vibrations of very high frequency (usually above 30 000 Hz).
Ureterolithotomy	Surgical removal of a stone from a ureter.
Urethrocele	Prolapse of the urethra, usually into the anterior vaginal wall.
Vagolytic	A drug (e.g. atropine) which neutralizes the effect of a stimulated vagus nerve (e.g. bradycardia).
Vagotomy	Surgical division of vagus nerves done in association with pyloroplasty of the stomach in the treatment of peptic ulcer.
Valgus	Displacement or angulation away from the midline of the body e.g. hallux valgus.
Varicocele	Varicosity of the veins of the spermatic cord.

Vasoconstrictor | Any drug which causes a narrowing of the lumen of blood vessels (e.g. Methoxamine).

Vasodilator | Any drug which causes a widening of the lumen of blood vessels (e.g. sodium nitroprusside).

Volvulus | A twisting of a section of bowel, thus occluding the lumen.

Xerostomia | A dry mouth.

Yttrium^{90} | A substance emitting beta particles with a half-life of 64 hours. These are implanted in the pituitary fossa after hypophysectomy for breast cancer.

Zygoma | Cheek bone.

Index